HEART CELL COUPLING AND IMPULSE PROPAGATION IN HEALTH AND DISEASE

BASIC SCIENCE FOR THE CARDIOLOGIST

1. B. Swynghedauw (ed.): *Molecular Cardiology for the Cardiologist.* Second Edition. 1998   ISBN 0-7923-8323-0

2. B. Levy, A. Tedgui (eds.): *Biology of the Arterial Wall.* 1999
   ISBN 0-7923-8458-X

3. M.R. Sanders, J.B. Kostis (eds.): *Molecular Cardiology in Clinical Practice.* 1999   ISBN 0-7923-8602-7

4. B.Ostadal, F. Kolar (eds.): *Cardiac Ischemia: From Injury to Protection.* 1999
   ISBN 0-7923-8642-6

5. H. Schunkert, G.A.J. Riegger (eds.): *Apoptosis in Cardiac Biology.* 1999
   ISBN 0-7923-8648-5

6. A. Malliani, (ed.): *Principles of Cardiovascular Neural Regulation in Health and Disease.* 2000   ISBN 0-7923-7775-3

7. P. Benlian: *Genetics of Dyslipidemia.* 2001   ISBN 0-7923-7362-6

8. D. Young: *Role of Potassium in Preventive Cardiovascular Medicine.* 2001
   ISBN 0-7923-7376-6

9. E. Carmeliet, J. Vereecke: *Cardiac Cellular Electrophysiology.* 2002
   ISBN 0-7923-7544-0

10. C. Holubarsch: *Mechanics and Energetics of the Myocardium.* 2002
    ISBN 0-7923-7570-X

11. J.S. Ingwall: *ATP and the Heart.* 2002   ISBN 1-4020-7093-4

12. W.C. De Mello, M.J. Janse: *Heart Cell Coupling and Impuse Propagation in Health and Disease.* 2002   ISBN 1-4020-7182-5

KLUWER ACADEMIC PUBLISHERS – DORDRECHT/BOSTON/LONDON

HEART CELL COUPLING AND IMPULSE PROPOGATION IN HEALTH AND DISEASE

by

Walmor C. De Mello

and

Michiel J. Janse

KLUWER ACADEMIC PUBLISHERS
Boston / Dordrecht / London

Distributors for North, Central and South America:
Kluwer Academic Publishers
101 Philip Drive
Assinippi Park
Norwell, Massachusetts 02061 USA
Telephone (781) 871-6600
Fax (781) 681-9045
E-Mail: kluwer@wkap.com

Distributors for all other countries:
Kluwer Academic Publishers Group
Post Office Box 322
3300 AH Dordrecht, THE NETHERLANDS
Telephone 31 786 576 000
Fax 31 786 576 474
E-Mail: services@wkap.nl

 Electronic Services < http://www.wkap.nl >

Library of Congress Cataloging-in-Publication Data

A C.I.P. Catalogue record for this book is available
from the Library of Congress.   ISBN 1-4020-7182-5

Heart Cell Coupling and Impulse Propagation in Health and Disease.
Edited by: W.C. De Mello and M.J. Janse

The Publisher offers discounts on this book for course use and bulk purchases. For further information, send email to melissa.ramondetta@wkap.com.

CONTENTS

Contributing Authors

Anumonwo JMB
Department of Pharmacology
SUNY Upstate Medical University
Syracuse NY, USA

Arnsdorf, Morton F.
Section of Cardiology
Department of Medicine
Pritzker Medical School
Chicago, IL, USA

Barker, RJ
Medical University of South Carolina
Charleston, SC, USA

Berenfield, Omer
Department of Pharmacology
SUNY Upstate Medical University
Syracuse, NY, USA

Beyer, Eric C.
Department of Pediatrics
Section of Hematology/Oncology
And Stem Cell Transplantation
University of Chicago
Chicago, IL, USA

Boyett, Mark R
University of Leeds
Leeds, UK

De Mello, Walmor C.
Department of Pharmacology
Medical Sciences Campus
University of Puerto Rico
San Juan, PR., USA

Dekker Lukas, RC
Department of Clinical Medicine
and Experimental
Medicine of Amsterdam.
The Netherlands

Dhaman, Amit
Department of Pharmacology
SUNY Upstate Medical University
Syracuse NY,USA

Gourdie, Robert G.
Medical University of South
Carolina
Charleston, SC, USA

Hayrapetyan, Volodya
Krannert Institute of Cardiology
Indiana University
School of Medicine
Indianapolis, IN, USA

Hirosawa, Nobue
Department of Physiology
School of Medicine
Fukuoka University
Fukuoka, Japan

Honjo, Haruo
Research Institute of Environmental
Medicine,
Nagoya University,
Nagoya, Japan

Imanaga, Issei
Department of Physiology
Fukuoka University
Fukuoka, Japan

Jalife, Jose
Department of Pharmacology
SUNNY Upstate Medical University
Syracuse, NY, USA

Janse, Michiel
Department of Clinical and
Experimental Cardiology
Academic Medical Center
University of Amsterdam
The Netherlands

Kleber, Andre G
Department of Physiology
University of Bern
Switzerland

Kodama, Itsuo
Research Institute of Environmental
Medicine,
Nagoya University
Nayoya, Japan

Lee, Peter
Department of Medicine
Section of Cardiology
University of Illinois
Chicago, IL, USA

Lin, Hai
Department of Physiology
School of Medicine
Fukuoka University
Fukuoka, Japan

Matsamura, Takashi
Department of Physiology
School of Medicine
Fukuoka University
Fukuoka, Japan

Mayama, Ken
Department of Physiology
School of Medicine
Fukuoka University
Fukuoka, Japan

Moreno, Alonso
Krannert Institute of Cardiology
Indiana University
School of Medicine
Indianapolis, IN. USA

Sakamoto, Yasuji
Department of Physiology
School of Medicine
Fukuoka University
Fukuoka, Japan

Servers, Nicholas
National Heart and Lung Institute
Faculty of Medicine
Imperial College
London, UK

Seul, Kyung H
Department of Pediatrics
Section of Hematology/Oncology
and Stem Cell Transplantation
University of Chicago,
Chicago, IL, USA

Spray, David
Department of Neurosciences
Albert Einstein College of Medicine
New York, USA

Suadicani, Sylvia
Department of Neurosciences
Albert Einstein College of Medicine
New York, USA

Takagishi, Yoshiko
Research Institute of Environmental
Medicine,
Nagoya University
Nayoya, Japan

Tan, Hanno L.
Department of Clinical and
Experimental Cardiology
Academic Medical Center
University of Amsterdam
The Netherlands

Veenstra, Richard D
SUNNY Upstate Medical University
Syracuse, NY,USA

Wagner, Mary B.
Emory University
Atlanta, GA, USA

Zhang, Henggui
Research Institute of Environmental
Medicine,
Nagoya University
Nayoya, Japan

Zhong, Guogiang
Krannert Institute of Cardiology
Indiana University
School of Medicine
Indianapolis, IN, USA

Introduction

Walmor C. De Mello

The present publication is an up-to-date review of the most relevant aspects of heart cell communication in health and disease written by distinguished colleagues, each one expert in his own field. It represents, in certain way, the culmination of more than a century of studies dedicated to heart cell biology and in particular to heart cell coupling.

One can say that during this difficulty trajectory, some moments were critical. The conceptualization of cardiac muscle as a physiological but not as an anatomical syntitium, was decisive for the development of our present stage of knowledge. Like in neurophysiology with the introduction of the neuronal theory of Ramon y Cajal, the conceptualization of heart muscle as formed by isolated cells surrounded by a membrane, created an enormous difficulty for the understanding of how the electrical impulse crosses from cell-to-cell. The ulterior demonstration that apposing heart cells are interconnected by intercellular junctions and that no chemical synapses are present among the cardiomyocytes, solved this crucial problem.

During the 50's and 60's intercellular low resistant pathways were described in cardiac fibers but initially considered as permanent structures without any modulatory function. The demonstration in the 70's and 80's that the gap junction conductance can be modulated by different factors like calcium, pH and cyclic nucleotides, etc, opened a fruitful field of investigation. During these two decades, some discrepant results concerning the characteristics of cell coupling in different tissues, were difficult to understand because it was thought that the process of cell communication must follow the rule of uniformity. It is well known, however, that evolution also creates diversity. Indeed, depending on the type of connexin involved, the characteristics of cell coupling change with consequent variations on the value of conduction velocity. Connexin 43, for instance is more abundant in the adult mammalian myocardium while in the sinoatrial node and other areas of the specialized conductive tissue, the expression of connexin 40 and 45 is appreciably enhanced providing explanation for slow conduction (Verheick et al,2000; Davies et al,1994; Simon et al,1998). A fundamental problem remains: how plastic is the role of the different connexins on the establishment of functional channels during normal or pathological conditions.

Although the presence of connexins, in itself, is not a necessary evidence of permeant intercellular channels, the progress in molecular biology of gap junction proteins, provided an important tool for the understanding of important aspects of gap junctional communication. The development of transgenic mice lacking Cx43 or Cx40, for instance, helped to demonstrate the role of these proteins on the process of intercellular communication (Simon et al,1998). The possible role of connexins in other biological processes inside the cells is not well known creating the possibility of misinterpretation of some of the results obtained with immunological methods.

We are far from understanding other aspects of gap junction communication such as the intricacies of chemical coupling and metabolic cooperation between heart cells and its possible implication for heart cell pathology. Future studies on this area will open a new field of research helping to understand better the integrative role of gap junctions.

The present volume is an effort to reorganize our knowledge of heart cell communication at the beginning of 2002 and led us hope it can be of benefit for those young investigators who decided to put on a full effort.

References

Davis LM,Kanten HL,Beyer EG,Saffitz JE (1994) Distinct gap junction protein phenotypes in cardiac tissue with diaparate conduction properties. J. Am Cell Cardiol. 24:11241-11320

Simon AM,Goodenough DA, Paul DL (1998) Mice lacking connexin 40 have cardiac conduction abnormalities characteristic of atrioventricular block and bundle branch block Curr Biol 26:295-298

Verheijck EE, van Kempen MJ, Veerschild M,Luivink L, Jongsma HY, Bouman LN (2001) Electrophysiological features of mouse sinoatrial node in relation to connexin distribution. Cardiovasc. Res 52: 40-50

1

THE CARDIAC SYNCYTIUM; AN OVERVIEW

Walmor C. De Mello

Department of Pharmacology, Medical Science Campus, UPR

The heart muscle was initially conceptualized as an anatomical syncytium. Indeed, at the beginning of the century, intercalated discs were interpreted as sarcomere differentiation or even as contraction artifacts (Ebner 1900;Heidenhain 1891; Godlewisky (1902). In morphological studies Godlewisky's observations emphasized the absence of cell boundaries. Quoting his original words:

> "… einen Tangentialschnitt durch the Herzwand
> eines drei-tagigen Entenembryos vorstellt. Nun ist
> allerdings richtig, dass sich damals trotz genauer
> Untersuchungen keine Zellengrenzen fanden".

These findings confirmed previous results of Fredericq (1875) using embryonic heart muscle. He concluded: "Examiné a un grossissement 500 il se montré composé de mêmes elements que les muscles volontaires: une masse granuleuse protoplasmique dans lequelle se trouvant plonges des nombreaux noyau. Ici egalement les cellules embryonaires parissent s'être fusioneés".

To avoid the concept of isolated cell Purkinje fibers were initially described as composed of grains (Körnchen) with a "Zwichensubstanz" between the Körnchen (Purkinje,1845). Although the studies of Werner (1910) recognized that the heart muscle consists of "territories with clear boundaries" the cellular nature of cardiac muscle was only accepted with the development of electronmicroscopy and the work of Sjostrand and Andersson, (1954). These authors showed that heart cells are enveloped by a membrane what demonstrated that the cardiac muscle is composed of isolated cells.

This finding certainly represented a serious problem for the explanation of how the electrical impulse propagates throughout the heart. The same question was a central point of controversy in neurophysiology with the neuronal theory of Ramon y Cajal (1895) because the nervous system was classically visualized as a net-like structure which is the reticular theory of Gerlach (1877). With the work of Loewi (1921), Dale (1935) and Katz (1935) the possibility of electrical synaptic transmission was discarded. As emphasized by Katz (1966) the impedance of nerve endings and the skeletal muscle fiber are mismatched, indicating that the electrical mechanism of synaptic transmission is not correct. Indeed, the end-plate potential was due to the removal of charge from the postsynaptic membrane which was found to be thousands of time larger than any removal process caused by presynaptic action current alone (Fatt,Katz 1951).

It was then conceivable that the release of some chemical transmitter by the myocyte might induce the depolarization of the neighboring cell. Contrary to the neurons, however, a chemical machinery necessary for the synthesis and the storage of transmitters into synaptic vesicles does not exist in cardiac muscle.

The classical observations of van Bremen (1953), Moore and Ruska, (1957), Poche and Lindner (1955) and Sjostrand and Andersson (1954), however, indicated that the plasma cell membrane is modified at the intercellular region showing junctional specializations like macula adherents (demosomes), fasciae adherents and nexuses (see Fig. 1). In desmosome the apposing plasma cell membranes are separated by a gap of

250-300 A while at the nexus the cell membranes are in intimate contact (Fig. 1). Using the electron opaque lanthanum hydroxide to mark the extracellular space Revel and Karnovsky (1967) showed, however, that at the nexus or "gap junction" there is gap of 2 nm between the two plasma cell membranes (see also Fig. 1.). In addition, these observations suggested that gap junctions are composed of membrane particles organized like a plaque.

The gap junction membrane channel involves rigid structural support, a selective filter, a voltage sensor and physical gates within the pore.   Moreover, the cytoplasm of the apposing cell influence the molecular organization of the gap junction (Sosinsky ,2000).

Subsequent physiological and biophysical observations demonstrated that hydrophilic channels located at the center of nexus subunits, connect the interior of adjacent cardiac cells (Makowsky et al,1977). Recently, observations of Veenstra et al., (1995) are consistent with the view that the conventional simple aqueous pore model of a gap junction channel must be replaced by a new model for channel conductance permeability based electrostatic interaction (see Chapter 6).

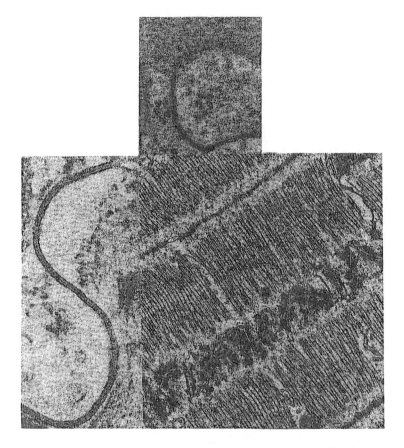

Fig 1.Top- shows extracellular space in gap junction marked with electron opaque lanthanum hydroxide. Bottom right-thin section electronmicrograph of gap junction showing internal structure. Left- electronmicroscopy of heart muscle showing intercalated disc. Kindly provided by Dr. JR Sommer, with permission.

An important information about the organization of cytoplasmic and external surfaces of gap junctions was achieved by using freeze –fracture-etch methods (Goodeneough, Gilula 1974). These and posterior studies indicated that each cell contributes to a hemi-channel or connexon (Sosinsky,2000) and that each connexon is composed of six protein subunits surrounding an aqueous pore (Figs. 2).Atomic force microscopy studies (Hoh et al,1993) indicated that the individual connexins protrude 14 A from the extracellular surface and have a pore of 38 A.

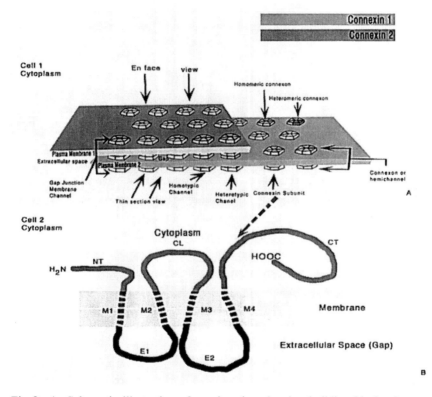

Fig 2   A -Schematic illustration of gap junction showing building block of connexin molecule. The half-channel is a hexamer of connexin subunits. Two connexons dock in the extracellular space to form the membrane channel. The diagram also shows homomeric and heteromeric connexons and hemotypic and heterotypic junctions.B-Topology diagram of the connexin primary sequence with three domains (cytoplasmic domain, membrane domain and extracellular domain).These domains each contain multiple stretches of amino acids(From Sosinsky 2000, with permission).

Cell communication assayed by electrical methods

The first evidence that heart fibers present cable properties was presented by Weidmann (1952). Applying one dimensional cable theory to cardiac Purkinje fibers he demonstrated that the data is well described by the cable theory. Indeed, when current is injected into a Purkinje cell appreciable changes in membrane potential can be seen in adjacent cell. These studies demonstrated that the core resistivity is quite low and the space constant (1.9 mm) is larger than the length of a single heart cell (125 μm). Moreover, Draper and Weidmann (1951) showed that the conduction velocity of the action potential in these fibers is 3-4 m/sec what means that a single myocyte is traversed in 3 μs. Since the action potential upstroke uses 0.3-0.5 ms it is possible to conclude that 10-15 cells participate simultaneously in the upstroke. As emphasized by Fozzard (1979) these observations support the view that the cells are electrically coupled because transmission through chemical synapses require longer times.

Using a method similar to that of Osterthout and Hill (1930) Barr et al, (1965) showed that the impulse conduction in atrial muscle is blocked by increasing the extracellular resistance in the central portion of a thin bundle (see Fig. 3). The blockade of the action potential was, however, reversed by connecting an appropriate resistance between both sides of the central gap (Fig. 3) what implies that low extracellular and intracellular resistances are both required for the propagation of the action potential.

The remaining question was whether intercellular junctions are necessary for the propagation of the impulse or was the electrical signal able to jump the gap between two apposing cells.

It is know since the work of Hodgkin (1937) that electrotonic potentials can jump across a short inexcitable zone. If the amplitude of the signal is not decreased to less than 1/5 across

old will be reached at the cell
ly a propagated action potential
nal membrane impedance falls
fiber diameter, it is easy to
tions like the septate axon, the
.... impulse across the seta is about 1/10
what means that the longitudinal propagation of the impulse is
"almost" possible even if we assume the absence of gap junctions
(Katz,1939). For cardiac fibers with a small diameter the
situation is quite different since the attenuation factor here is
extremely large and the possibility that the electrical impulse
cross the gap is impossible. This means that the hypothesis of
impulse propagation across intercellular gaps can be discarded
and the presence of intercellular channels is then required for the

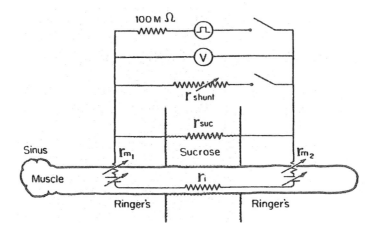

Fig 3 Diagram showing the experimental procedure followed by Barr et al., to
demonstrate the electrical coupling in frog atrial muscle, The central area of the bundle
was perfused with isotonic sucrose solution while the two peripheral regions were
bathed with Ringer's solution and separated from the central zone by a partition. From
Barr et al. 1965 , with permission.

intercellular spread of current. Indeed, experiments performed on
cultured heart cells indicated that the coupling resistance is high

(> 100 M Ω) at the moment of contact but starts falling immediately after reaching values of 20 M Ω at the moment electrical synchronization is achieved (Clapham et al,1980). Assuming a resistance of 10^{-10} Ω for a single hydrophilic channel, the rate of channel synthesis was found to be one channel per cell per minute (Clapham et al,1980). Furthermore, during the establishment of the gap junction, the conductance is increased by quantal steps suggesting a gradual increment in the number of channels (Loewenstein et al,1975).

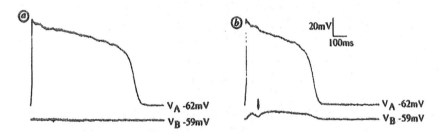

Fig. 4 Membrane potentials recorded from two heart cells in the process of coupling under current clamps conditions. A just offer the cells have been pushed together; B-7 minutes later. From Rook et at 1988, with permission.

When neonatal heart cells are pushed together and one of the cells is stimulated, an action potential is recorded in the stimulated cell but no response is detected in the other cell (Rook et al,1988). In about 5-15 minutes, however, the non-stimulated cell starts showing subthreshold depolarization and finally total cell communication is established (Fig.4).

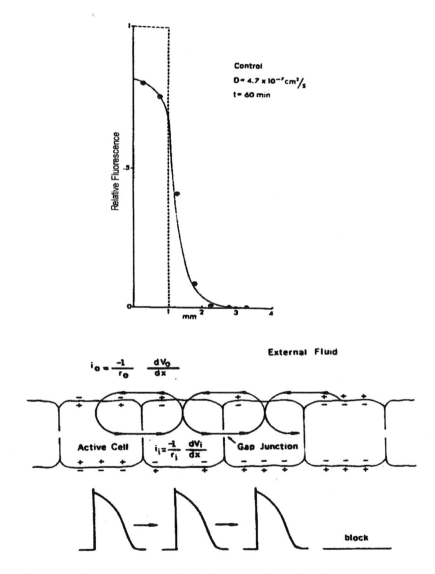

Figure 5. Top - longitudinal distribution of Lucifer Yellow along trabecula dissected from the right atrium of dog's heart. D = diffusion coefficient. From reference De Mello and van Loon, 1987 ,with permission. Bottom - diagram illustrating the flow of local current in a cardiac fiber and the role of gap junctions in the spread of propagated activity.

These and other findings lead to the conclusion that the mechanism of impulse propagation in the heart is through local current flow what means that current flows through the active areas along the myoplasm and gap junctions, outward through the resting adjacent cell membrane, back along the extracellular fluid and inward through the active region, so completing the local circuit (see Fig .) The potential change across the non-junctional membrane (Vm) is given by the difference between the potential on the inside (Vi) and the potential on the outside (Vo): Vo=(Vi-Vo). The current flowing along the outside of the membrane is io=(1/ro)(dVo/dx) where do/dx is the extra cellular potential gradient and ro the resistance per unit length of the extra cellular fluid. The current flowing along the core of the cardiac fiber is given by i $_i$= (-1/ri)(dVi/dx) where dVi/dx is the intracellular gradient and ri the intracellular resistance per unit length, which represents the myoplasmic and the junctional resistance in series. Contrary to nerve cells, the cardiac myocytes have a highly structured intracellular medium in which the sarcoplasmic reticulum occupies a quite large proportion of this space. Despite of this, the cytoplasm of the heart and other muscle fibers has a specific resistance similar to that of the extracellular fluid (Fatt, Katz1951; Falk,Fatt,1964).

The complex geometry of the myocardium has a great influence on the spread of current. In the rat atrium, for instance, the depolarization of one cell causes appreciable change in the membrane potential of adjacent cells (Woodbury,Crill,1961) but a steep decline of the electrotonic potentials was found (λ=130 μm) when an intracellular electrode was used to polarize the cell. An enormous decrement of the electrotonic potentials was due to the three dimensional characteristics of the rat trabecula and was not related to a high intracellular or extracellular resistance or to a low non-junctional membrane resistance. The decay of the electrotonic potential in this case is better fitted by a Bessel function (Woodbury, Crill 1961).

It is essential to recognize that the coupling coefficient (Cc) between two isopotential cells is given by the following ratio:

$$Cc= gj/gj +gjn$$

where gj is the junctional conductance and gjn is the conductance of the surface cell membrane. This means that an increased gjn will result in a smaller coupling coefficient.

In specialized fibers of the A-V node as well as in the sinoatrial node, for instance, acetylcholine causes a decline in the electrical coupling mainly through an increase of surface cell membrane conductance (De Mello,1977;1980).

In both tissues the spread of electrical current is limited by a small space constant (465 μm for the sinoatrial node (Bonke,1973) and 430 μm for the AV node (De Mello, 1977). Gap junctions have been identified between pacemaker cells (Masson-Pevet et al,1982) but their mean area is smaller than those found in the myocardium. In the sinoatrial node, for instance, the nexuses represent 0.2% of cell surface area which is about 10 times less than in working myocardial cells (Masson-Pevet et al,1982). In the AV node, a high intracellular resistance contributes to the small conduction velocity (De Mello,1977) and makes the cell-to-cell propagation greatly dependent on changes in non-junctional membrane resistance. Although it is known that a slower depolarizing mechanism in the AV node cell is also responsible for slow conduction, there is evidence that in atrial muscle appreciable amounts of Cx43, Cx40 and Cx45 can be found while the AV node and sinoatrial node are devoid of Cx43 (Davis, Kanter,1994).These observations highly suggest that the different expression of the connexins influences the junctional conductance and consequently the conduction velocity.

Studies of connexin expression revealed that Cx40 is present in the conduction system. Indeed, in mice lacking Cx40, conduction abnormalities characteristic of the first degree AV block has been described (Simon et al,1998). Recent studies showed strands of Cx43 and Cx40 positive atrial cell protruding into the Cx45 positive sinoatrial area while bands of connective tissue separates the nodal from the atrial tissue (Verheijck et al, 2001). The concept of the sinoatrial node as a heterogeneous structure is gradually emerging. The mosaic model involving a variable mix of atrial and sinoatrial node cells from periphery to center (see Boyett et al,2000), seems to indicate that multiple mechanisms allows the sinoatrial node to drive the atrium without being electrotonically suppressed. Moreover, via action potential duration gradient and conduction block, anterograde propagation from SA node to atrium prevents reentry (see Chapter 8).

Because gj is dependent upon Ca_i (De Mello,1975) the question of whether the junctional conductance is constant or changes during the cardiac cycle merits serious consideration. Measurements of intracellular resistance and space constant performed during diastolic depolarization in isolated Purkinje fibers indicated that the electrical coupling is gradually increased during diastole (De Mello,1986). The increment of electrical coupling is due to both a fall in the intracellular resistance (ri) and an increase of non -junctional membrane resistance (rm). According to these findings, the firing of the action potential coincides with the moment a maximal degree of cell coupling is achieved. Although the mechanism by which ri falls during diastole remains to be determined, it is known that epinephrine increases the electrical coupling during diastole depolarization (De Mello, 1986) suggesting that this phenomenon is enhanced by cAMP and possible phosphorylation of gap junction proteins (De Mello,1980).

Modulation of gap junctional conductance

Evidence that the junctional conductance can be modulated was presented in the 70's (De Mello,1975;Rose and Loewenstein 1975). It is known since Engelmann (1877) that "death of a cardiac cell does not result in the death of the neighboring cell". This important conclusion was based on the observation that the injury potential induced by lesion of cardiac muscle soon vanishes (healing-over)- a phenomenon that is not related to the depolarization of the surface cell membrane because a new lesion applied near the previous one re-establishes the injury potential (De Mello,1972). Although the possibility exists that a new surface cell membrane is quickly established sealing the damaged area(like that seen in skeletal muscle), that fact that no healing-over occurs in skeletal muscle in which the fibers are not communicated by gap junctions, rule out the possibility that the healing-over process be related to the reconstitution of the surface cell membrane (De Mello 1973).

It is known that the healing-over process is dependent on the presence of calcium ions in the extracellular medium (De Mello et al,1969) and that other ions like Ba or Mg had no effect on the sealing process (De Mello 1972).

In order to test the hypothesis that the healing-over process is related to an increase in gap junction resistance, calcium ions were injected electrophoretically inside normal cardiac cells and its effect on the electrical coupling was followed. The results indicated that an increase in free $Ca^{2+}i$ lead to a gradual decline of cell coupling (De Mello,1975; Noma, Tsuboi, 1987) while the input resistance is appreciably increased. Although calcium ions are a good cell decoupler when the cells are damaged, the role of calcium ions as a physiological modulator of gj is still disputed. This is in part due to the fact that it is very difficult to determine the calcium concentration near the gap junctions. Moreover, evidence exists that at calcium waves propagate from cell to-cell through the gap junctions-a phenomenom probable related to intercellular diffusion of IP$_3$ (see Chapter 5) .

Since Turner and Warner (1977) it is know that a fall in intracellular pH elicit a decline of gj. When H ions are injected electrophoretically inside heart cells the electrical coupling is abolished within seconds (De Mello,1980). Previous studies indicated that the healing-over process can be promoted by protons in absence of calcium ions but only if the pH falls to 5.5 (De Mello,1980). Clearly this is a pH that falls outside the pH range in a living heart cell. The healing-over process (which requires an appreciable increase in junctional resistance) is in agreement with the cable analysis data obtained in Purkinje fibers (Reber and Weingart, 1982). These authors found that an increase of intracellular resistance of only 30% when the pHi was changed from 7.3 to 6.8.These findings indicate that calcium ions are more important to the healing-over process than protons .

It is known that the influence of protons on gj in different cell systems varies. This is probably related to the fact that Cx43 is more sensitive to acidification than Cx32 (Liu et al 1993; Hermans et al,1995). The question whether protons changed gj directly or through an intermediary factor has been discussed (see Delmar 1995). A cytoplasmic mediator seems to to be required for the cell uncoupling (Nicholson et al,1998) and calmodulin inhibition has been found to prevent pH gating in Cx38-expressing oocyte pairs (Peracchia et al,1996).

The molecular mechanism of cell uncoupling due to acidification has been investigated. The truncation of the carboxyl terminal of Cx43,for instance, was found to impair pH gating (Liu et al,1993).

Phosphorylation of junctional proteins and the regulation of junctional communication

Initial electrophysiological studies indicated that epinephrine and theophylline which increment the intracellular cAMP concentration in heart muscle, increases the spread of electrotonic potentials (De Mello,1980). Moreover, the intracellular injection of cAMP or the administration of isobutyl-methyl-xanthine (a phosphodiesterase inhibitor) to the extracellular medium, increases the electrical coupling of cardiac cells (De Mello,1986). These observations lead to the view that phosphorylation of gap junction proteins is involved in the regulation of gj. A strong support for the phosphorylating hypothesis is the finding that dibutyryl-cAMP enhances the diffusion of Lucifer Yellow CH in cardiac fibers from 4×10^{-7} cm2/s to 2×10^{-6} cm2/s(De Mello, van Loon(1987). Similar results were found with isoproterenol (De Mello, van Loon,1987).Burt and Spray,1988 and De Mello (1986) found an increase in junctional conductance in heart cell pairs when the intracellular cAMP concentration is increased. Moreover, when the catalytic subunit of the protein kinase A was dialyzed inside the heart cell the gj was increased (De Mello,1991). Evidence is also available that in some cell lines exposed to dibutyryl-cAMP for several hours, there is an increased synthesis of intercellular channels (Flagg-Newton et al,1981).In isolated trabeculae from dogs treated chronically with ephedrine, the intercellular diffusion of Lucifer Yellow CH is enhanced, an effect seen even after elimination of the drug(De Mello,1988)

These observations indicate that cAMP has a short and a long-term effect on intercellular communication. Recently, it was found that PKA activation upregulates Cx43 in neonatal cardiomyocytes cultures (Darrow et al,1996). However, some authors found no influence of PKA activation on gj (Kwak, Jongsma 1996). This discrepance seems related to the presence of different types of connexins (Kwak, Jongsma 1996). For more information see Chapter 7.

Cell-to-cell coupling assayed by fluorescent probes

Further evidence that heart cells are intercommunicated was provided by studies of ion or dye- coupling. In 1966 Weidmann demonstrated that potassium ions diffuse through the gap junctions of sheep and calf ventricular muscle. Subsequent studies showed that Lucifer Yellow CH - a non-toxic substituted naphtalimide with two sulfonated groups, diffuses through the cytoplasm and gap junctions in heart fibers but does not cross the surface cell membrane (De Mello, van Loon,1987). As shown in Fig. 5 the introduction of Lucifer yellow CH into dog trabeculae with the cut-end method, was followed by its redistribution over distances larger than the length of a single cell. Considering that the permeability of the surface cell membrane to the dye is negligible, the results represent a strong evidence that the cardiac cells are connected by permeable channels. The diffusion coefficient (Dj) can be quantitatively evaluated by fitting the experimental results to theoretical points estimated using the Crank's equation for the diffusion in a cylinder assuming no loss of tracer through the surface cell membrane. Fluorescence microscopy showed indeed, Lucifer Yellow CH located exclusively inside the heart fibers. The average value of Dj for the dog trabeculae estimated by an interactive computer program for non-linear regression, was $4 \pm 0.63 \times 10^{-7}$ cm^2/s (De Mello and van Loon, 1987. For Lucifer Yellow CH the value of Dj is smaller than the diffusion coefficient of the dye in the sarcoplasm ($Ds=2 \times 10^{-6}$ cm^2/s) indicating that there its a restrictive diffusion at the gap junctions. Indeed, studies performed with other compounds not only supported this view but also indicated that the junctional permeability (Pj), which has the physical dimension of velocity (cm/s), is inversely proportional to the molecular weight of the compounds (Imanaga 1987). For Lucifer Yellow CH (mol.wt 473) $Pj= 3x 10^{-4}$ cm/s (De Mello, van Loon,1987),for TEA (mol.wt. 130) was 1.27×10^{-3} cm/s (Weingart,1974), for cAMP (mol.wt 328) was 1.33×10^{-6} (Tsien,Weingart,1976) and for K was 7.68×10^{-3} cm/s (Weidmann,1966). Not only the size of the molecule but its charge

influence   its   passage   through   the   intercellular   channel
(Imanaga,1974). Indeed, the permeability limit decreases with
increasing the negativity on the rhodamine or fluorescein dye
conjugates, what suggests that the gap junction pore has a fixed
negative charge (Brink Dewey 1980) (see Chapter 6). The diameter
of the pore connecting apposing cells was found to be 1-1.55 nm
while   Procion Yellow (mol. wt 397) - an elongated structure
measuring 0.5 x 2.7 nm, is the largest molecule to pass the channel
(Imanaga,1974)   It is important to add that the terms "ionic
permeability" and "ionic conductance" are not interchangeable
because   permeability is $P= (\mu B/d)(RT/F)$ where μ is electrical
mobility, B is the partition coefficient between solution and
membrane and d is thickness of the membrane. The two properties
are, however, in intimate relation.

**Bioenergetics and cell communication; cell uncoupling seen as
a protective mechanism.**

Cardiac cells are chemical machines in which the chemical energy
is obtained from oxidation. The cardiac fibers can be visualized as
formed by energy compartments connected through low barrier
pathways. Under normal conditions the stimulation and consequent
depolarization of one cell lead to the generation of an action
potential which results in a decrease in its "free energy" and
consequent production of work. When cells are coupled, the
spread of current from cell-to-cell can be visualized as a cascade
reaction with consequent fall in free energy.

In the diseased heart in which some cells have a reduced amount of
chemical energy, cell uncoupling might be seen as having an
important biological importance providing the sick cell an
opportunity to rest and re-establishes its chemical energy.

When the rate of ATP resynthesis between apposing heart cells
was reduced by dialysing 2-4 dinitrophenol (0.01 mM), an
uncoupler of oxidative phosphorylation into just one of the cells of

the pair, the value of junctional conductance was unchanged for at least 8 min if the "normal" cell was pulsed at very low rate (0.04 Hz) but the increment in rate of pulsing to 4 Hz caused a decrease (13%) of gj within 30 sec. If the pacing was interrupted the change in gj was spontaneously reversed indicating that if time of rest is provided to this dialyzed cell, the electrical coupling is re-established (De Mello,1992).

References

Barr L, Dewey MM, Berger M(1965). Propagation of action potentials and the structure of the nexus in cardiac muscle. J Gen Physio 48:797-823.

Bonke EIM (1973). Electrotonic spread in the sinoatrial node of the rabbit heart.Pflugers Arch 339:17-24

Boyett MR, Honjo H, Kodama I (2000) The sinoatrial node, a heterogeneous pacemaker structute Cardiovasc Res 47: 458-487

Brink PR, Dewey MM (1980) Evidence for fixed charge in the nexus. Nature 285:101-102

Burt J, Spray DC(1988) Inotropic agents modulate gap junction conductance between cardiac myocytes. Am J. Physiol. 254: H1206-H1210

Clapham DE, Shrier A and DeHaan RL (1980). Junctional resistance and action potential delay between embryonic heart cell aggregates. J Gen Physiol 75:633- 66.

Dale HH (1935). Pharmacology and nerve endings. Proc R Soc Med 28; 319-332.

Darrow BJ, Fast VG, Kleber AG, Beyer EC, Saffitz JE (1996) Functional and structural assessment of intercellular communication. Increased conduction velocity and enhanced connexin expression in dibutyryl-cAMP- treated cultured cardiac myocytes. Circ. Res. 79:174-183

Davis LM,.Kanter HL, Beyer EG and Saffitz JE (1994) Distinct gap junction protein phenotypes in cardiac tissues with disparate conduction properties. J Am Cell Cardiol 24:1124-11320

Delmar M, Liu S, Morey GE,Ek JF, Anumonwo JMB, Taffet SM (1995) Toward a molecular model for the pH regulation of intercellular communication in the heart. In : Cardiac Electrophysiology. From Cell to Bed Side (Zipes D, Jalife J, eds) pp 135-143 WB Saunders, Philadelphia

De Mello WC (1972) The healing-over process in cardiac and other muscle Fibers. In: Electrical Phenomena in the Heart (De Mello WC, ed) pp 323-351. New York Academic Press.

De Mello WC (1973) Membrane sealing in frog skeletal muscle Fibers.Proc Natl Acad Sci USA 70: 982-984

De Mello WC (1975) Effect of intracellular injection of calcium and strontiumon cell communication in heart. J Physiol (London) 50:231-2450

De Mello WC (1977). Passive electrical properties of the atrioventricular node. Pflugers Arch Ges Physiol 371:135-139.

De Mello WC (1980) The influence of pH on the healing-over of mammalian cardiac muscle. J. Physiol (London) 339:299-307

De Mello WC (1980). Intercellular communication and Junctional permeability In-Membrane Structure and Function (EE Bittar, ed) Vol 13, pp 125-164 Wiley, NewYork

De Mello WC (1986) Interaction of cAMP and calcium in the control of electrical coupling in heart fibers. Biochem Biophys Acta 888:91-99

De Mello WC (1986) Increased spread of electrotonic potentials during diastolic depolarization in cardiac muscle. J Mol Cell Cardiol 18:23-29

De Mello WC (1986) Interaction of cAMP and calcium in the control of electrical coupling in heart fibers. Biochem. Biophys. Acta 888:91-99

De Mello WC(1988) Cyclic nucleotides and gap junction permeability. Braz J Med 21:1225-1230

De Mello WC (1991) Further studies on the influence of cAMP-dependent protein kinase on junctional conductance in isolated heart cell pairs. J. Mol Cell Cardiol 23: 371-379

De Mello WC (1992) Bioenergetics and cell communication; cell uncoupling seen as a protective mechanism in cardiac muscle. Cell Biol Int Rep. 16:625-637

De Mello WC, Motta G and Chapeau M (1969) A study on the healing-over of myocardial cells of toads. Circ. Res. 4:475-487

De Mello WC and van Loon P (1987) Further studies on the influence of cyclic nucleotides on junctional permeability in heart. J Mol Cell Cardiol. 19:763-771

Draper H and Weidmann S (1951). Cardiac resting and action potentials recorded with an intracellular electrode, J Physiol (London), 115:74-94.

Ebner V (1900). Ueber die Kittlinien der Hermuskelfasern Sitzungsber. Wien Akad Math Nat Kl, 109, 3.

Engelmann TW (1877)   Vergleichende Untersuchungen zur Lehere von der
    Muskel-und-Nerveelectriktat.Pflug Arch ges Physiol 15:116-148

Falk G and Fatt P (1964) Linear electrical properties of striated fibres observed
    with intracellular electrodes. Proc Roy Soc London Ser B 160:69-123

Fatt P and Katz (1951). An analysis of the end-plate potential recorded with an
    intracellular rnicroelectrode. J Physiol (London) 115: 320-370.

Flagg-Newton JL, Dahl G, Loewenstein WR(1981) Cell junctions and cyclic
    AMP: Upregulation of junctional membrane permeability and junctional
    membrane particles by administration of cyclic nucleotide or
    phosphodiesterase inhibitor. J. Memb. Biol 63: 105-121

Fozzard H (1979). Conduction of the action potential. In Handbook of
    Physiology, Section 2 Vol I pp 335-355 (Berne M , Sperelakis N and
    Geiger   SR, eds) American Physiological Society, Washington.

Fredericq L (1875). Generation et structure du tissu musculaire.Bruxelles.

Gerlach J (1877). Von dem Ruckenmarke. In: Handbuch der Lehre von den
    Gweben. Bd 2, (S Stricker, ed).

Godlewisky E (1902). Die Entiwicklung des Skelet-und Herzmuskelgewebes
    der Saugthiere. Arch Mikros Anat 60:111.

Goodenough DA Gilula NB (1974). The splitting of hepatocyte gap junctions
    and zonnulae occludents with hypertonic solution. J Cell Biol 61:575-
    591

Heidenhain M(1891). Ueber die Structur des menschlichen Hermuskels. Anat
    Anz 20:33.

Hermans MM, Kontekaas P, Jongsma HJ, Rook MB (1995) pH
    sensitivity of the cardiac gap junction protein connexin 45 and 43.
    Pflugers Arch 431: 138-140

Hodgkin A (1937). Evidence for electrical transmission in nerve. J Physiol
    (London) 90:183-232.

Hoh J, Sosinsky GE, Revel JP, Hansma PK (1993) Structure of the extracellular
    surface of gap junctions by atomic force microscopy. Biophys. JU. 65:
    149-163

Imanaga I (1974) Cell-to-cell diffusion of procion yellow in sheep and calf
    Purkinje fibers. J Memb Biol 16:381-388

Katz B (1935). The transmission of impulses from nerve to muscle and the
    subcellular unit of synaptic action. Proc Roy Soc (London) Ser B
    155:455-477.

Katz B (1939). Electric excitation of nerve. Oxford University, Press, London.

Katz (1966). Nerve, muscle, and Synapse. McGraw-Hill Inc

Kwak BR, Jongsma HJ (1996) Regulation of gap junction channel permeability and conductance by several phosphorylating conditions. Mol Cell Biochem 157:93-99

Liu S, Taffet SM, Stoner L, Delmar M, Vallano ML, Jalife J (1993) A structural basis of unequal sensitivity of the major cardiac and liver gap junctions to intracellular acidification. Biophys. J 54: 1422-1433

Loewenstein WR, Kanno Y and Socolar SJ (1975). Quantum jumps of conductance during formation of membrane channels at cell-cell junction. Nature, London, 274:133-136.

Loewi O (1921). Ueber humorale Ubertragbarkeit der Herzenwirkung. Pflug. Arch. ges. Physlol. 189:239-242.

Makowsky L, Caspar DLD, Phillips C and Goodenough DA (1977). Gap junction structures II. Analysis of the X-ray diffraction data. J Cell Biol 74: 629-645.

Masson-Pevet M, Beeker WK, Besselsen E, Mackaay JC, Jongsma HJ and Bouman LN (1982)On the ultrastructural identification of pacemaker cell types within the sinus node. In. Cardiac rate and Rhythm, (Boumnan LN and Jongsma HJ, eds) pp 19-34, Martinus Nijihoff Publishers, Boston.

Moore D and Ruska H (1957). Electron microscope study of mammalian cardiac muscle cells. J Biophys Biochem Cytol 3:261-269.

Nicholson BJ, Zhou L, Cao F,Zhu H,Chen Y(1998) Diverse molecular mechanisms of gap junction channel gating. In : Gap Junctions (Werner R, ed) pp 3-7 IOS Press, Amsterdam

Noma A, Tsuboi N (1987) Dependence of junctional conductance on proton, calcium and magnesium ions in cardiac paired cells of the guinea pig. J. Physiol. (London) 382:193-211

Osterhout WJV and Hill SE (1930) Salt bridges and negative variations. J Ge Physiol 13 :547-553

Peracchia C,Wang X, Li L, Peracchia LL (1996) Inhibition of calmodulin-expression prevents low pH-induced gap junction uncoupling in Xenopus oocytes. Pflugers Arch ges. Physiol 431: 379-387

Perkins GA,Goodenough DA,Sosinsky GE (1997) Three dimensional structure of the gap junction connexon Biophys.J 72: 533-544

Poche R and Lindner E (1955). Untersuchungen zur Frage der Glanzstreifen des Hermuskelgewebes beim Warmbluttér und beim Kaltblutter. Z. Zellforch Mikrosk Anat 43:104-105.

Purkinje JE (1845).Mikroskopisch-neurologische Beobachtungen. Arch Anat Physiol. Leipzig, 281.

Ramon y Cajal S (1895). Les nouvelles idées sur la structure du Systéme nerveux chez l'homme et chez les vertebres Reinwald, Paris.

Reber W, Weingart R (1982) Ungulate cardiac Purkinje fibers: the influence of intracellular pH on electrical cell-to-cell coupling J. Physiol (London) 328:87-104

Revel JP and Karnovsky MJ (1967). Hexagonal arrays of subunits in intercellular junctions of the mouse heart and liver. J Cell Biol 33:C7-C12.

Rook B, Jongsma HY and Van Ginnecken ACG (1988). Properties of single gap junctional channels between isolated neonatal rat heart cells. Am J Physiol 255:H770-H752

Rose B and Loewenstein WR(1975) Calcium ion distribution in cytoplasm visualized by aequorin: diffusion in cytosol restricted by energized sequestering Science 190:1204-1206

Simon AM, Goodeneough DA, Paul DL (1998) Mice lacking connexin 40 have cardiac conduction abnormalities characteristic of atrioventricular block and bundle branch block. Curr Biol 26:295-298

Sjostrand FS and Andersson KE (1954). Electron microscopy of the intercalated disks of cardiac muscle tissue. Experientia 10, 369-371.

Sosinsky G (2000) Gap Junction Structure : New Structures and New Insights In:Gap Junctions (C. Peracchia, ed) pp 1-22, Academic Press, San Diego, CA

Tsien R and Weingart R (1976) Inotropic effect of cyclic AMP in calf ventricular muscle studied by a. cut-end-method. J Physiol (London) 260:117-141.

Turin L, Warner AE (1977) Carbon dioxide reversibly abolishes ionic communication between cells of early amphybian embryo. Nature 270:56-57

van Bremen (1953). Intercalated discs in heart muscle studied with the electron microscope. Anat Rec 117: 49-54.

Veenstra RD,Wang HZ, Beblo DA,Chilton MG, Harris AL,Beyer EG, Brink PR (1995). Selectivity of connexin-specific gap junctions does not correlate with channel conductance. Circ. Res 77:1156-1165

Verheijck EE,van Kempen MJ, Veereschild M, Luivink L, Jongsma HJ, Bouman LN (2001) Electrophysiological features of mouse sinoatrial node in relation to connexin distribution. Cardiovasc Res 52: 40-50

Weidmann S (1952). The electrical constants of Purkinje fibers. J Physiol (London), 118:348-360.

Weidmann S (1966) The diffusion of radiopotassium across intercalated discs of
        mammalian cardiac muscle, J Physiol (London) 18:323-342
Weingart R (1974) The permeability to tetraethylammonium ions of the surface
        membrane and the intercalated disks of the sheep and calf myocardium.
        J Physiol (London) 240:741-762
Werner M(1910). Besteht die Hermuskulatur der Saugethiere Ausallseitz scharf
        begrentzen Zellen oder nicht? Arch Mikrosk Anat 71:101.
Woodbury YW and Crill WE(1961). On the problem of impulse conduction in
        the atrium. In: Nervous Inhibition (F1orey, L ed) Plenum, pp 24-35, New
        York.

2

CONNEXIN INTERACTING PROTEINS

Ralph J. Barker and Robert G. Gourdie
Medical University of South Carolina, Charleston, SC 29425

INTRODUCTION

The list of connexin-interacting proteins continues to grow along with the complexity of potential roles for these factors in gap junctional function and regulation. A recent study using a pull down assay with the carboxy terminal tail of connexin 43 (Cx43) as bait indicated that at least a dozen proteins may bind to this region of the molecule (Giepmans et al., 2001). A similarly large group of Cx43 binding partners was also indicated from yeast two hybrid studies (Giepmans et al., 1998; Jin et al., 2000). Together, these data indicate that a complex of proteins and a variety of regulatory interactions may exist at the cytoplasmic surface of the Cx43-containing gap junctional plaque. This level of regulatory control by connexin interacting proteins may permit subtle differences in function and distribution which may allow for fine tuning of gap junctional intercellular communication (GJIC). Although some connexin-binding partners are known, many others have yet to be identified and characterized. This task will be important for the next generation of researchers as it is increasingly becoming clear that gap junctional binding proteins are critical for many essential functions of tissues and cells.

The purpose of this review is to familiarize the reader with the known protein-protein interactions in which connexins may participate. As gap junctional channels are comprised of connexin-connexin interactions, one possible mechanism for regulating gap junctional properties is through the assembly of channels with variable connexin composition (Falk et al., 1997; Yeager et al., 1998). Heteromeric channels possess characteristics differing from homomeric channels with the same connexin subtypes, such as changes in channel gating by altering intracellular pH (Francis et al., 1999). Although connexin-connexin interactions are important in increasing the functional variation found within gap junctions (Stergiopolis et al., 1999), this review will focus on the direct interactions between connexins and other non-connexin proteins (summarized on table 1), with a special emphasis on Cx43 binding partners.

Table 1. **Connexin interacting proteins.** Summarized below are proteins known to directly interact with connexins, the connexin subtype with which they have been shown to interact, a proposed function for the interaction, and an appropriate reference.

Connexin Subtype(s)	Interacting Protein	Proposed Function	Reference
Cx32	calmodulin	responses to calcium, pH changes	Peracchia et al., 2000 Welsh et al., 1982
Cx43	PKC-α	decreased GJIC; phosphorylation mediated by other kinases	Bowling et al., 2001
Cx43	PKC-ε	decreased GJIC; direct phosphorylation on serine	Doble et al., 2000 Bowling et al., 2001
Cx46	PKC-γ	decreased GJIC; direct phosphorylation	Saleh et al., 2001
Cx43	v-src, c-src	decreased GJIC; direct phosphorylation on Y247, Y265	Kanemitsu et al., 1997 Toyofuku et al., 2001
Cx32	occludin	unknown	Kojima et al., 1999
Cx43	β-tubulin	stabilizing microtubular network	Giepmans et al., 2001

Cx43, Cx45, Cx46, Cx50	ZO-1	targeting, stabilization, aggregation, internalization, trafficking	Toyofuku et al., 1998 Nielsen et al., 2001 Laing et al., 2001 Barker et al., 2002
Cx43	β-catenin*	modulation of gene expression	Ai et al., 2000
Cx43	p120 catenin[#]	regulation of cell motility	Xu et al., 2001

*β-catenin has been shown through immunoprecipitation to interact, directly or indirectly, with Cx43.

[#]p120 catenin has been shown to co-localize with Cx43 in neural crest cells.

GAP JUNCTIONS AND CALMODULIN

One of the first proteins reported to interact with the connexin family of proteins was calmodulin (Welsh et al., 1982), a nearly ubiquitous calcium-binding protein known to regulate the function of a variety of different channel types (reviewed Saimi et al., 1994). Two putative calmodulin-binding domains were found to exist in the Cx32 amino acid sequence (Torok et al., 1997), and the binding of calmodulin to gap junctions was shown to be involved in mediating gap junctional responses to changes in calcium concentration (Torok et al., 1997; Toyama et al., 1994). Calmodulin was subsequently shown to be directly involved in the gating of Cx32-containing gap junctional channels by binding to the connexon subunit, possibly via physical blockade of the intercellular channel (Peracchia et al., 2000). The effects of lowered cytosolic pH in reducing cell-cell coupling through gap junctions may be mediated through calmodulin activity (Peracchia et al., 1996), and may potentially involve connexin phosphorylation (Arellano et al., 1990). In addition to the effects of calmodulin on channel gating, there is also a potential role for this protein in the assembly and targeting of connexons. A synthetic calmodulin-binding protein was capable of reversibly inhibiting the assembly of Cx32 into connexons (Ahmad et al., 2001). When a Cx32 protein with a deletion of the putative calmodulin binding site was transiently expressed in COS-7 cells, connexon formation was adversely affected and functional gap junctions were unable to form from these proteins (Ahmad et al., 2001).

A detailed picture of gap junction regulation through the extensive use of connexin binding proteins is beginning to emerge. Calmodulin is but one component in the dynamic interplay between various signaling pathways and structural proteins that have subsequently been characterized which may function to coordinate gap junction distribution and activity in cells and tissues (Saez et al., 1990; Watterson et al., 1984).

CONNEXIN-KINASE INTERACTIONS

Most connexins are phosphoproteins, and processes such as gap junction gating, trafficking, turnover, distribution, and assembly are likely to be regulated by phosphorylation of connexin subunits by a variety of protein kinases (reviewed Lampe and Lau, 2000; Lau et al., 1996; Laird, 1996). In the case of Cx43, the connexon hexamers found in functional gap junctions contain at least two major connexin phospho-isoforms (Musil et al., 1991). Correlations have been made between the phosphorylation status of Cx43 and its insolubility in Triton X-100 (Musil et al., 1991), indicating that changes in cytoskeletal involvement may accompany phosphorylation events. During formation, connexins assembled into functional gap junctions at the membrane are more phosphorylated and are less soluble in detergent solutions than those found at cytoplasmic sites (Atkinson et al., 1995; Musil et al., 1991). Connexin phosphorylation is likely to be an important component in the formation of gap junction channels, as Cx43 is phosphorylated on serine and threonine residues prior to insertion into functional gap junctional channels (Musil et al., 1991). Regulation of assembly and turnover may also occur through phosphorylation. Increases in phosphorylation by PKA, PKC,

MAPK, and tyrosine kinases can inhibit or enhance gap junction intercellular communication (reviewed Lau et al., 1996). In addition, redistribution of Cx43 from the cell membrane to cytoplasmic sites has been correlated with the phosphorylation of Cx43 in some cell types (Guan et al., 1995; Barker et al., 2002; Lampe et al., 1998).

Among the most potent regulators of gap junctional activity are a variety of protein kinases that have been shown to directly interact with the Cx43 molecule (reviewed Lampe and Lau, 2000). These kinases are likely to be responsible, in part or in whole, for the basal level of phophorylation that allows for normal gap junction function and activity. This group of proteins is known to include c-src, PKC-α, PKC–ε, and PKC-γ, and there are certain to be many others whose function in gap junction regulation remain to be discovered. This field is made more complicated by the observation that there has been a consistent lack of correlation between the phosphorylation status of the Cx43 protein and changes in GJIC or specific signal transduction pathways between different cell types. It is likely that a great deal of variability exists between the different cell types in the connexins expressed, the kinases that are involved, and the downstream effectors of these kinases. The cross-talk between signaling pathways that is known to occur also makes exploring kinase function in gap junctions a challenging area of study (Bowling et al., 2001; Zhou et al., 1999).

The PKC Family of Protein Kinases

Members of the PKC family of kinases have been show to interact with, and phosphorylate, Cx43 in a variety of tissues and cell lines. In general, PKC phosphorylation has been shown to decrease GJIC (Lampe et al., 2000), while PKA activity has been associated with an increased cell-cell coupling, although many exceptions to this rule have been observed. PKA activity and increases in cAMP are reported to increase gap junction permeability (van Rijen et al., 2000; Sakai et al., 1992), enhance gap junction assembly (Albright et al., 2001; Paulson et al., 2000) and decrease gap junction removal from the membrane (Saez et al., 1989). The constrasting activity of these two kinase systems along with MAP kinase are in part responsible for moderating the function of gap junctions in most cells.

12-O-tetradecanoylphorbol-13-acetate (TPA) has been used to probe the activity of PKC in cells and has been shown to be a potent inhibitor of GJIC (Ruch et al., 2001; Lampe et al., 2000; Kwak et al., 1996), although much variability has been reported. In fibroblasts, total PKC activity could not be correlated with phosphorylation of Cx43 or changes in GJIC (Cruciani et al., 2001), which suggests that the activity of specific PKC isoforms might be more important than overall PKC activation. Thus, many groups have focused on determining how the activity of specific PKC isoforms may affect gap junctional function. For example, in lens, PKC-γ has been shown to phosphorylate and interact with Cx46 (Saleh et al., 2001). In heart, Cx43 co-immunoprecipitates with PKC-α and -ε, and this level of interaction is increased in failing ventricle (Doble et al., 2000; Bowling et al., 2001), a condition which induces changes in the function and distribution of myocardial gap junctions (reviewed Severs et al., 1999; Matsushita et al., 1997; Huang et al., 1999). Both kinases may increase the phosphorylation of connexins and reduce GJIC, but PKC-ε directly phosphorylates Cx43 (Bowling et al., 2001). PKC-α phosphorylation, though not direct, was suggested to occur by the action of other kinases, such as mitogen-associated protein kinase (MAPK), in downstream events (Bowling et al., 2001). Overlap between the function of PKCs and MAP kinases in regulating cell-cell coupling has been reported in other systems (Rivedahl et al., 2001). In cultured neonatal myocytes, PKC-ε was directly involved in phosphorylating Cx43, which was necessary for the inhibitory effects of FGF-2 on GJIC (Doble et al., 2000). ERK activation may occur following the interaction of Cx43 with PKC isoforms (Ruch et al., 2001). The interaction of connexins with multiple PKCs hints at the presence of a larger regulatory complex that may be the key to moderating the operation of gap junction channels.

Src and Cx43

Tyrosine phosphorylation of Cx43 has been associated with a decrease in GJIC (Zhang YW 1999; Toyofuku et al., 2000). Two members of the src family of non-receptor tyrosine kinases, c-src and v-src, have been shown to interact directly with and phosphorylate Cx43 in vitro and in vivo (Lau et al., 1996; Lampe et al., 2000; Toyofuku et al., 2001). v-src directly phosphorylates Cx43 (Lin et al., 2001), and the two proteins can be co-immunoprecipitated (Kanemitsu et al., 1997; Loo et al., 1999), indicating that phosphorylation may be related to binding of the two proteins. Proline rich regions of Cx43 may be involved in src association (Kanemitsu et al., 1997).

Tyrosine phosphorylation by src appears to form the basis for Cx43 binding. The SH2 and SH3 domains of v-src are thought to contain the regions which interact with Cx43, and this binding enables v-src to directly phosphorylate Cx43 on residues Y265 and Y247 (Lin et al., 1997). v-Src was unable to disrupt GJIC in mutants containing phenylalanine in place of the tyrosine residues, and mutations in SH2 and SH3 domains of v-src inhibited binding with Cx43 (Kanemitsu et al., 1997).

Src activity may also be related to the interaction between Cx43 and zonula occludens-1 (ZO-1), a scaffolding protein which may be involved in connexin distribution and function (Toyofuku et al., 2001; Giepmans et al., 2001). An in vitro binding assay showed that tyrosine phosphorylation of Cx43 on residue 265 enhanced binding to c-src and inhibited the interaction between Cx43 and ZO-1 (Toyofuku et al., 2001). ZO-1 and a mutant Cx43 lacking the tyrosine at 265 failed to be co-precipitated following c-src association (Giepmans et al., 2001). In HEK293 cells, constitutively active c-src (Y527F) appeared to reduce levels of cell surface-located Cx43. The interaction of these two proteins occurred between c-src's SH2 domain and a region on Cx43 other than the known ZO-1 binding site (Toyofuku et al., 2001). Constitutively activated c-src was a better binding partner for Cx43 than the wild-type protein, and kinase activity of c-src could be correlated with the level of Cx43 association (Giepmans et al., 2001). The functional consequences of decreased GJIC was observed in a hamster model of congestive heart failure, where tyrosine phosphorylation of Cx43 by c-src was correlated with decreased gap junctional conductance (Toyofuku et al., 1999). The mechanisms behind how tyrosine phosphorylation decreases GJIC in physiological or pathological conditions remains to be determined.

MICROTUBULES

Giepmans et al. (2001) has recently shown that one of at least a dozen potential proteins that can be pulled down by the carboxy terminus of Cx43 is β-tubulin, a component of microtubules. Co-sedimentation experiments confirmed these results and indicated that the binding was direct. A potential tubulin binding motif was found within the amino acid sequence of Cx43 and this motif was lacking in other connexin isoforms examined. Elegant fluorescence and immuno-electron microscopy indicate that these proteins are co-localized in about half of the gap junctional plaques examined, with microtubular structures terminating at the gap junction. No function consequence of microtubule disruption on GJIC was noted upon treatment of Rat-1 cells with nocodazole, a microtubular de-polymerizer. However, it is possible that microtubules may be important in the trafficking of connexons to specific regions of the cell, such as the cell membrane or cytoplasmic areas. Formation of gap junctions in chick retina was inhibited with treatment of colchicine (Meller et al., 1981), a pharmacological agent known to cause microtubular depolymerization. In apparent contrast, rat hepatocytes treated with colchicine formed gap junctions that were increased in size and formed a greater proportion of total surface area of the cell, with annular gap junctions more frequently observed in the cytoplasm (Rassat et al., 1982). The authors of these reports suggested that the localization of gap junctions may be dependent on an intact and functional microtubular system. It has also been suggested that Cx43 may act as a capping protein by preventing depolymerization at the plus ends of the microtubule (Giepmans et al., 2001). It was proposed that Cx43-gap junctions have a role in stabilizing the established microtubular network, although this remains to be determined. Another interesting hypothesis is that Cx43 may work in concert with cadherins to regulate cell motility using microtubular machinery (Xu et al., 2001). A Cx43 protein lacking a small portion of this putative microtubular binding motif was capable of inhibiting motility of 3T3 cells (Moorby et al., 2000). On the other hand, other studies indicate that microtubules may not be an important component for either gap junction removal or assembly (Feldman et al., 1997). More studies of Cx43 and tubulin interaction are necessary to determine the nature of the association between microtubules and gap junctions.

TIGHT AND ADHESIVE-ASSOCIATED JUNCTIONAL PROTEINS

Catenins and Occludin

Evidence suggests that the localization and function of gap junctions may be linked to components initially identified in two other junction types, the adherens junction and the tight junction. β-catenin, a structural and signaling component of the adherens junction, and Cx43 were co-localized both in cultured neonatal myocytes (Ai et al., 2000) and in neural crest cells (Xu et al., 2001). β-catenin and Cx43 can be induced to interact in neonatal myocytes in culture by exposure to lithium, an agent that mimics signaling by the Wnt family of secreted proteins (Ai et al., 2000). This interaction may be one mechanism for regulating Cx43 transcription, as β-catenin bound to gap junctions at the membrane is unable to participate in the transactivation of the Cx43 promoter. In this manner, Wnt activity and β-catenin interaction may modulate both expression of Cx43 and accumulation of gap junctional plaques at the membrane. Another member of the catenin family, p120 catenin, from the armadillo family of proteins, has been shown to colocalize with Cx43 in migrating neural crest cells (Xu et al., 2001). This binding represents a mechanism by which Cx43 may act to modulate the motility of these cells.

Occludin is a transmembrane protein integral to the structure of the junction structure (Tsukita et al., 1997). In immunoprecipitation studies, occludin was shown to interact directly with Cx32 in transfected mouse hepatocytes (Kojima et al., 1999). Occludin and Cx32 were partially co-localized both at the cell membrane and within the cytoplasm, and co-localization within the cytoplasm was maintained after treatment with brefeldin A (Kojima et al., 1999), an agent inhibiting Cx32 targeting to the membrane (Kojima et al., 1996). These results are indicative of an important association between the components of connexin-containing gap junctions and other junction types. A potential link between the interaction of these components may be mediated through the scaffolding protein, ZO-1. In MDCK cells, ZO-1 was found to link occludin to the actin cytoskeleton (Fanning et al., 1998). ZO-1 is also associated with the structure of cadherin based adherens junctions by virtue of its ability to bind α-catenin directly. Thus, ZO-1 may interact indirectly with β-catenin (Itoh et al., 1997). In addition, ZO-1 has also been shown to interact with connexins 43 and 45 (Toyofuku et al., 1998; Giepmans et al., 1998; Laing et al., 2001). The expression of a deletion mutant of occludin in a murine epithelial cell line altered gap junction distribution and induced an association between gap junctions and components of the tight junction (Bamforth et al., 1999). The interrelationships between proteins involved in the regulation of tight and adherens junctions with gap junctions indicate a potential for the convergence of signaling pathways utilized by these junctions.

ZO-1

Originally discovered in association with the cytoplasmic plaque at tight junctions, ZO-1 is one member of a family of proteins which function in protein targeting, signal transduction, and determination of cell polarity (reviewed Anderson et al., 1995). These proteins are known as MAGUKs because members are characterized by a region of homology to membrane associated guanylate kinase and by the presence of three protein domains of about 90 amino acids termed the PDZ domain (for PDZ95/DlgA/ZO-1 homology domain). This domain has been shown to function in protein binding to specialized consensus regions on target proteins (Itoh et al., 1991; Goodenough et al.,1999; Toyofuku et al, 1998). The known MAGUKs have been consistently found associated with the cell membrane at sites of cell-cell contact, where they are thought to regulate junctional properties and organize contacts for signal propagation. MAGUKs have been implicated in facilitating lateral aggregation of membrane proteins into functional domains (Sheng et al, 1997). Other findings suggest that previously hypothesized functions for MAGUK proteins (e.g. ZO-1, dlg, PSD-95, PSD-93) in protein targeting and aggregation may need re-evaluation or expansion to consider other possible functions for these proteins (Migaud et al., 1998; McGee et al., 2000; Barker et al., 2002).

ZO-1 is thought to function in the organization and maintenance of intercellular junctions. In tight junctions, ZO-1 is known to interact with both occludin and ZO-2 through its PDZ domains (Goodenough et al., 1999), and is linked to the cytoskeleton via the direct and indirect interaction with F-actin (Fanning et al., 1998). Itoh et al. (1991) found that ZO-1 was associated with the undercoat of cadherin based cell adhesion plaques in both epithelial and non-epithelial cell types. Further studies showed that ZO-1 indirectly associates with cadherins via direct interaction with alpha-catenin, and may stabilize adherens junctions and link these junctions to the cytoskeleton through an interaction with actin and α-spectrin (Itoh et al., 1997). ZO-1 may also be involved in regulating assembly and localization of adherens junctions (Collares-Buzato et al., 1998).

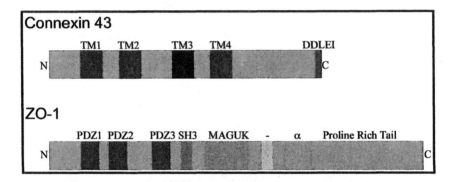

Figure 1. **Structural domains contained within connexin 43 and zonula occludens – 1.** Connexin proteins are composed of four transmembrane domains, a cytosolic amino and carboxy terminus, one intracellular linker domain, and two extracellular linker regions. The carboxy and intracellular linker region are unique to each of the connexins, and are the primary determinants of connexin size and interaction specificity. The last five amino acid residues of Cx43, DDLEI, have been shown to bind directly to the second PDZ domain of ZO-1. ZO-1, a 220 kiloDalton member of the MAGUK family of signaling proteins, contains three PDZ domains which are known to function in multiple molecular interactions. In addition, it also contains an SH3 domain, a region of homology to membrane associated guanylate kinase (MAGUK), an acid rich region designated as (-), an alternative splice site (α), and a proline rich tail.

Co-localization of Cx43 and ZO-1 has been reported in a variety of cells and tissues including uterine myocytes (Day et al., 1998), testis (Batias et al., 1999), thyroid (Guerrier et al., 1995), and neonatal myocardial cells (Toyofuku et al., 1998). Using a yeast two-hybrid assay with the cytosolic carboxy region of Cx43, the last five amino acids (DDLEI) of Cx43 was shown to bind the second PDZ domain of ZO-1 (Giepmans et al., 1998; see figure 1). In transfected COS7 cells, rat fibroblasts, HEK 293 cells (Toyofuku et al., 1998), and adult cardiomyocytes (Barker et al.,

2002), ZO-1 was co-immunoprecipitated with Cx43. In addition, expression of the amino terminus region of ZO-1 containing the second PDZ domain was reported to cause a redistribution of Cx43 to cytoplasmic structures and a loss of electrical coupling in cultured neonatal myocytes (Toyofuku et al., 1998), suggesting an involvement of ZO-1 in targeting or turnover of Cx43. Furthermore, it was reported that ZO-1, Cx43, and α-spectrin were co-localized at the area of membrane between these cells (Toyofuku et al., 1998). It is possible that ZO-1 serves to link Cx43 to cytoskeletal structures and acts to target Cx43 to the intercalated disc region in cardiac myocytes (Toyofuku et al., 1998). Further studies indicated that c-src may be capable of mediating the interaction between ZO-1 and Cx43 through tyrosine phosphorylation (Toyofuku et al., 2001) and by directly binding the gap junctional subunit (see the previous section on kinases for more on src and Cx43). A Cx43-ZO-1 interaction may not be necessary for connexons to assemble into gap junction plaques at the membrane, as mutant Cx43 proteins lacking the ZO-1/PDZ binding region have been shown to form functional gap junctions (Dunham et al., 1992). It remains to be seen whether normal Cx43 localization is dependent on a stable interaction between Cx43 and ZO-1.

ZO-1 may also play an important role in the localization of other connexin subtypes. A recent study showed that Cx45 and ZO-1 interact in osteoblastic cells and could be co-localized at the cell membrane using immunofluorescence microscopy (Laing et al., 2001). High levels of ZO-1 expression has been observed in lens, where ZO-1 was shown to interact with both Cx46 and Cx50 (Nielsen et al., 2001). Binding of Cx43 to ZO-1 was suggested to occur on regions similar to the binding domain originally discovered within Cx43. Whether the functional consequences of ZO-1 binding are similar among the connexin subtypes remains to be determined.

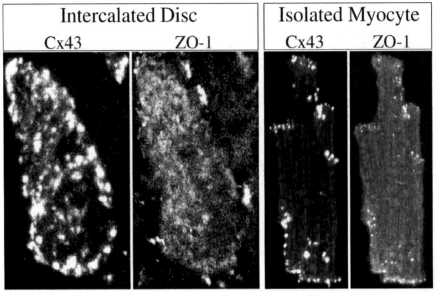

| Intercalated Disc | | Isolated Myocyte | |
| Cx43 | ZO-1 | Cx43 | ZO-1 |

Figure 2. **Co-localization of Cx43 and ZO-1 in the intercalated disc of intact myocardium vs. isolated myocytes.** Disc from adult myocardium showed low to moderate levels of co-localization. A higher level of co-localization was observed upon isolation of myocytes in internalized gap junction, suggesting an increase in the interaction between Cx43 and ZO-1.

Our own studies of the function of ZO-1 in cardiac myocytes suggests that the role of ZO-1 may need to be revised or expanded to include the possibility of ZO-1-Cx43 interaction occurring during dynamic gap junctional events involving the internalization of gap junctions and formation of annular gap junctions. We have shown that the co-distribution of these proteins, as detected by immunofluorescence and immuno-electron microscopy, is limited to a low to moderate level in the discs of normal adult cardiomyocytes (Barker et al., 2002). The lack of correspondence between the distribution of the two proteins is evident in three dimensional projections through "en face" discs (see figure 2). However, the co-localization and degree of interaction (as assessed by ratio of co-immunoprecipitated ZO-1 per unit of Cx43 – see figure 3b) can be increased in myocytes and WBF344 rat liver epithelial cells by treatments inducing the formation of subsarcolemmal and annular gap junctions (see figure 2). The specific method by which we have affected the endocytosis of gjs has been enzymatic treatment to dissociate cells (rat myocardium or WBF344 cell cultures) or exposure to TPA, a phorbol esther known to activate PKCs (see the section on kinases for more information). However, other conditions which are known cause changes in gap junctional distribution may also induce this change in Cx43 – ZO-1 association. For example, ZO-1 was shown to co-localize with Cx43 in the cytoplasm of epithelial 42GPA9 Sertoli cells after treatment with lindane (Defamie et al, 2001), a toxin which reduces GJIC and causes internalization of gap junctions (Guan et al., 1995).

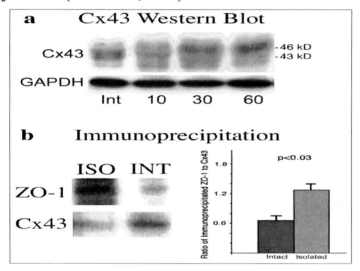

Figure 3. **Cx43 Western blots and immunoprecipitation studies.** (a) Western blots indicate a change in relative mobility of the Cx43 protein following isolation of myocytes that may be indicative of a change in phosphorylation status. **Int**=Intact Myocardium. **10, 30, 60**=minutes after isolation of mycoytes. (b) Immunoprecipitation studies in-dicate that more ZO-1 can be immuno-precipitated in isolated myocytes (**ISO**) vs. intact myocardium (**INT**). The difference in ratio between immuno-recipitated proteins (graph in **b**) was significant (p<0.03).

Acting can be found in the undercoat of gap junctions (Watanabe et al., 1988) and has been implicated in the endocytosis of these structures (Larsen et al., 1979). Recent studies have shown that acting is involved in the endocytosis of vesicles from the cell membrane (Merrifield et al., 1999), including during annular gap junction formation in SW-13 adrenal cortical tumor cells (Murray et al., 1997). Cytochalasin B, an actin depolymerizer, inhibited the formation of annular gap junctions in this cell type, indicating the participation of actin in removal of gap junction plaques from the membrane. As a link between membrane proteins and the actin-based cytoskeleton (Itoh et al., 1997; Fanning et al., 1998), a potential role exists for ZO-1 in the remodeling of gap junctions during a variety of processes known to involve the formation of annular gap junctions. We have noted that annular gap junctions can be observed in two areas in which we have been actively investigating: development of the heart and myocardial pathology. Given that ZO-1 may play a crucial role in the remodeling of gap junction distribution in these areas, we are in the process of characterizing the interaction between Cx43 and ZO-1.

Annular gap junctions can be observed in vivo during development of the mammalian myocardium (Legato et al., 1979; Chen et al., 1989). In the adult heart, gap junctions and cell adhesion junctions can be found predominantly at the area of membrane at the ends of myocytes known as the intercalated disc (Gourdie et al., 1992). The targeting of gap junctions to this area of the cell membrane remains an area of active investigation. A hypothesis which was originally proposed by our lab is that the regulation of gap junctional assembly and turnover may be the primary factor in determining the distribution of gap junctions in polarized cells such as these. During the postnatal development of mammalian heart, myocardial gap junctions undergo an extensive change in distribution (Gourdie et al., 1992; Fromaget et al., 1992) that may be related to differential rates of gap junctional turnover at the cell membrane. In the neonate, confocal microscopy indicates that gap junctions are distributed relatively uniformly throughout the membranes of myocytes. During early postnatal development, gap junctions and cell adhesion junctions gradually become polarized to the ends of cardiomyocytes at the intercalated disc.   We have proposed that gap junctions at the ends of the cardiomyocyte are being turned-over more slowly than those at the lateral borders of the cell. The rate of gap junctional turnover may be related to a reduction in shear stress upon the gap junctional plaque by virtue of its proximity to stabilizing fascia adherens and desmosomes found at the cardiac intercalated disc. The outcome is an accumulation of gap junctions at the disc. One finding that can be predicted by this hypothesis is that a lag exists between the developmental points in which the adherens junctions and the gap junctions become localized primarily at the disc (Angst et al, 1997).   Thus, assembly and turnover may be an essential   component   in   the   regulation   of   gap   junctional distribution and cell-cell coupling.

In several types of heart disease such as myocardial ischemia, gap junctions are known to become remodeled to resemble the distribution typically found in the neonatal myocardium (Severs et al., 1994; Sepp et al., 1997; Smith 1991; Matsushita et al., 1999). During this period of redistribution, gap junctions are rapidly endocytosed to form annular gap junctions, and this process may be an essential component of generating deranged gap junctional distribution (Peters et al., 1993; Uzzaman et al., 2000).   These changes in coupling geometry are thought to be a predisposing factor in the generation of re-entrant arrhythmia and other conduction abnormalities (Spach et al., 2000; Wilders, 2000). The role of ZO-1 in mediating an interaction between Cx43 and the cytoskeleton may be important in determining how gap junctions distribution becomes altered.   One model of ischemia indicates that ZO-1 shifts from a soluble to insoluble (cytoskeletal) pool upon ATP-depletion (Tsukamoto et al., 1997). A similar shift by a complex of proteins including ZO-1 and Cx43 may explain how or why gap junction redistribution may accompany ischemia. this understanding of how patterns of gap junction distributions are generated during development may be helpful in the development of future therapeutics aimed at reducing morbidity and mortality associated with altered coupling. We have shown that ZO-1 may be involved in removing gap junctions from the membrane upon isolation of adult cardiomyocytes (Barker et al., 2002), and similarities in gap junctional remodeling occurring during ischemia indicate that gap junctional removal from the membrane in these cells may occur in a similar fashion. The parallels that we have observed between gap junctional redistribution in these systems indicate a potential for convergence upon common or related remodeling mechanisms.

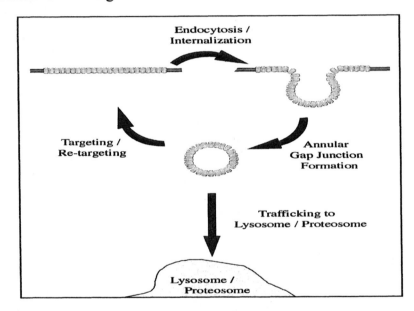

Figure 4. **Proposed processes in which gap junctions may interact with ZO–1.** ZO-1 has been suggested to function in the targetingof Cx43-containing gap junctions to the cell membrane (Toyofuku et al., 1998), but may also participate in the endocytosis, formation, or trafficking of gap junctions from the cell membrane to sites of degradation such as the lysosome or proteosome. In addition, re-targeting of annular gap junctions back to the cell membrane remains a possibility. The interaction between connex-ins and ZO-1 remains an active area of research and may be regulated through tyrosine phosphorylation by c-src.

Based on the evidence indicating that Cx43 and ZO-1 interaction is increased in internalized gap junctions, we have proposed that ZO-1, via its ability to bind simultaneously to gap junctional proteins and cytoskeletal elements (Fanning et al., 1998;

Toyofuku et al., 1998; Itoh et al., 1997; Giepmans et al., 1998), may act in the internalization, endocytosis, or trafficking of gap junctions (Barker et al., 2002). In addition, ZO-1 may also function as a scaffold for enhancing and stabilizing the interaction between Cx43 and regulatory proteins, such as kinases and transcription factors. The possible involvement of ZO-1 in regulating the removal of gap junction from the cell membrane has many implications, considering that the formation of annular gap junctions from cell surface located gap junctions may be a common cellular process as well (Laird et al., 2001). The mechanisms behind the association between Cx43 and ZO-1 may be one component in modulating gap junction distribution between cells.

REFERENCE

Ahmad S, Martin PE, and Evans WH. (2001) Assembly of gap junction channels: mechanism, effects of calmodulin antagonists and identification of connexin oligomerization determinants. Eur J Biochem 268:4544-4552. Ai Z, Fischer A, Spray DC, Brown AMC, and Fishman GI. (2000) Wnt-1 regulation of connexin43 in cardiac myocytes. J Clin Invest 105:161-171.

Albright CD., Kuo J, and Jeong S. (2001) cAMP enhances Cx43 gap junction formation and function and reverses choline deficiency apoptosis. Exp Mol Pathol 71:34-39.

Angst BD, Khan LU, Severs NJ, Whitely K, Rothery S, Thompson RP, Magee AI, Gourdie RG. (1997) Dissociated spatial patterning of gap junctions and cell adhesion junctions during postnatal differentiation of ventricular myocardium. Circ Res 80:88-94.

Arellano RO, Rivera A, and Ramon F. (1990) Protein phosphorylation and hydrogen ions modulate calcium-induced closure of gap junction channels. Biophys J 57:363-367.

Atkinson MM, Lampe PD, Lin HH, Kollander R, Li XR, and Kiang DT. (1995) Cyclic AMP modifies the cellular distribution of connexin43 and induces a persistent increase in the junctional permeability of mouse mammary tumor cells. J Cell Sci 108:3079-3090.

Bamforth SD, Kniesel U, Wolburg H, Engelhardt B, and Risau W. (1999) A dominant mutant of occludin disrupts tight junction structure and function. J Cell Sci 112:1879-1888.

Barker RJ, Price RL, and Gourdie RG. (2002) Increased Association of ZO-1 with Connexin43 During Remodeling of Cardiac Gap Junctions. Circ Res 90:317-324.

Batias C, Defamie N, Lablack A, Thepot D, Fenichel P, Segretain D, and Pointis G. (1999) Modified expression of testicular gap junction connexin 43 during normal spermatogenic cycle and in altered spermatogenesis. Cell Tissue Res 298:113-121.

Bowling N, Huang X, Sandusky GE, Fouts RL, Mintze K, Esterman M, Allen PD, Maddi R, McCall E, and Vlahos CJ. (2001) Protein kinase C-α and –ε modulate connexin-43 phosphorylation in human heart. J Mol Cell Cardiol 33:789-798.

Chen L, Goings GE, Upshaw-Earley J, and Page E. (1989) Cardiac gap junctions and gap junction-associated vesicles: ultrastructural comparison of in situ negative staining with conventional positive staining. Circ Res 64:501-514.

Collares-Buzato CB, Jepson MA, Simmons NL, and Hirst BH. (1998) Increased tyrosine phosphorylation causes redistribution of adherens junction and tight junction proteins and perturbs paracellular barrier function in MDCK epithelia. Eur J Cell Biol 76: 85-92.

Cruciani V, Husoy T, and Mikalsen S. (2001) Pharmocological evidence for system dependent involvement of prtotein kinase C isoenzymes inphorbol esther-suppressed gap junctional communication. Exp Cell Res 268:150-161.

Day WE, Bowen J, Barhoumi R, Bazer FW, and Burghardt RC. (1998) Endometrial connexin expression in the mare and pig – evidence for the suppression of cell-cell communication in the uterineluminal epithelium. Anat Rec 251:277-285.

Defamie N, Mograbi B, Roger C, Cronier L, Malassine A, Brucker-Davis F, Fenichel P, Segretain D, and Pointis G. (2001) Disruption of gap junctional intercellular communication by lindane is associated with aberrant localization of connexin43 and zonula occludens-1 in 42GPA9 Sertoli cells. Carcinogenesis. 22:1537-1542.

Doble BW, Ping P, and Kardami E. (2000) The ε subtype of protein kinase C is required for cardiomyocyte connexin-43 phosphorylation. Circ Res 86:293-301.

Dunham B, Liu S, Taffet S, Trabka-Janik E, Delmar M, Petryshyn R, Zheng S, Perzova R, Vallano ML. (1992) Immunolocalization and expression of functional and nonfunctional cell-to-cell channels from wild-type and mutant rat heart connexin43 cDNA. Circ Res 70:1233-1243.

Falk MM, Buehler LK, Kumar NM, and Gilula NB. (1997) Cell-free synthesis and assembly of connexins into functional gap junction membrane channels. EMBO J 16:2703-2716.

Fanning AS, Jameson BJ, Jesaitis LA, and Anderson JM. (1998) The tight junction protein ZO-1 establishes a link between the transmembrane protein occludin and the actin cytoskeleton. J Biol Chem 273:29745-29753.

Feldman PA, Kim J, and Laird DW. (1997) Loss of gap junction plaques and inhibition of intercellular communication in ilimaquinone-treated BICR-M1Rk and NRK cells. J Membr Biol 155:275-287.

Fromaget C, el Aoumari A, and Gros D. (1992) Distribution pattern of connexin 43, a gap junctional protein, during the differentiation of mouse heart myocytes. Differentiation 51:9-20.

Giepmans BNG and Moolenaar WH. (1998) The gap junction protein connexin43 interacts with the second PDZ domain of the zona occludens-1 protein. Curr Biol 8:931-934.

Giepmans BNG, Verlaan I, Hengeveld T, Janssen H, Calafat J, Falk MM, and Moolenaar WH. (2001) Gap junction protein connexin-43 interacts directly with microtubules. Curr Biol 11:1364-1368.

Gourdie RG, Green CR, Severs NJ, and Thompson RP. (1992) Immunolabelling patterns of gap junction connexins in the developing and mature rat heart. Embryology (Berl) 185:363-78.

Goodall H and Maro B. (1986) Major loss of junctional coupling during mitosis in early mouse embryos. J Cell Biol 102(2):568-575.

Goodenough DA. (1999) Plugging the leaks. PNAS USA 96:319-321.

Gu H, Ek-Vitorin JF, Taffet SM, and Delmar M. (2000) Co-expression of connexins 40 and 43 enhances the pH sensitivity of gap junctions: a model for synergistic interactions among connexins. Circ Res 86:E98-E103.

Guan X, Ruch RJ. (1996) Gap junction endocytosis and lysosomal degradation of connexin43-P2 in WB-F344 rat liver epithelial cells treated with DDT and lindane. Carcinogenesis17:1791-1798.

Guerrier A, Fonlupt P, Morand I, Rabilloud R, Audebet C, Krutovskikh V, Gros D, Rousset B, and Munari-SilemY. (1995) Gap junctions and cell polarity: connexin32 and connexin43 expressed in polarized thyroid epithelial cells assemble into separate gap junctions, which are located in distinct regions of he lateral plasma membrane domain. J Cell Sci 108:2609-2617.

Huang XD, Sandusky GE, and Zipes DP. Heterogeneous loss of connexin43 protein in ischemic dog hearts. Journal of Cardiovascular Electrophysiology 10:79-91, 1999.

Itoh M, Nagafuchi A, Moroi S, and Tsukita S. (1997) Involvement of ZO-1 in cadherin based cell adhesion through its direct binding to alpha catenin and actin filaments. J Cell Biol 138:181-192.

Itoh M, Yonemura S, NagafuchiA, Tsukita S, and Tsukita S. (1991) A 220-kD undercoat-constitutive protein: its specific localization at cadherin-based cell-cell adhesion sites. J Cell Biol 115:1449-1469.

Jin C, Lau AF, and Martyn KD. (2000) Identification of connexin-interacting proteins: application of the yeast two hybrid screen. Methods 20:219-231.

Kanemitsu MY, Loo LW, Simon S, Lau AF, and Eckhart W. (1997) Tyrosine phosphorylation of connexin 43 by v-Src is mediated by SH2 and SH3 domain interactions. J Biol Chem 272:22824-22831.

Kwak BR and Jongsma HJ. (1996) Regulation of cardiac gap junction channel permeability and conductance by several phosphorylating conditions. Mol Cell Biochem 157:93-99.

Kojima T, Sawada N, Chiba H, Kokai Y, Yamamoto M, Urban M, Lee GH, Hertzberg EL, Mochizuki Y, and Spray DC. (1999) Induction of tight junctions in human connexin 32 (hCx32)-transfected mouse hepatocytes: connexin 32 interacts with occludin. Biochem Biophys Res Commun 266:222-229.

Kojima T, Yamamoto M, Tobioka H, Mizuguchi T, Mitaka T, and Mochizuki Y. (1996) Changes in cellular distribution of connexins 32 and 26 during formation of gap junctions in primary cultures of rat hepatocytes. Exp Cell Res 223:314-326.

Laing JG, Manley-Markowski RN, Koval M, Civitelli R, and Steinberg TH. (2001) Connexin45 interacts with zonula occludens-1 and connexin43 in osteoblastic cells. J Biol Chem 276:23051-23055.

Laird DW, Jordan K, Shao Q. (2001) Expression and imaging of connexin-GFP chimeras in live mammalian cells. Methods Mol Biol 154:135-142.

Laird DW. (1996) The life cycle of a connexin: gap junction formation, removal, and degradation. J Bioenerg Biomembr 28:311-318.

Lampe PD, TenBroek EM, Burt JM, Kurata WE, Johnson RG, and Lau AF. (2000) Phosphorylation of connexin43 on serine 368 by protein kinase C regulates gap junction communication. J Cell Biol 149:1503-1512.

Lampe PD and Lau AF. (2000) Regulation of Gap Junctions by Phosphorylation of Connexins. Arch Biochem Biophys 384:205-215.

Lampe PD, Kurata WE, Warn-Cramer BJ, and Lau AF. (1998) Formation of a distinct connexin43 phosphoisoform in mitotic cells is dependent upon p34cdc2 kinase. J Cell Sci 111:833-841.

Lau AF, Kurata WE, Kanemitsu MY, Loo LW, Warn-Cramer BJ, Eckhart W, and Lampe PD. (1996) Regulation of connexin43 function by activated tyrosine protein kinases. J Bioenerg Biomembr 28:359-368.

Larsen WJ, Tung HN, Murray SA, and Swenson CA. (1979) Evidence for the participation of actin microfilaments and bristle coats in the internalization of gap junction membrane. J Cell Biol 83:576-87.

Legato MJ. (1979) Cellular mechanisms of normal growth in the mammalian heart. II. A quantitative and qualitative comparison between the right and left ventricular myocytes in the dog from birth to five months of age. Circ Res 44:263-279.

Lin R, Warn-Cramer BJ, Kurata WE, and Lau AF. (2001) v-Src phosphorylation of connexin 43 on Tyr247 and Tyr265 disrupts gap junctional communication. J Cell Biol 154:815-827.

Loo LWM, Kanemitsu MY, and Lau AF. (1999) In vivo association of pp60 (v-src) and the gap junction protein connexin 43 in v-src transformed fibroblasts. Mol Carcinog 25:187-195.

Matsushita T and Takamatsu T. (1997) Ischaemia-induced temporal expression of connexin43 in rat heart. Virchows Arch 431:453-458.

McGee AW, Topinka JR, Hahimoto K, Petrailia RS, Kakizawa S, Kauer F, Aguilera-Moreno A, Wenthold RJ, Kano M, Bredt DS. (2001) PSD-93 knock-out mice reveal that neuronal MAGUKs are not required for development or function of parallel fiber synapses in cerebellum. J Neurosci 21:3085-3091.

Meller K. (1981) Effects of colchicine on gap junction formation during retinal neurogenesis. Anat Embryol 163: 321-330.

Merrifield CJ, Moss SE, Ballestrem C, Imhof BA, Giese G, Wunderlich I, and Almers W. (1999) Endocytic vesicles move at the tips of actin tails in cultured mast cells. Nat Cell Biol 1:72-74.

Migaud M, Charlesworth P, Dempster M, Webster LC, Watabe AM, Makhinson M, He Y, Ramsay MF, Morris RG, Morrison JH, O'Dell TJ, Grant SG. (1998) Enhanced long-term potentiation and impaired learning in mice with mutant postsynaptic density-95 protein. Nature 396:433-9.

Moorby CD. (2000) A connexin 43 mutant lacking the carboxyl cytoplasmic domain inhibits both growth and motility of mouse 3T3 fibroblasts. Mol Carcinog 28:23-30.

Murray SA, Williams SY, Dillard CY, Narayanan SK, and McCauley. (1997) Relationship of cytoskeletal filaments to annular gap junction expression in human adrenal cortical tumor cells in culture. J Exp Cell Res 234:398-404.

Musil LS. Goodenough DA. (1991) Biochemical analysis of connexin43 intracellular transport, phosphorylation, and assembly into gap junctional plaques. J Cell Biol 115:1357-1374.

Nielsen PA, Baruch A, Giepmans BNG, and Kumar NM. Characterization of the Association of Connexins and ZO-1 in the Lens. Cell Communication and Adhesion, 2001. In Press.

Paulson AF, Lampe PD, Meyer RA, TenBroek E, Atkinson MM, Walseth TF, and Johnson RG. (2000) Cyclic AMP and LDL trigger a rapid enhancement in gap junction assembly through a stimulation of gap junction trafficking. J Cell Sci 113:3037-3049.

Peracchia C, Sotkis A, Wang XG, Peracchia LL, and Persechini A. (2000) Calmodulin directly gates gap junction channels. J Biol Chem 275:26220-26224.

Peracchia C, Wang X, Li L, and Peracchia LL. (1996) Inhibition of calmodulin expression prevents low-pH-induced gap junction uncoupling in Xenopus oocytes. Pflugers Arch – Eur J of Physiol 431:379-387.

Peters NS, Green CR, Poole-Wilson PA, and Severs NJ. (1993) Reduced content of connexin43 gap junctions in ventricular myocardium from hypertrophied and ischemic human hearts. Circulation 88:864-875.

Rassat J, Robenek H, and Themann H. (1982) Alterations of tight and gap junctions in mouse hepatocytes following administration of colchicine. Cell Tissue Res 223:187-200.

Rivedahl E and Opsahl, H. (2001) Role of PKC and MAP kinase in EGF- and TPA-induced connexin43 phosphorylation and inhibition of gap junction intercellular communication in rat liver epithelial cells. Carcinogenesis 22:1543-1550.

Ruch RJ, Trosko JE, and Madhukar BV. (2001) Inhibition of connexin43 gap junctional intercellular communication by TPA requires ERK activation. J Cell Biochem 83:163-169.

Saez JC, Nairn AC, Czernik AJ, Spray DC, Hertzberg EL, Greengard P, and Bennett MV. (1990) Phosphorylation of connexin 32, a hepatocyte gap-junction protein, by cAMP-dependent protein kinase, protein kinase C and Ca2+/calmodulin-dependent protein kinase II. Eur J Biochem 192:263-273.

Saez JC, Gregory WA, Watanabe T, Dermietzel R, Hertzberg EL, Reid L, Bennett MV, and Spray DC. (1989) cAMP delays disappearance of gap junctions between pairs of rat hepatocytes in primary culture. Am J Phys 257:C1-C11.

Saimi Y and Kung C. (1994) Ion channel regulation by calmodulin binding. FEBS Lett 350: 155-158.

Sakai N, Blennerhassett MG, and Garfield RE. (1992) Intracellular cyclic AMP concentration modulates gap junction permeability in parturient rat myometrium. Canadian J Physiol Pharmacol 70:358-364.

Saleh SM, Takemoto LJ, Zoukhri D, and Takemoto DJ. (2001) PKC-gamma phosphorylation of connexin 46 in the lens cortex. Mol Vision 7:240-246.

Sepp R, Severs NJ, and Gourdie RG. (1996) Altered patterns of intercellular junction distribution in hypertrophic cardiomyopathy. Heart 76:412-417.

Severs NJ. (1999) Cardiovascular disease. Novartis Found Symp 219:188-206.

Severs NJ. (1994) Pathophysiology of gap junctions in heart disease. J Cardiovasc Electrophysiol 5: 462-475.

Sheng M and Wyszynski M. (1997) Ion channel targeting in neurons. Bioessays 19:847-853.

Smith JH, Green CR, Peters NS, Rothery S, and Severs NJ. (1991) Altered patterns of gap junction distribution in ischemic heart disease. An immunohistochemical study of human myocardium using laser scanning confocal microscopy. Am J Pathol 139:801-821.

Stein LS, Boonstra J, and Burghardt RC. (1992) Reduced cell-cell communication between mitotic and non-mitotic coupled cells. Exp Cell Res 198:1-7.

Torok K, Stauffer K, and Evans WH. (1997) Connexin 32 of gap junctions contains two calmodulin binding domains. Biochem J 326:479-483.

Toyama J, Sugiura H, Kamiya K, Kodama I, Terasawa M, and Hidaka H. (1994) Ca(2+)-calmoduolin mediated modulation of the electrical coupling of ventricular myocytes isolated from guinea pig hearts. J Mol Cell Cardiol 26:1007-1015.

Toyofuku T, Yabuki M, Otsu K, Kuzuya T, Hori M,and Tada M. (1998) Direct association of the gap junction protein connexin 43 with ZO-1 in cardiac myocytes. J Biol Chem 273:12725-12731.

ToyofukuT, Yabuki M, Otsu K, Kuzuya T, Tada M, and Hori M. (1999) Functional role of c-Src in gap junctions of the cardiomyopathic heart. Circ Res 85:672-681.

Toyofuku T, Akamatsu Y, Zhang H, Kuzuya T, Tada M, and Hori M. (2001) c-Src regulates the interaction between connexin-43 and ZO-1 in cardiac myocytes. J Biol Chem 276:1780-1788.

Tsukita S, Furuse M, and Itoh M. (1997) Molecular architecture of tight junctions: occludin and ZO-1. Soc Gen Physiol Ser 52:69-76.

Uzzaman M, Honjo H, Takagishi Y, Emdad L, Magee AI, Severs NJ, and Kodama I. (2000) Remodeling of gap junctional coupling in hypertrophied right ventricles of rats with monocrotaline-induced pulmonary hypertension. Circ Res 86:871-878.

van Rijen HV, van Veen TA, Hermans MM and Jongsma HJ. (2000) Human connexin40 gap junction channels are modulated by cAMP. Cardiovasc Res 45:941-951.

Watanabe H, Washioka H, and Tonosaki A. (1988) Gap junction and its cytoskeletal undercoats as involved in invagination-endocytosis. Tohoku J Exp Med 156:175-190.

Watterson DM, Burgess WH, Lukas TJ, Iverson D, Marshak DR, Schleicher M, Erickson BW, Fok KF, and Van Eldik LJ. (1984) Towards a molecular and atomic anatomy of calmodulin and calmodulin-binding proteins. Adv Cyc Nucleot Protein Phosphoryl Res 16:205-226.

Welsh MJ, Aster JC, Ireland M, AlcalaJ, and Maisel H. (1982) Calmodulin binds to chick lens gap junction protein in a calcium-independent manner. Science 216:642-644.

Wilders R, Wagner MB, Golod DA, Kumar R, Wang YG, Goolsby WN, Joyner RW, and Jongsma HJ. (2000) Effects of anisotropy on the development of cardiac arrhythmias associated with focal activity. Pflugers Arch 441:301-312.

Xie H, Laird DW, Chang TH and Hu VW. (1997) A mitosis-specific phosphorylation of the gap junction protein connexin43 in human vascular cells: biochemical characterization and localization. J Cell Biol 137:203-210.

Xu X, Li WE, Huang GY, Meyer R, Chen T, Luo Y, Thomas MP, Radice GL, and Lo CW. (2001) Modulation of mouse neural crest cell motility by N-cadherin and connexin 43 gap junctions. J Cell Biol 154:217-230.

Yeager M, Unger VM, and Falk MM. Synthesis, assembly and structure of gap junction intercellular channels. Curr Opin Struct Biol 8:517-524, 1998.

Zhang YW, Morita I, Ikeda M, Ma KW, and Murota S. (2001) Connexin43 supresses proliferation of osteosarcoma U2OS cells through post-transcriptional regulation of p27. Oncogene 20:4138-4149.

Zhou L, Kasperek EM, and Nicholson BJ. (1999) Dissection of the molecular basis of pp60(v-src) induced gating of connexin 43 gap junction channels. J Cell Biol 144:1033-1045.

3

CARDIOVASCULAR CONNEXINS: MOLECULAR COMPOSITION AND BIOCHEMICAL REGULATION

Eric C. Beyer and Kyung Hwan Seul
Department of Pediatrics, Section of Hematology/Oncology and Stem Cell Transplantation, University of Chicago, Chicago, Il 60637

Gap junctions are plasma membrane specializations containing channels which permit the intercellular exchange of ions and small molecules. Gap junction channels are of central importance in electrically excitable tissues such as myocardium where cell-to-cell passage of ions allows propagation of action potentials. Gap junctions are also present in many non-excitable cells (for example endothelial cells) where they may facilitate intercellular exchange of nutrients, metabolites, and signaling molecules as well as ions. This review will focus on molecular biological and biochemical studies that have enhanced our understanding of the molecular composition of cardiac and vascular gap junction channels and the regulation of the subunit proteins that form them.

Electrical coupling of cardiac cells through such low resistance intercellular pathways was first proposed by Weidmann (1952) who applied linear cable theory to the spread of electrotonic potentials in cardiac Purkinje fibers. Barr *et al.* (1965) subsequently demonstrated that a closely apposed region of adjacent plasma membranes, termed the nexus or gap junction, was the functional site of electrical contact between heart cells; they showed that disruption of such structures by hypertonic solutions also blocked action potential conduction. In thin-section electron micrographs, the gap junction appeared as a pair of parallel membranes separated by a narrow 20 Angstrom extracellular gap spanned by hexagonally arranged protein subunits (Revel and Karnovsky, 1967; Robertson, 1963). Each protein bridge was postulated to consist of a pair of hemichannels (or connexons), one from each cell, which align and join to form a continuous aqueous cell-to-cell passageway insulated from the extracellular space it traverses (Loewenstein, 1966). Micrographs of cardiovascular gap junctions are shown in figure 1.

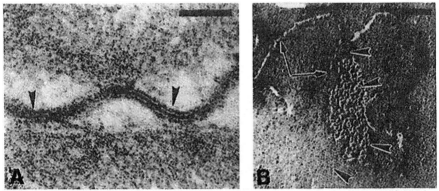

Figure 1. Electron micrographs showing gap junctions between cultured cells. (A) Thin-section view of gap junction (arrowheads) between two rat ventricular myocytes, cultured as in Eid *et al.* (1992). (B) Freeze-fracture replica of gap (arrowheads) and tight (arrows) junctions between two bovine brain microvascular endothelial cells, cultured as in Larson, *et al.* (1987). Note P-face particles and E-face pits in gap junction. Bars = 0.1 μm.

1. Gap junction structure

In the 1970's, procedures were developed for the isolation of gap junctions from liver (Evans and Gurd, 1972; Goodenough and Stoeckenius, 1972). These isolated gap junctions were studied by x-ray diffraction and electron microscopy to develop a low resolution (25 A) structural model (Figure 2A) (Caspar et al., 1977; Makowski et al., 1977; Unwin and Zampighi, 1980). The model shows that a gap junction plaque is composed of from tens to thousands of channels. Each channel is composed of a hexameric structure (connexon) composed of six integral membrane subunits (connexins) which surround a central pore. The connexon joins in mirror symmetry with a connexon in the plasma membrane of the adjacent cell. While they have been studied less, cardiac gap junctions are believed to have a generally similar structure except for larger cytoplasmic domains (Manjunath et al., 1984; Yeager and Gilula, 1992). Recent studies by Unger *et al.* (1997, 1999) examining expressed gap junctions derived from cloned material have supported and refined this model.

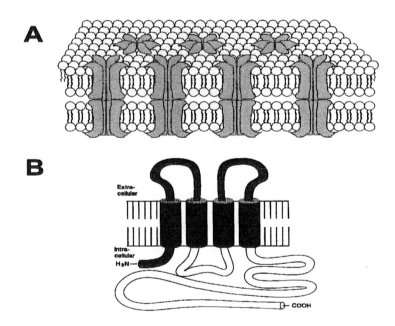

Figure 2. A. Model of the structure of a gap junction based on analyses of isolated liver and expressed Cx43 (truncated) gap junctions (Caspar et al., 1977; Makowski et al., 1977; Unwin and Zampighi, 1980; Unger *et al.* 1997, 1999)). B. Topology of the connexin protein relative to the junctional plasma membrane. Shaded regions represent sequences within the polypeptide that are conserved among all connexins while unshaded regions are unique.

In addition to the liver junctions, methods were developed for the isolation of myocardial gap junctions (Kensler et al., 1979; Manjunath et al., 1984) and of lens fiber plasma membranes which contain 5-10%

gap junction profiles (Alcala et al., 1975; Bloemendal et al., 1972; Goodenough, 1979). SDS-PAGE of these preparations showed that the isolated liver gap junctions are composed primarily of a 27 kDa polypeptide, accompanied by proteolysis fragments, aggregates, and a 21 kDa polypeptide (Hertzberg and Gilula, 1979). Isolated myocardial gap junctions contain a 43-47 kDa polypeptide, cleaved by endogenous proteases to 34, 32, and 29 kDa bands (Manjunath et al., 1984, 1987a; Manjunath and Page, 1985). Isolated bovine and ovine lens fiber plasma membranes contain a number of polypeptides including one of 70 kDa (MP70) (Kistler et al., 1985). N-terminal sequencing of these proteins by Edman degradation has demonstrated that the liver 27 kDa and 21 kDa proteins (Nicholson et al., 1987), the heart 43-47 kDa protein and its degradation products (Gros et al., 1983; Nicholson et al., 1985; Manjunath et al., 1987b), and the lens 70 kDa protein (Kistler et al., 1988)are homologous proteins.

2. Connexin cloning and diversity

Availability of isolated gap junction proteins, development of antibodies, and acquisition of some sequence information allowed the molecular cloning of sequences encoding gap junction proteins. Beginning in the late 1980s, various molecular strategies were used to clone cDNAs and genomic DNAs encoding the subunit gap junction proteins. Paul (1986) cloned a cDNA for the rat liver 27 kDa protein by antibody screening of a bacteriophage expression library, and Kumar and Gilula (1986)cloned a cDNA for its human counterpart by hybridization screening with an amino-terminal oligonucleotide. Both cDNAs encode a polypeptide of 32 kDa. Paul (1986)demonstrated by RNA blotting that mRNA hybridizing to this cDNA was also present in brain, stomach, and kidney, but was not detectable in heart or lens. Beyer *et al.* (1987)isolated a related sequence from a rat heart cDNA library by screening with the rat liver cDNA at reduced stringency. The rat heart cDNA codes for a polypeptide of 43 kDa which contains 43% identical amino acids to the protein cloned from rat liver. The amino terminal sequence predicted from the heart clone matches that determined by Edman degradation of the major protein in isolated rat heart gap junctions (Manjunath et al., 1987b; Nicholson et al., 1985). Morphological proof that these proteins are components of gap junctions has been provided by immunocytochemistry using antibodies directed against bacterially-expressed fusion proteins (Paul, 1986)or against synthetic peptides based on the predicted polypeptidespecific anti-peptide antisera (Beyer et al., 1989; Yancey et al., 1989); functional proof that they can form intercellular channels has come from expression of the cloned cDNAs in *Xenopus* oocytes (Dahl et al., 1987; Swenson et al., 1989; Werner et al., 1989)or stably transfected cells (Eghbali et al., 1990; Veenstra et al., 1992).

Subsequent cloning studies have demonstrated there is a large family of related subunit gap junction proteins which are now called *connexins*. Many of these proteins are not uniquely expressed in a single tissue. Moreover, the mobilities of these proteins on SDS-PAGE may vary with electrophoresis conditions (Green et al., 1988). Therefore, previous descriptions of gap junction proteins based on tissue of origin or electrophoretic mobility were abandoned, and an operational nomenclature was developed using the generic term connexin (abbreviated as Cx) for the protein family, with an indication of species (as necessary) and a numeric suffix designating the molecular mass in kiloDaltons, predicted from the derived polypeptide sequence (Beyer et al., 1987, 1988, 1990) . According to this system, the 27 kDa protein from rat liver is termed rat Cx32, the 43 kDa protein from rat heart is termed rat Cx43, and the lens MP70 is termed rat Cx46. Recently, this system has gotten somewhat awkward and potentially confusing . For example, the identification of additional family members has necessitated the use of decimal points to distinguish connexins (e.g Cx31 vs.Cx31.1 or Cx30 vs. CX30.2 vs. Cx30.3). Moreover, orthologs in different species may have different names (e.g. mouse Cx40 corresponds to chicken CX42; human CX46 corresponds to bovine Cx44 and chicken CX56). Despite these problems, this nomenclature continues in general use, since researchers in the field have been unable to agree on a better system.

Table I shows the connexin sequences that have been identified in the human genome and the corresponding mouse sequences.

Table I. Identified human connexin genes and mouse orthologs

Human	Mouse	Human	Mouse
hCX25		hCX37	mCx37
hCX26	mCx26	hCX40	mCx40
hCX30	mCx30	hCX40.1	mCx39
hCX30.2	mCx29	hCX43	mCx43
hCX30.3	mCx30.3	hCX45	mCx45
hCX31	mCx31	hCX46	mCx46
hCX31.1	mCx31.1	hCX46.6	mCx47
hCX31.9	mCx30.2	hCX50	mCx50
hCX32	mCx32	hCX58	
	mCx33	hCX62	mCx57
hCX36	mCx36		

Connexin sequences were identified by cDNA or genomic cloning or by examination of the human and mouse genomes. Most of these sequences have been published and/or deposited in the GenBank or EMBL databases, but some identified by genomic sequencing gazing were presented at the 2002 International Gap Junction meeting. Orthologs were identified by similarities in expression patterns or channel properties as well as extensive sequence identity. For some connexins (hCX25, mCx33, hCX58), no orthologous sequence in the other species is apparent.

The amino acid sequences derived from the cloned cDNAs have been used to predict the structures of the connexins. Hydropathy plots of all members of the family suggest four hydrophobic domains (Paul, 1986). These predictions, together with the results of proteolysis studies of isolated junctions, have been used to construct a topology model for the relation of these polypeptides to the junctional plasma membrane, assuming that each hydrophobic domain represents a transmembrane segment of the molecule (Beyer et al., 1987, 1988) (Figure 2B). The model has been tested by examining the protease sensitivity of isolated liver gap junctions and by the mapping of site-specific antisera by immunocytochemistry. The controlled proteolytic cleavage has demonstrated that both the N- and C-termini of Cx32 face the cytoplasm, and that an additional cytoplasmically-accessible proteolytic site is located between the second and third transmembrane segments (Hertzberg et al., 1988; Zimmer et al., 1987). Antisera have been raised against synthetic oligopeptides representing various segments of several connexins and have been used to map the topology in the electron microscope (Goodenough et al., 1988; Milks et al., 1988; Beyer et al., 1989; Yancey et al., 1989; Yeager and Gilula, 1992) , showing that the amino-terminus, the carboxyl terminus and a loop in the middle of the protein are all located on the cytoplasmic face of the junctional membrane. To the degree that the harsh experimental conditions do not alter the protein topology, they also demonstrate that the predicted extracellular connexin domains can be detected on the extracellular surfaces of the junctional membranes.

The availability of cloned connexin sequences has made it possible to express the proteins encoded by the different sequences and to examine the properties of the channels produced. Two major strategies have been utilized extensively: injection of *Xenopus* oocytes with *in vitro* transcribed connexin mRNAs (Dahl et al., 1987; Swenson et al., 1989; Werner et al., 1989) and stable transfection of communication-deficient cell lines with connexin DNAs (Eghbali et al., 1990; Veenstra et al., 1992). Data derived from some of these studies will be examined in more detail elsewhere (see chapter by Veenstra), but they can be summarized by concluding that each of the connexins forms channels with unique characteristics, including unitary conductance, gating by voltage or pH, and selectivity/permeability (Barrio et al., 1992; Spray et al., 1992; Veenstra et al., 1992; Liu et al., 1993; Elfgang et al., 1995; Veenstra et al., 1995).

All connexin genes appear to be single copy genes. However, in humans, a Cx43 pseudogene has been identified (Fishman et al., 1990).

The gene structures have been determined for a number of connexins by comparison of genomic and cDNA sequences or by other strategies including DNA blotting , genomic polymerase chain reaction (PCR), and RT-PCR (Miller et al., 1988; Hennemann et al., 1992a; Sullivan et al., 1993; Seul et al., 1997; Yu et al., 1994; Seul and Beyer, 2000b; Jacob and Beyer, 2001). Most connexins (including Cx37, Cx40, and Cx43) have a similar gene structure with a small first exon containing only 5'-untranslated sequences and a large second exon containing the complete coding region as well as all remaining untranslated sequences (Fig. 3). The size of the intron can vary substantially; it is 11 to 14 kb in Cx40 and Cx43, but only 1 kb in Cx37 (Sullivan et al., 1993; Seul et al., 1997; Seul and Beyer, 2000b).

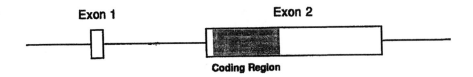

Figure 3. Connexin gene structure. The protein coding region is represented by the shaded region, and the rest of the exons are represented by open boxes.

A few exceptions to this structure have been determined. In Cx36, there are two exons, but the coding region is interrupted by an intron, since the first exon contains 72 nucleotides of coding sequence as well as 5'-UTR (Condorelli et al., 1998). Cx45, has one exon containing a small amount of 5'-UTR, the coding region and all of the 3'UTR; however, it has two additional exons of 5'UTR (Jacob and Beyer,

2001). Rapid amplification of cDNA ends shows that parts of these 5' exons are differentially used, allowing the production of heterogenous Cx45 mRNAs with differing 5' UTR. In Cx32, there are alternative first exons which allow differential transcription in different tissues (Neuhaus et al., 1995; Sohl et al., 1996).

The basal promoters of Cx43, Cx40 and Cx37 have been characterized. All three genes have TATA boxes with transcriptional start sites in close proximity (Sullivan et al., 1993; Seul et al., 1997; Groenewegen et al., 1998; Seul and Beyer, 2000b). However, identification of regulatory factors that control transcription of cardiovascular connexins is still preliminary. Reporter gene transfections of various cell lines have identified several enhancer or repressor elements within the Cx43 gene implicated in estrogen responsiveness (Yu et al., 1994), myometrial-specific regulation (Chen et al., 1995), or regulation by protein kinase C (Geimonen et al., 1996). The Cx40 gene contains a negative regulatory element near the beginning of the intron (Seul et al., 1997). Cx40 transcription may also be regulated by the homeobox gene Nkx 2.5.

3. Connexin distribution in the cardiovascular system

The cloned connexin sequences or anti-connexin antibodies have been used to examine the distribution of different connexins in various organs, tissues, and cell types. Connexin-specific DNA or RNA probes have been used for hybridization to RNA blots prepared from organ or cell culture homogenates or for *in situ* hybridization studies of tissue sections. Antibodies raised against connexin-specific synthetic peptides or bacterially-expressed polypeptides representing the unique cytoplasmic domains have been used for immunoblots and immunohistochemical localization studies.

3.1 *Connexins in the heart.*

By various of these techniques, up to six connexins (Cx37, Cx40,

Cx43, Cx45, Cx46, and Cx50) have been detected in the mammalian heart. RNA blots show hybridization of Cx37, Cx40, Cx43, Cx45, and Cx46 probes to corresponding mRNAs in total RNA prepared from heart homogenates (Beyer et al., 1987, 1992; Paul et al., 1991; Willecke et al., 1991; Haefliger et al., 1992; Hennemann et al., 1992b), but only Cx40, Cx43, and Cx45 have been unambiguously detected in RNA from cardiac myocytes (Kanter et al., 1992). Cx37 was cloned from endothelial cell cDNA (Reed et al., 1993) (among other sources), and those cells are presumably the source of Cx37 in the heart. The cardiac source of Cx46 expression has not been defined. Cx50 mRNA has not been detected in heart, but Harfst et al. (1990) found immunostaining in heart valves using a monoclonal antibody directed against the ovine orthologue of Cx50, MP70.

While Cx40, Cx43, and Cx45 have all been detected in cardiac myocytes, immunohistochemistry and *in situ* hybridization studies have shown that these myocyte connexins have different distributions in different cardiac regions. Davis *et al.* (1994, 1995) have surveyed the distribution of different connexins within different regions of the canine and human heart (Table II) Cx45 is present in all cardiac regions examined. Cx43 is abundant in atrium, ventricle, and in Purkinje fibers, but is not detectable in the canine sinus or atrio-ventricular nodes or the proximal His-Purkinje system. Cx40 is abundant in atrium, bundle branches and Purkinje fibers, present in the sinus and A-V nodes and scarce in ventricular myocardium. The differential distribution of Cx40 and Cx43 is illustrated by the immunofluorescent staining of a frozen section of mouse heart shown in Figure 5. The distribution of Cx40, Cx43, and, in some cases Cx45, have also been examined in other mammalian species including human, mouse, rat, rabbit, and guinea pig (76-80) showing similar patterns of expression. In addition to differences in the patterns of connexins expressed, different cardiac tissues also differ in the size and number of their gap junctions (see Table II). The absolute amounts of different connexins in cardiac myocytes have not been determined; rather, different abundances have been considered based on the intensity of immunostaining. This has led to some debate regarding the significance of levels of Cx45 in ventricular myocardium (Coppen et al., 1999; Johnson et al., 2002).

In cardiac cells that contain two or more connexins, those connexins appear to be in the same gap junctions. Double label immunohistochemistry has been performed using a mouse monoclonal antibody to Cx43 and polyclonal antibodies directed against Cx40 or Cx45. Analysis of immunoreactive material in frozen sections or in isolated myocytes with immunofluorescence microscopy and double label immunoelectron microscopy has revealed an identical distribution of both proteins in gap junctions (Davis et al., 1994; Kanter et al., 1993).

Table II. Gap Junction Structure and Connexin Phenotypes of Cardiac Regions

Cardiac Tissue	Connexin Phenotype			Gap Junction Structure	
	Cx40	Cx43	Cx45	Size	Number
Sinus node	scant	absent	scant	small	few
Right Atrium	abundant	abundant	moderate	large	many
AV Node and Proximal His Bundle	scant	absent	scant	small	few
Distal His Bundle and Purkinje Fibers	abundant	abundant	moderate	large	moderate
Ventricle	absent	abundant	moderate	moderate	many

These data are based on the analyses of human and dog hearts by Davis *et al.* (1994,1995).

While the patterns of connexin expression appear rather similar in multiple mammalian species (van Kempen et al., 1995), they apparently differ in birds (and perhaps other vertebrates). Chicken cardiac myocytes predominantly contain Cx42 (a connexin most closely related to the mammalian Cx40 sequence) and only little Cx43 (Beyer, 1990; Minkoff et al., 1993). Changes in levels of connexins during cardiac development are considered in other chapters.

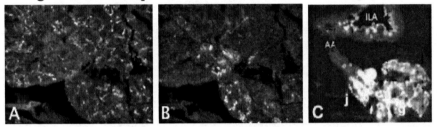

Figure 4. Localization of connexins by immunofluoescence in a frozen section of mouse heart (A,B) or mouse kidney (C). A. Anti-Cx43 antibodies predominantly label gap junctions between ventricular myocytes. B. Anti-Cx40 antibodies label only sub-endocardial Purkinje fiber cells. There is some overlap of Cx40 and Cx43 immunoreactivity. C. Anti-Cx40 antibodies show extensive, but heterogeneous localization of Cx40 in renal blood vessels. The endothelium (e) of the interlobular artery (ILA) and glomerulus (g) are contain abundant Cx40; in contrast, Cx40 staining is scanty in the endotheliium (e) of the afferent arteriole (AA). The smooth muscle of the juxtaglomerular apparatus (j) contains abundant Cx40 abundantly, but other vascular smooth muscle (s) in ILA or AA does not.

3.2 *Connexin distribution in blood vessels*

Several ultrastructural studies have shown gap junctions between endothelial cells or between smooth muscle cells in the vascular wall (reviewed by Dejana, *et al.*, 1995 and Christ *et al.*, 1996)). Heterocellular gap junctions between endothelial cells and pericytes or smooth muscle cells have also been demonstrated (Cuevas et al., 1984; Spagnoli et al., 1982). Assessments of dye or electrical transfer *in vivo* have confirmed the presence of functional intercellular communication (Beny and Pacicca, 1994; Little et al., 1995b).

In 1990, Larson *et al.* (1990) surveyed a wide variety of cultured endothelial cells, smooth muscle cells and pericytes from several species and determined that they all expressed Cx43 mRNA. In addition, freshly isolated preparations of bovine aortic endothelium and smooth muscle each contained Cx43 mRNA. Subsequently,

Beyer *et al.* (1992) cloned Cx40 from rat genomic DNA and showed that this connexin was expressed in A7r5 cells (a cell line derived from rat aortic smooth muscle) and cultured bovine aortic smooth muscle cells. Reed *et al.* (1993), cloned human Cx37 from a human umbilical vein endothelial cell library and demonstrated expression in human and bovine endothelial cells including freshly isolated bovine aortic endothelium, but not in cultured smooth muscle cells. Subsequent investigations by a variety of groups using DNA or antibody probes to screen for connexins have demonstrated substantial variability in expression *in vivo* and in culture, depending on vascular bed and species (see extensive list of these references in Beyer et al., 1998).

In general, all types of vessel wall cells express Cx43, *in vivo* and *in vitro*. *In vivo*, Cx40 mRNA or protein have been demonstrated in large and small vessel endothelium and in smooth muscle from several species but not others. Cx40 is a major gap junction protein of endothelial cells of the adult vasculature in most organs (Little et al., 1995a; van Kempen and Jongsma, 1999), but it shows heterogeneous expression along the vasculature (Seul and Beyer, 2000a) (Fig. 4). The differential distribution of Cx37 and Cx43 suggests that they are involved in more dynamic processes. However, interpretations of their patterns of expression along vessel walls are controversial. Cx43 is highly localized to sites of disturbed flow in rat aortic endothelium, but Cx37 and Cx40 are more uniformly distributed (Gabriels and Paul, 1998). The patterns of expression of connexins among endothelial and smooth muscle cells are modulated under pathologic conditions ((Haefliger et al., 2000; Haefliger and Meda, 2000).

Cx37 has been less extensively studied; however, it has been shown in various endothelia but not in smooth muscle in vivo or in culture. Interestingly, Larson *et al.* (1997) have shown that Cx37 is expressed at high levels in confluent endothelial cells (in vivo and in vitro) yet it is barely detectable in subconfluent cultured cells. The relatively small amount of information on vascular pericytes suggests an expression pattern similar to that of smooth muscle cells, as might be expected.

An additional connexin, Cx45, has been identified in one smooth muscle line, A7r5 (Laing et al., 1994).

Cx37 and Cx43 are regulated differentially by cell density, growth, and TGF-beta 1 in cultured bovine aortic endothelial cells (Larson et al., 1997). Both Cx37 and Cx43 are increased in regenerating endothelium after vessel injury (Yeh et al., 2000). Using PymT-transformed mouse endothelial cell lines, Kwak et al. (2001) found that mechanical wounding increased expression of Cx43 and decreased expression of Cx37 at the site of injury. Transcripts of Cx43 are decreased and those of Cx37 are increased by shear stress in cultured HUVECs. Cx43 between smooth muscle cells is upregulated after balloon catheter injury in the rat carotid artery (Yeh et al., 2000) and during early stages of human coronary atherosclerosis (Blackburn et al., 1995); Cx37, but not Cx40 or Cx43, is induced in vascular smooth muscle cells during coronary arteriogenesis (Cai et al., 2001).

3.3 Connexin distribution in leukocytes

Circulating leukocytes are usually given as an example of one of the cell types that does not make gap junctions and this is apparently true. Once they stop circulating, however, a few studies have shown the capability of these cells to transfer intercellular tracers or have demonstrated the expression of Cx43. Polacek *et al.* (1993) have shown Cx43 expression in macrophage foam cells in human atherosclerotic lesions but not in peripheral mononuclear cells. Beyer and Steinberg (1991,1993) have demonstrated expression of Cx43 by macrophage-like cell lines and changes in its expression in response to treatment with cytokines.   Jara *et al.* (1995)have found that leukocytes, directly stimulated with lipopolysaccharide, or peritoneal macrophages from lipopolysaccharide-stimulated hamsters express Cx43 *de novo* while untreated cells do not. Other examples, such as the reports of dye transfer by lymphocytes during penetration of endothelial monolayers (Guinan et al., 1988), suggest that functional gap junction expression in leukocytes may be necessary for extravasation or subsequent activities in extravascular tissues. Several reports have indicated that precursor cells have gap junctions, are functionally coupled, or express Cx43 in the bone marrow (Dorshkind et al., 1993; Rosendaal et al., 1994; Krenacs and Rosendaal, 1998; Montecino-Rodriguez et al., 2000; Montecino-Rodriguez and Dorshkind, 2001;).

4. Mixing of connexins

The expression of multiple connexins within an organism and within a single tissue or cell implies that gap junctional plaques may not all be composed only of a homogenous population of channels composed of a single connexin. Rather, connexins may potentially intermingle or mix with each other. The co-expression of multiple connexins in cardiac myocytes and vascular cells suggests that connexin mixing might influence cardiovascular intercellular communication.

There are many examples of co-expression of two connexins within the same cell. This was first documented for Cx26 and Cx32 in hepatocytes (Traub et al., 1989). In many cases, immunocytochemistry experiments show colocalization to the same gap junction plaques, as we have seen in canine or rat ventricular myocytes and cell lines (Kanter et al., 1993; Darrow et al., 1995; Laing et al., 1994). A number of electrophysiologic experiments have shown the presence of multiple different channel sizes in cells which express multiple connexins.

One kind of mixing of connexins within gap junction channels is the formation of *heterotypic* channels. This would occur if two adjacent cells expressed different connexins and formed junctional channels with each hemi-channel formed homogeneously of a single connexin. The formation of heterotypic channels *in vitro* has been examined extensively by the pairing of *Xenopus* oocytes injected with RNAs for two different connexins (Swenson et al., 1989; Werner et al., 1989). The two connexins may sometimes form heterotypic channels with complicated, novel gating properties (Barrio et al., 1991; Verselis et al., 1994). Not all connexins are compatible partners for the formation of heterotypic channels in this expression system; the second extracellular loop in the connexin molecules may contribute to the specificity of these interactions (White et al., 1995). Heterotypic gap junctions might allow for the interaction of different cells or tissues in vivo and might contribute to the formation of communication compartments with borders determined by the expression of incompatible connexins.

In a cell which co-expresses two connexins, the two proteins might mix within a single hemi-channel, forming *heteromeric* hemi-channels. If two co-expressed connexins are freely capable of mixing and forming heteromeric hemichannels, then in any individual cell there might be 2^6 or 64 possible hemichannels which could result in the formation of 4096 different full channels. If a six-fold symmetry axis is assumed then the predicted number of different hemichannels and complete channels are 14 and 196 respectively. This large number of different heteromeric mixtures might lead to a large variety of channels. Immunocytochemistry experiments do not have the resolution to detect heteromeric channels. Our own recent data suggest that Cx43 can form heteromeric channels with Cx37, Cx40, or Cx45 when these connexins are co-expressed in established cell lines (Brink et al., 1997; Elenes et al., 2001; Valiunas et al., 2001).

5. Gap junction synthesis and degradation

The development of specific anti-connexin antibody probes has made possible *in vitro* studies of connexin biosynthesis by metabolic labeling and immunoprecipitation. Rather few studies of the synthesis, post-translational modification, assembly, and degradation of connexins and gap junctions have been performed in cardiovascular cells (Laird et al., 1991;Laing et al., 1998). However, there have been extensive studies of these subjects in other systems. Many studies have examined Cx43 synthesis or degradation in established cell lines that endogenously express Cx43 or in cells transfected with connexins containing fluorescent protein tags ((Falk, 2000a; Falk and Lauf, 2001; Jordan et al., 1999; Laird et al., 2001). Other cardiovascular connexins appear to follow similar biosynthetic processes to Cx43, but they have been less extensively studied (Laing et al., 1994; Larson et al., 2000). Detailed discussions of the modification of connexins by phosphorylation have been presented by Saez et al., (1993, 1998), Lau *et al.* (1996), and by Warn-Cramer et al., 2001).

5.1. *Serine phosphorylation of Cx43.*

Pulse chase studies have demonstrated that Cx43 is initially synthesized as a 42 kDa polypeptide which subsequently is post-translationally modified to forms with slightly slower mobility on SDS-PAGE by the addition of phosphate to serine residues (Crow et al., 1990; Filson et al., 1990; Musil et al., 1990a). There are multiple phosphates added to each mole of Cx43. At least some of this phosphorylation may occur in a serine-rich sequence near the carboxyl-terminus containing multiple potential phosphorylation sites (Lampe et al., 2000; TenBroek et al., 2001). Other connexins (including Cx37, Cx40, Cx45, and Cx46) contain similar sequences and have also been demonstrated to be phosphoproteins (Hertlein et al., 1998; Laing et al., 1994; Larson et al., 2000; van Veen et al., 2000).

The kinase(s) responsible for Cx43 phosphorylation have not all been determined, however, protein kinase C is strongly implicated in at least some of the phosphorylation events since treatment of a number of different cell lines with phorbol esters produces an increase in the phosphorylation of Cx43 and a decrease in intercellular coupling (Lampe, 1994; Lampe et al., 2000). Lau and colleagues have demonstrated changes in Cx43 phosphorylation due to mitogen activated kinase or epidermal growth factor stimulation (Lau et al., 1996; Warn-Cramer et al., 1996; Lampe et al., 1998; Warn-Cramer et al., 1998).

Musil *et al.* (1990b) have investigated some biological consequences of the serine phosphorylation of Cx43. They demonstrated that Cx43 was present in the non-communicating cell lines L929 and S180, but it was not present in cell surface gap junctional plaques; rather it accumulated intercellularly. The Cx43 was incompletely phosphorylated. However, transfection of S180 cells with the cell adhesion molecule E-cadherin restored gap junctional communication, full phosphorylation of Cx43, and expression in cell surface gap junctions. These findings suggest a relation between the ability of cells to fully phosphorylate Cx43 and the ability to form communicating junctions. They also suggest a hierarchy of events in the formation of intercellular junctions: a primary cell adhesion event is required prior to formation of gap junctions. Similar observations regarding the requirement of cadherin-mediated cell adhesion for development of gap junctions have also been made in epidermal cells (Jongen et al., 1991). Fujimoto *et al.*(1997) used electron microscopy to show co-localization of connexins with E-cadherin or alpha-catenin during gap junction formation in regenerating liver. Meyer *et al.* (1992) have shown that antibodies to extracellular epitopes in Cx43 or N cadherin will inhibit gap junction formation by Novikoff hepatoma cells. However, Wang and Rose (1997) have shown inhibition of communication in L cells transfected with N-cadherin and increases in communication between Morris hepatoma H5123 cells by the same treatment, suggesting that a cell type-specific effect. Musil and Goodenough (1991) have extended their original observations in NRK cells by showing the presence of extracellularly accessible Cx43 (in the non-phosphorylated form) and a correlation between phosphorylation of Cx43 and acquisition of insolubility in Triton-X-100, suggesting a role for phosphorylation in gap junction formation.

5.2. *Connexin trafficking and gap junction assembly.*

Based on these studies and many more (reviewed by Laird (1996) and Yeager (1998)), a scheme for post-translational processing of Cx43 and its assembly is emerging. Cx43 is synthesized and undergoes some phosphorylation in the endoplasmic reticulum. Musil and Goodenough (1993) suggest that formation of hexamers (connexons) occurs in the Golgi or TGN, but other investigators believe that oligomerization occurs in the endoplasmic reticulum (Falk et al., 1997; Falk, 2000b; Das et al., 2001; George et al., 1999). Connexons are delivered to the plasma membrane by vesicular carriers (Jordan et al., 1999). This process may involve microtubules (Giepmans et al., 2001). Connexons are inserted into the cell membrane in a shut configuration, perhaps at regions of cadherin-mediated adhesion or near tight junctions. Formation of plaques of channels requires docking of the connexons with connexons from the adjacent cell and correlates with resistance to solubilization in Triton X-100 and with additional phosphorylation.

5.3. *Tyrosine phosphorylation of Cx43.*

A large body of data demonstrating that intercellular communication is abolished in fibroblasts infected with Rous sarcoma virus (RSV) (Atkinson et al., 1981; Azarnia et al., 1988)has led several investigators to investigate the effects of pp60^{src} on Cx43-expressing cells. Crow *et al.* (1990) demonstrated that RSV infection uncoupled vole fibroblasts and lead to the incorporation of phosphate in Cx43 tyrosine residues. Filson *et al.* (1990) extended these observations by showing that each molecule of phosphorylated Cx43 contained both phosphoserine and phosphotyrosine and by showing that the ability of *src* variants to abolish cellular communication correlated with tyrosine phosphorylation of Cx43. Swenson *et al.* (1990) showed that in a *Xenopus* oocyte expression system coexpression of pp60^{v-src} with Cx43 reduced cell-cell coupling and lead to tyrosine phosphorylation of Cx43. But, site-directed mutagenesis of Tyr265 in Cx43 eliminated the tyrosine phosphorylation and the depression of communication. More recently, Loo *et al.* (1995, 1999) have demonstrated that the induced tyrosine phosphorylation is even more complex, resulting in modification of multiple residues. The role of activation of serine kinases by *src* is debated (Zhou et al., 1999). Other oncogenes may have similar effects on intercellular communication and connexin phosphorylation (Atkinson and Sheridan, 1988; Kurata and Lau, 1994).

5.4 *Connexin associated proteins.*

Until relatively recently, no proteins had been unambiguously identified as associated with gap junctions within cells. This deficiency may have been in part due to the harsh detergent conditions required for gap junction isolation.

Some studies have suggested an association between connexins and calmodulin (Zimmer et al., 1987). Such interactions might explain observed of calcium or calmodulin on gap junction channels (Peracchia et al., 2000).

The most convincing evidence shows an association between the peripheral membrane protein ZO-1 and Cx43 (Giepmans and Moolenaar, 1998; Toyofuku et al., 1998) or Cx45 (Laing et al., 2001). ZO-1 is also a component of tight junctions and adherens junctions. It has multiple binding partners (especially in epithelial cells) (Gonzalez-Mariscal et al., 2000). Mutational analysis has shown that the second PDZ domain of ZO-1 interacts with the carboxy terminus of Cx43 (Giepmans and Moolenaar, 1998; Toyofuku et al., 1998); this interaction can be regulated by the *src* oncogene (Toyofuku et al., 2000).

5.5. *Degradation of gap junctions.*

Gap junctions are apparently rather labile structures; Fallon and Goodenough (1981)have estimated that the half-life of metabolically-labeled liver junctions *in vivo* is about 5 hours. Electron microscopic studies suggest that entire gap junctions are internalizationed into endosomes (forming so-called annular gap junctions) followed by degradation in lysosomal, multivesicular body, or autophagosomal compartments (Ginzberg and Gilula, 1979; Larsen et al., 1979; Larsen and Tung, 1978; Severs et al., 1989; Traub et al., 1983). However, the abundance or importance of annular gap junctions may differ under different conditions; these structures are primarily found *in vivo* following pathological insults such as ischemia or during tissue remodeling. Cell fractionation and immunoelectron microscopic studies have also shown an association of connexins with lysosomes in cultured cells (Dermietzel et al., 1991; Naus et al., 1993; Rahman et al., 1993). Studies of GFP-labeled connexins also suggest endosomal internalization of gap junctions to annular gap junctions (Jordan et al., 2001). Dispersal of channels may also be an important event in gap junction degradation. Laing and colleagues (1995, 1997) demonstrated that inhibition of proteasomal degradation extended the half-life of Cx43 in cultured cells; they also suggest a role for ubiquitination in connexin proteolysis. The proteasome likely is important for "proof-reading" of mis-folded or mis-assembled connexins (Musil et al., 2000), but it may also be involved in the degradation of gap junction plaques.

A diagram of the major events in gap junction synthesis and degradation is presented in Fig. 5.

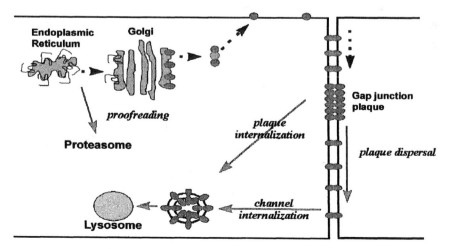

Figure 5. Diagram illustrating the steps in the synthesis and degradation of a gap junction.

6. Molecular interventional approaches to the study of cardiac intercellular communication

The availability of the cloned connexin sequences has made possible strategies to alter the abundance of the various connexins in cultured cells and in animals to test the involvement of gap junctions in cardiovascular development and physiology. Reaume *et al.* (1995) have developed a Cx43 "knock out" mouse, and they have found that homozygous null animals are cyanotic and die soon after birth apparently due to right ventricular outflow tract obstruction. These observations implicate Cx43 in cardiac development. Animals that are heterozygous for the Cx43 null mutation contain only half as much Cx43 protein as wild type littermates and exhibit slowed ventricular (but not atrial) conduction (Guerrero et al., 1997; Thomas et al., 1998). These data directly demonstrate the importance of connexin abundance as a determinant of cardiac conduction. An endothelial cell-specific Cx43 knock out mouse shows hypertension (Liao et al., 2001). The Cx40 null mouse shows bundle branch block (likely due to the absence of this connexin from the atrio-ventricular conduction pathways) (Bevilacqua et al., 2000; Kirchhoff et al., 2000; Simon et al., 1998; van Rijen et al., 2001)and may have defects in propagation of vasomotor responses. The Cx45 null mouse dies during embryonic development likely due to deficient vasculogenesis (perhaps related to the absence of smooth muscle cell Cx45) (Kruger et al., 2000; Kumai et al., 2000). While the Cx37 null mouse has no cardiovascular phenotype (it does show female infertility related to abnormal ovarian follicle maturation (Simon et al., 1997), Cx40/Cx37 double null animals die as embryos and have apparent abnormalities of endothelial integrity (Simon and Goodenough, unpublished data). Several Cx43 transgenics have implicated the importance of Cx34 in the function of cardiac neural crest (Huang et al., 1998a; Huang et al., 1998b; Sullivan et al., 1998; Xu et al., 2001)

All of these "knock out" and transgenic studies confirm the importance of cardiovascular connexins.

REFERENCE

Alcala,J., Lieska,N., and Maisel,H. (1975). Protein composition of bovine lens cortical fiber cell membranes. Exp. Eye Res. *21*, 581-589.

Atkinson,M.M., Menko,A.S., Johnson,R.G., Sheppard,J.R., and Sheridan,J.D. (1981). Rapid and reversible reduction of junctional permeability in cells infected with a temperature-sensitive mutant of avian sarcoma virus. J. Cell Biol. *91*, 573-578.

Atkinson,M.M. and Sheridan,J.D. (1988). Altered junctional permeability between cells transformed by v- ras, v-mos, or v-src. Am. J. Physiol. *255*, C674-C683.

Azarnia,R., Reddy,S., Kmiecik,T.E., Shalloway,D., and Loewenstein,W.R. (1988). The cellular src gene product regulates junctional cell- to-cell communication. Science *239*, 398-401.

Barr,L., Dewey,M.M., and Berger,W. (1965). Propagation of action potentials and the structure of the nexus in cardiac muscle. J. Gen. Physiol. *48*, 797-823.

Barrio,L.C., Suchyna,T., Bargiello,T., Xu,L.X., Roginski,R.S., Bennett,M.V., and Nicholson,B.J. (1991). Gap junctions formed by connexins 26 and 32 alone and in combination are differently affected by applied voltage. Proc. Natl. Acad. Sci. U. S. A. *88*, 8410-8414.

Barrio,L.C., Suchyna,T., Bargiello,T., Xu,L.X., Roginski,R.S., Bennett,M.V., and Nicholson,B.J. (1992). Gap junctions formed by connexins 26 and 32 alone and in combination are differently affected by applied voltage. Proc. Natl. Acad. Sci. U. S. A. *89*, 4220.

Beny,J.L. and Pacicca,C. (1994). Bidirectional electrical communication between smooth muscle and endothelial cells in the pig coronary artery. Am. J. Physiol. *266*, H1465-H1472.

Bevilacqua,L.M., Simon,A.M., Maguire,C.T., Gehrmann,J., Wakimoto,H., Paul,D.L., and Berul,C.I. (2000). A Targeted Disruption in Connexin40 Leads to Distinct Atrioventricular Conduction Defects. J. Interv. Card Electrophysiol. *4*, 459-567.

Beyer,E.C. (1990). Molecular cloning and developmental expression of two chick embryo gap junction proteins. J. Biol. Chem. *265*, 14439-14443.

Beyer,E.C., Goodenough,D.A., and Paul,D.L. (1988). The connexins, a family of related gap junction proteins. Mod. Cell Biol. *7*, 167-175.

Beyer,E.C., Kistler,J., Paul,D.L., and Goodenough,D.A. (1989). Antisera directed against connexin43 peptides react with a 43-kD protein localized to gap junctions in myocardium and other tissues. J. Cell Biol. *108*, 595-605.

Beyer,E.C., Paul,D.L., and Goodenough,D.A. (1987). Connexin43: a protein from rat heart homologous to a gap junction protein from liver. J. Cell Biol. *105*, 2621-2629.

Beyer,E.C., Paul,D.L., and Goodenough,D.A. (1990). Connexin family of gap junction proteins. J. Membr. Biol. *116*, 187-194.

Beyer,E.C., Reed,K.E., Westphale,E.M., Kanter,H.L., and Larson,D.M. (1992). Molecular cloning and expression of rat connexin40, a gap junction protein expressed in vascular smooth muscle. J. Membr. Biol. *127*, 69-76.

Beyer,E.C., Seul,K.H., and Larson,D.M. (1998). Cardiovascular gap junction proteins: molecular characterization and biochemical regulation. In Heart Cell Communication in Health and Disease, W.C.De Mello and M.J.Janse, eds. (Norwell, MA: Kluwer Academic Publishers), pp. 45-72.

Beyer,E.C. and Steinberg,T.H. (1991). Evidence that the gap junction protein connexin-43 is the ATP- induced pore of mouse macrophages. J. Biol. Chem. *266*, 7971-7974.

Beyer,E.C. and Steinberg,T.H. (1993). Connexins, gap-junction proteins, and ATP-induced pores in macrophages. In Gap Junctions (Progress in Cell Reserach, Vol. 3), J.E.Hall, G.Zampighi, and R.M.Davis, eds. (Amsterdam: Elsevier), pp. 55-58.

Blackburn,J.P., Peters,N.S., Yeh,H.I., Rothery,S., Green,C.R., and Severs,N.J. (1995). Upregulation of connexin43 gap junctions during early stages of human coronary atherosclerosis. Arterioscler. Thromb. Vasc. Biol. *15*, 1219-1228.

Bloemendal,H., Zweers,A., Vermorken,F., Dunia,I., and Benedetti,E.L. (1972). The plasma membrane of eye lens fibers. Biochemical and structural characterization. Cell Differ. *1*, 91-106.

Brink,P.R., Cronin,K., Banach,K., Peterson,E., Westphale,E.M., Seul,K.H., Ramanan,S.V., and Beyer,E.C. (1997). Evidence for heteromeric gap junction channels formed from rat connexin43 and human connexin37. Am. J. Physiol. (Cell Physiol.) *273*, C1386-C1396.

Cai,W.J., Koltai,S., Kocsis,E., Scholz,D., Schaper,W., and Schaper,J. (2001). Connexin37, not Cx40 and Cx43, is induced in vascular smooth muscle cells during coronary arteriogenesis. J Mol. Cell Cardiol. *33*, 957-967.

Caspar,D.L.D., Goodenough,D.A., Makowski,L., and Phillips,W.P. (1977). Gap junction structures. I. Correlated electron microscopy and X-ray diffraction. J. Cell Biol. *74*, 605-628.

Chen,Z.Q., Lefebvre,D., Bai,X.H., Reaume,A., Rossant,J., and Lye,S.J. (1995). Identification of two regulatory elements within the promoter region of the mouse connexin 43 gene. J. Biol. Chem. *270*, 3863-3868.

Christ,G.J., Spray,D.C., El-Sabban,M., Moore,L.K., and Brink,P.R. (1996). Gap junctions in vascular tissues: evaluating the role of intercellular communication in the modulation of vasomotor tone. Circ. Res. *79*, 631-646.

Condorelli,D.F., Parenti,R., Spinella,F., Salinaro,A.T., Belluardo,N., Cardile,V., and Cicirata,F. (1998). Cloning of a new gap junction gene (Cx36) highly expressed in mammalian brain neurons. Eur. J. Neurosci. *10*, 1202-1208.

Coppen,S.R., Kodama,I., Boyett,M.R., Dobrzynski,H., Takagishi,Y., Honjo,H., Yeh,H.I., and Severs,N.J. (1999). Connexin45, a major connexin of the rabbit sinoatrial node, is co- expressed with connexin43 in a restricted zone at the nodal-crista terminalis border. J. Histochem. Cytochem. *47*, 907-918.

Crow,D.S., Beyer,E.C., Paul,D.L., Kobe,S.S., and Lau,A.F. (1990). Phosphorylation of connexin43 gap junction protein in uninfected and Rous sarcoma virus-transformed mammalian fibroblasts. Mol. Cell Biol. *10*, 1754-1763.

Cuevas,P., Gutierrez-Diaz,J.A., Reimers,D., Dujovny,M., Diaz,F.G., and Ausman,J.L. (1984). Pericyte endothelial gap junctions in human cerebral capillaries. Anat. Embryol. *170*, 155.

Dahl,G., Miller,T., Paul,D., Voellmy,R., and Werner,R. (1987). Expression of functional cell-cell channels from cloned rat liver gap junction complementary DNA. Science *236*, 1290-1293.

Darrow,B.J., Laing,J.G., Lampe,P.D., Saffitz,J.E., and Beyer,E.C. (1995). Expression of multiple connexins in cultured neonatal rat ventricular myocytes. Circ. Res. *76*, 381-387.

Das,S.J., Meyer,R.A., Wang,F., Abraham,V., Lo,C.W., and Koval,M. (2001). Multimeric connexin interactions prior to the trans-Golgi network. J Cell Sci. *114*, 4013-4024.

Davis,L.M., Kanter,H.L., Beyer,E.C., and Saffitz,J.E. (1994). Distinct gap junction phenotypes in cardiac tissues with disparate conduction properties. J. Am. Coll. Cardiol. *24*, 1124-1132.

Davis,L.M., Rodefeld, M.E., Green,K., Beyer, E.C., and Saffitz, J.E. (1995). Gap junction protein phenotypes of the human heart and conduction system. J. Cardiovasc. Electrophysiol. *6*, 813-822.

Dejana,E., Corada,M., and Lampugnani,M.G. (1995). Endothelial cell-to-cell junctions. FASEB J. *9*, 910-918.

Dermietzel,R., Hertberg,E.L., Kessler,J.A., and Spray,D.C. (1991). Gap junctions between cultured astrocytes: immunocytochemical, molecular, and electrophysiological analysis. J. Neurosci. *11*, 1421-1432.

Dorshkind,K., Green,L., Godwin,A., and Fletcher,W.H. (1993). Connexin-43-type gap junctions mediate communication between bone marrow stromal cells. Blood *82*, 38-45.

Eghbali,B., Kessler,J.A., and Spray,D.C. (1990). Expression of gap junction channels in communication-incompetent cells after stable transfection with cDNA encoding connexin 32. Proc. Natl. Acad. Sci. U. S. A. *87*, 1328-1331.

Eid,H., Larson,D.M., Springhorn,J.P., Attawia,M.A., Nayak,R.C., Smith,T.W., and Kelly,R.A. (1992). Role of epicardial mesothelial cells in the modification of phenotype and function of adult rat ventricular myocytes in primary coculture. Circ. Res. *71*, 40-50.

Elenes,S., Martinez,A.D., Delmar,M., Beyer,E.C., and Moreno,A.P. (2001). Heterotypic docking of cx43 and cx45 connexons blocks fast voltage gating of cx43. Biophys. J. *81*, 1406-1418.

Elfgang,C., Eckert,R., Lichtenberg-Frate,H., Butterweck,A., Traub,O., Klein,R.A., Hulser,D.F., and Willecke,K. (1995). Specific permeability and selective formation of gap junction channels in connexin-transfected HeLa cells. J. Cell Biol. *129*, 805-817.

Evans,W.H. and Gurd,J.W. (1972). Preparation and properties of nexuses and lipid enriched vesicles from mouse liver plasma membranes. Biochem. J. *128*, 691-700.

Falk,M.M. (2000a). Biosynthesis and structural composition of gap junction intercellular membrane channels. Eur. J. Cell Biol. *79*, 564-574.

Falk,M.M. (2000b). Cell-free synthesis for analyzing the membrane integration, oligomerization, and assembly characteristics of gap junction connexins. Methods *20*, 165-179.

Falk,M.M., Buehler,L.K., Kumar,N.M., and Gilula,N.B. (1997). Cell-free synthesis and assembly of connexins into functional gap junction membrane channels. EMBO J. *16*, 2703-2716.

Falk,M.M. and Lauf,U. (2001). High resolution, fluorescence deconvolution microscopy and tagging with the autofluorescent tracers CFP, GFP, and YFP to study the structural composition of gap junctions in living cells. Microsc. Res Tech. *52*, 251-262.

Fallon,R.F. and Goodenough,D.A. (1981). Five-hour half-life of mouse liver gap-junction protein. J. Cell Biol. *90*, 521-526.

Filson,A.J., Azarnia,R., Beyer,E.C., Loewenstein,W.R., and Brugge,J.S. (1990). Tyrosine phosphorylation of a gap junction protein correlates with inhibition of cell-to-cell communication. Cell Growth Differ. *1*, 661-668.

Fishman,G.I., Spray,D.C., and Leinwand,L.A. (1990). Molecular characterization and functional expression of the human cardiac gap junction channel. J. Cell Biol. *111*, 589-598.

Fujimoto,K., Nagafuchi,A., Tsukita,S., Kuraoka,A., Ohokuma,A., and Shibata,Y. (1997). Dynamics of connexins, E-cadherin and alpha-catenin on cell membranes during gap junction formation. J. Cell Sci. *110*, 311-322.

Gabriels,J.E. and Paul,D.L. (1998). Connexin43 is highly localized to sites of disturbed flow in rat aortic endothelium but connexin37 and connexin40 are more uniformly distributed [see comments]. Circ. Res. *83*, 636-643.

Geimonen,E., Jiang,W., Ali,M., Fishman,G.I., Garfield,R.E., and Andersen,J. (1996). Activation of protein kinase C in human uterine smooth muscle induces *connexin-43* gene transcription through an AP-1 site in the promoter sequence. J. Biol. Chem. *271*, 23667-23674.

George,C.H., Kendall,J.M., and Evans,W.H. (1999). Intracellular trafficking pathways in the assembly of connexins into gap junctions. J. Biol. Chem. *274*, 8678-8685.

Giepmans,B.N. and Moolenaar,W.H. (1998). The gap junction protein connexin43 interacts with the second PDZ domain of the zona occludens-1 protein. Curr. Biol. *8*, 931-934.

Giepmans,B.N., Verlaan,I., Hengeveld,T., Janssen,H., Calafat,J., Falk,M.M., and Moolenaar,W.H. (2001). Gap junction protein connexin-43 interacts directly with microtubules. Curr. Biol. *11*, 1364-1368.

Ginzberg,R.D. and Gilula,N.B. (1979). Modulation of cell junctions during differentiation of the chicken otocyst sensory epithelium. Dev. Biol. *68*, 110-129.

Gonzalez-Mariscal,L., Betanzos,A., and Avila-Flores,A. (2000). MAGUK proteins: structure and role in the tight junction. Semin. Cell Biol. *11*, 315-324.

Goodenough,D.A. (1979). Lens gap junctions: a structural hypothesis for nonregulated low- resistance intercellular pathways. Invest. Ophthalmol. Vis. Sci. *18*, 1104-1122.

Goodenough,D.A., Paul,D.L., and Jesaitis,L. (1988). Topological distribution of two connexin32 antigenic sites in intact and split rodent hepatocyte gap junctions. J. Cell Biol. *107*, 1817-1824.

Goodenough,D.A. and Stoeckenius,W. (1972). The isolation of mouse hepatocyte gap junctions. Preliminary chemical characterization and x-ray diffraction. J. Cell Biol. *54*, 646-656.

Green,C.R., Harfst,E., Gourdie,R.G., and Severs,N.J. (1988). Analysis of the rat liver gap junction protein: clarification of anomalies in its molecular size. Proc. R. Soc. Lond. [Biol]. *233*, 165-174.

Groenewegen,W.A., van,V.T., van der Velden HM, and Jongsma,H.J. (1998). Genomic organization of the rat connexin40 gene: identical transcription start sites in heart and lung. Cardiovasc. Res. *38*, 463-471.

Gros,D.B., Nicholson,B.J., and Revel,J.P. (1983). Comparative analysis of the gap junction protein from rat heart and liver: is there a tissue specificity of gap junctions? Cell *35*, 539-549.

Guerrero,P.G., Schuessler,R.B., Davis,L.M., Beyer,E.C., Johnson,C.M., Yamada,K.A., and Saffitz,J.E. (1997). Slow ventricular conduction in mice heterozygous for a connexin43 null mutation. J. Clin. Invest. *99*, 1991-1998.

Guinan,E.C., Smith,B.R., Davies,P.F., and Pober,J.S. (1988). Cytoplasmic transfer between endothelium and lymphocytes: quantitation by flow cytometry. Am. J. Pathol. *132*, 406-409.

Haefliger,J.A., Bruzzone,R., Jenkins,N.A., Gilbert,D.J., Copeland,N.G., and Paul,D.L. (1992). Four novel members of the connexin family of gap junction proteins. Molecular cloning, expression, and chromosome mapping. J. Biol. Chem. *267*, 2057-2064.

Haefliger,J.A. and Meda,P. (2000). Chronic hypertension alters the expression of Cx43 in cardiovascular muscle cells. Braz. J. Med. Biol. Res. *33*, 431-438.

Haefliger,J.A., Polikar,R., Schnyder,G., Burdet,M., Sutter,E., Pexieder,T., Nicod,P., and Meda,P. (2000). Connexin37 in normal and pathological development of mouse heart and great arteries. Dev. Dyn. *218* , 331-344.

Harfst,E., Severs,N.J., and Green,C.R. (1990). Cardiac myocyte gap junctions: evidence for a major connexon protein with an apparent relative molecular mass of 70,000. J. Cell Sci. *96*, 591-604.

Hennemann,H., Kozjek,G., Dahl,E., Nicholson,B., and Willecke,K. (1992a). Molecular cloning of mouse connexins26 and -32: similar genomic organization but distinct promoter sequences of two gap junction genes. Eur. J. Cell Biol. *58*, 81-89.

Hennemann,H., Suchyna,T., Lichtenberg Frate,H., Jungbluth,S., Dahl,E., Schwarz,J., Nicholson,B.J., and Willecke,K. (1992b). Molecular cloning and functional expression of mouse connexin40, a second gap junction gene preferentially expressed in lung. J. Cell Biol. *117*, 1299-1310.

Hertlein,B., Butterweck,A., Haubrich,S., Willecke,K., and Traub,O. (1998). Phosphorylated carboxy terminal serine residues stabilize the mouse gap junction protein connexin45 against degradation. J. Membr. Biol. *162*, 247-257.

Hertzberg,E.L., Disher,R.M., Tiller,A.A., Zhou,Y., and Cook,R.G. (1988). Topology of the Mr 27,000 liver gap junction protein. Cytoplasmic localization of amino- and carboxyl termini and a hydrophilic domain which is protease-hypersensitive. J. Biol. Chem. *263*, 19105-19111.

Hertzberg,E.L. and Gilula,N.B. (1979). Isolation and characterization of gap junctions from rat liver. J. Biol. Chem. *254*, 2138-2147.

Huang,G.Y., Cooper,E.S., Waldo,K., Kirby,M.L., Gilula,N.B., and Lo,C.W. (1998a). Gap Junction-mediated Cell-Cell Communication Modulates Mouse Neural Crest Migration. J. Cell Biol. *143*, 1725-1734.

Huang,G.Y., Wessels,A., Smith,B.R., Linask,K.K., Ewart,J.L., and Lo,C.W. (1998b). Alteration in connexin 43 gap junction gene dosage impairs conotruncal heart development. Dev. Biol. *198*, 32-44.

Jacob,A. and Beyer,E.C. (2001). Mouse connexin 45: genomic cloning and exon usage. DNA Cell Biol. *20*, 11-19.

Jara,P.I., Boric,M.P., and Saez,J.C. (1995). Leukocytes express connexin43 after activation with lipopolysaccharide and appear to form gap junctions with endothelial cells after ischemia-reperfustion. Proc. Natl. Acad. Sci. USA *92*, 7011-7015.

Johnson,C.M., Kanter,E.M., Green,K.G., Laing,J.G., Betsuyaku,T., Beyer,E.C., Steinberg,T.H., Saffitz,J.E., and Yamada,K.A. (2002). Redistribution of connexin45 in gap junctions of connexin43-deficient hearts. Cardiovasc. Res *(in press)*.

Jongen,W.M., Fitzgerald,D.J., Asamoto,M., Piccoli,C., Slaga,T.J., Gros,D., Takeichi,M., and Yamasaki,H. (1991). Regulation of connexin 43-mediated gap junctional intercellular communication by Ca2+ in mouse epidermal cells is controlled by E- cadherin. J. Cell Biol. *114*, 545-555.

Jordan,K., Chodock,R., Hand,A.R., and Laird,D.W. (2001). The origin of annular junctions: a mechanism of gap junction internalization. J Cell Sci. *114*, 763-773.

Jordan,K., Solan,J.L., Dominguez,M., Sia,M., Hand,A., Lampe,P.D., and Laird,D.W. (1999). Trafficking, assembly, and function of a connexin43-green fluorescent protein chimera in live mammalian cells. Mol. Biol. Cell *10*, 2033-2050.

Kanter,H.L., Laing,J.G., Beyer,E.C., Green,K.G., and Saffitz,J.E. (1993). Multiple connexins colocalize in canine ventricular myocyte gap junctions. Circ. Res. *73*, 344-350.

Kanter,H.L., Saffitz,J.E., and Beyer,E.C. (1992). Cardiac myocytes express multiple gap junction proteins. Circ. Res. *70*, 438-444.

Kensler,R.W., Brink,P.R., and Dewey,M.M. (1979). The septum of the lateral axon of the earthworm: a thin section and freeze-fracture study. J. Neurocytol. *8*, 565-590.

Kirchhoff,S., Kim,J.S., Hagendorff,A., Thonnissen,E., Kruger,O., Lamers,W.H., and Willecke,K. (2000). Abnormal cardiac conduction and morphogenesis in connexin40 and connexin43 double-deficient mice. Circ. Res. *87*, 399-405.

Kistler,J., Christie,D., and Bullivant,S. (1988). Homologies between gap junction proteins in lens, heart and liver. Nature *331*, 721-723.

Kistler,J., Kirkland,B., and Bullivant,S. (1985). Identification of a 70,000-D protein in lens membrane junctional domains. J. Cell Biol. *101*, 28-35.

Krenacs,T. and Rosendaal,M. (1998). Connexin43 gap junctions in normal, regenerating, and cultured mouse bone marrow and in human leukemias: their possible involvement in blood formation. Am. J. Pathol. *152*, 993-1004.

Kruger,O., Plum,A., Kim,J., Winterhager,E., Maxeiner,S., Hallas,G., Kirchhoff,S., Traub,O., Lamers,W.H., and Willecke,K. (2000). Defective vascular development in connexin 45-deficient mice. Development *127*, 4179-4193.

Kumai,M., Nishii,K., Nakamura,K., Takeda,N., Suzuki,M., and Shibata,Y. (2000). Loss of connexin45 causes a cushion defect in early cardiogenesis. Development *127*, 3501-3512.

Kumar,N.M. and Gilula,N.B. (1986). Cloning and characterization of human and rat liver cDNAs coding for a gap junction protein. J. Cell Biol. *103*, 767-776.

Kurata,W.E. and Lau,A.F. (1994). p130gag-fps disrupts gap junctional communication and induces phosphorylation of connexin43 in a manner similar to that of pp60v-src. Oncogene 9, 329-335.

Kwak,B.R., Pepper,M.S., Gros,D.B., and Meda,P. (2001). Inhibition of endothelial wound repair by dominant negative connexin inhibitors. Mol. Biol. Cell 12, 831-845.

Laing,J.G. and Beyer,E.C. (1995). The gap junction protein connexin43 is degraded via the ubiquitin proteasome pathway. J. Biol. Chem. 270, 26399-26403.

Laing,J.G., Manley-Markowski,R.N., Koval,M., Civitelli,R., and Steinberg,T.H. (2001). Connexin45 interacts with zonula occludens-1 and connexin43 in osteoblastic cells. J Biol. Chem. 276, 23051-23055.

Laing,J.G., Tadros,P.N., Green,K., Saffitz,J.E., and Beyer,E.C. (1998). Proteolysis of connexin43-containing gap junctions in normal and heat- stressed cardiac myocytes. Cardiovasc. Res. 38, 711-718.

Laing,J.G., Tadros,P.N., Westphale,E.M., and Beyer,E.C. (1997). Degradation of connexin43 gap junctions involves both the proteasome and the lysosome. Exp. Cell Res. 236, 482-492.

Laing,J.G., Westphale,E.M., Engelmann,G.L., and Beyer,E.C. (1994). Characterization of the gap junction protein connexin45. J. Membr. Biol. 139, 31-40.

Laird,D.W. (1996). The life cycle of a connexin: gap junction formation, removal, and degradation. J. Bioenerg. Biomemb. 28, 311-318.

Laird,D.W., Jordan,K., and Shao,Q. (2001). Expression and imaging of connexin-GFP chimeras in live mammalian cells. Methods Mol. Biol. 154, 135-142.

Laird,D.W., Puranam,K.L., and Revel,J.P. (1991). Turnover and phosphorylation dynamics of connexin43 gap junction protein in cultured cardiac myocytes. Biochem. J. 273, 67-72.

Lampe,P.D. (1994). Analyzing phorbol ester effects on gap junctional communication: a dramatic inhibition of assembly. J. Cell Biol. 127, 1895-1905.

Lampe,P.D., Kurata,W.E., Warn-Cramer,B.J., and Lau,A.F. (1998). Formation of a distinct connexin43 phosphoisoform in mitotic cells is dependent upon p34cdc2 kinase. J. Cell Sci. 111, 833-841.

Lampe,P.D., TenBroek,E.M., Burt,J.M., Kurata,W.E., Johnson,R.G., and Lau,A.F. (2000). Phosphorylation of connexin43 on serine368 by protein kinase C regulates gap junctional communication. J. Cell Biol. 149, 1503-1512.

Larsen,W.J. and Tung,H.N. (1978). Origin and fate of cytoplasmic gap junctions in rabbit granulosa cells. Tissue Cell 10, 585-598.

Larsen,W.J., Tung,H.N., Murray,S.A., and Swenson,C.A. (1979). Evidence for the participation of actin microfilaments in the internalization of gap junction membrane. J. Cell Biol. 83, 576-587.

Larson,D.M., Carson,M.P., and Haudenschild,C.C. (1987). Junctional transfer of small molecules in cultured bovine brain microvascular endothelial cells and pericytes. Microvasc. Res. *34*, 184.

Larson,D.M., Haudenschild,C.C., and Beyer,E.C. (1990). Gap junction messenger RNA expression by vascular wall cells. Circ. Res. *66*, 1074-1080.

Larson,D.M., Seul,K.H., Berthoud,V.M., Lau,A.F., Sagar,G.D.V., and Beyer,E.C. (2000). Functional expression and biochemical characterization of an epitope-tagged connexin37. Mol. Cell Biol. Res. Commun. *3* , 115-121.

Larson,D.M., Wrobleski,M.J., Sagar,G.D.V., Westphale,E.M., and Beyer,E.C. (1997). Differential regulation of connexin43 and connexin37 in endothelial cells by cell density, growth, and TGF-beta1. Am. J. Physiol. (Cell Physiol.) *272*, C405-C415.

Lau,A.F., Kurata,W.E., Kanemitsu,M.Y., Loo,L.M., Warn-Cramer,B.J., Eckhart,W., and Lampe,P.D. (1996). Regulation of connexin43 function by activated tyrosine protein kinases. J. Bioenerg. Biomemb. *28*, 357-365.

Liao,Y., Day,K.H., Damon,D.N., and Duling,B.R. (2001). Endothelial cell-specific knockout of connexin 43 causes hypotension and bradycardia in mice. Proc. Natl. Acad. Sci. U. S. A *98*, 9989-9994.

Little,T.L., Beyer,E.C., and Duling,B.R. (1995a). Connexin43 and connexin40 gap junction proteins are present in arteriolar smooth muscle and endothelium in vivo. Am. J. Physiol. *268*, H729-H739.

Little,T.L., Xia,J., and Duling,B.R. (1995b). Dye tracers define differential endothelial and smooth muscle coupling patterns within the arterial wall. Circ. Res. *76*, 498-504.

Liu,S., Taffet,S., Stoner,L., Delmar,M., Vallano,M.L., and Jalife,J. (1993). A structural basis for the unequal sensitivity of the major cardiac and liver gap junctions to intracellular acidification: the carboxyl tail length. Biophys. J. *64*, 1422-1433.

Loewenstein,W.R. (1966). Permeability of membrane junctions. Ann. N. Y. Acad. Sci. *137*, 441-472.

Loo,L.W., Berestecky,J.M., Kanemitsu,M.Y., and Lau,A.F. (1995). pp60src-mediated phosphorylation of connexin 43, a gap junction protein. J. Biol. Chem. *270*, 12751-12761.

Loo,L.W., Kanemitsu,M.Y., and Lau,A.F. (1999). In vivo association of pp60v-src and the gap-junction protein connexin 43 in v-src-transformed fibroblasts. Mol. Carcinog. *25*, 187-195.

Makowski,L., Caspar,D.L.D., Phillips,W.C., and Goodenough,D.A. (1977). Gap junction structures. II. Analysis of the X-ray diffraction data. J. Cell Biol. *74*, 629-645.

Manjunath,C.K., Goings,G.E., and Page,E. (1984). Cytoplasmic surface and intramembrane components of rat heart gap junctional proteins. Am. J. Physiol. *246*, H865-H875.

Manjunath,C.K., Goings,G.E., and Page,E. (1987a). Human cardiac gap junctions: isolation, ultrastructure, and protein composition. J. Mol. Cell Cardiol. *19*, 131-134.

Manjunath,C.K., Nicholson,B.J., Teplow,D., Hood,L., Page,E., and Revel,J.P. (1987b). The cardiac gap junction protein (Mr 47,000) has a tissue- specific cytoplasmic domain of Mr 17,000 at its carboxy- terminus. Biochem. Biophys. Res. Commun. *142*, 228-234.

Manjunath,C.K. and Page,E. (1985). Cell biology and protein composition of cardiac gap junctions. Am. J. Physiol. *248*, H783-H791.

Meyer,R.A., Laird,D.W., Revel,J.P., and Johnson,R.G. (1992). Inhibition of gap junction and adherens junction assembly by connexin and A-CAM antibodies. J. Cell Biol. *119*, 179-189.

Milks,L.C., Kumar,N.M., Houghten,R., Unwin,N., and Gilula,N.B. (1988). Topology of the 32-kd liver gap junction protein determined by site-directed antibody localizations. EMBO J. *7*, 2967-2975.

Miller,T., Dahl,G., and Werner,R. (1988). Structure of a gap junction gene: rat connexin-32. Biosci. Rep. *8*, 455-464.

Minkoff,R., Rundus,V.R., Parker,S.B., Beyer,E.C., and Hertzberg,E.L. (1993). Connexin expression in the developing avian cardiovascular system. Circ. Res. *73*, 71-78.

Montecino-Rodriguez,E. and Dorshkind,K. (2001). Regulation of hematopoiesis by gap junction-mediated intercellular communication. J Leukoc. Biol. *70*, 341-347.

Montecino-Rodriguez,E., Leathers,H., and Dorshkind,K. (2000). Expression of connexin 43 (Cx43) is critical for normal hematopoiesis. Blood *96*, 917-924.

Musil,L.S., Beyer,E.C., and Goodenough,D.A. (1990a). Expression of the gap junction protein connexin43 in embryonic chick lens: molecular cloning, ultrastructural localization, and post-translational phosphorylation. J. Membr. Biol. *116*, 163-175.

Musil,L.S., Cunningham,B.A., Edelman,G.M., and Goodenough,D.A. (1990b). Differential phosphorylation of the gap junction protein connexin43 in junctional communication-competent and -deficient cell lines. J. Cell Biol. *111*, 2077-2088.

Musil,L.S. and Goodenough,D.A. (1991). Biochemical analysis of connexin43 intracellular transport, phosphorylation, and assembly into gap junctional plaques. J. Cell Biol. *115*, 1357-1374.

Musil,L.S. and Goodenough,D.A. (1993). Multisubunit assembly of an integral plasma membrane channel protein, gap junction connexin43, occurs after exit from the ER. Cell *74*, 1065-1077.

Musil,L.S., Le,A.C., VanSlyke,J.K., and Roberts,L.M. (2000). Regulation of Connexin Degradation As a Mechanism to Increase Gap Junction Assembly and Function. J. Biol. Chem.

Naus,C.C., Hearn,S., Zhu,D., Nicholson,B.J., and Shivers,R.R. (1993). Ultrastructural analysis of gap junctions in C6 glioma cells transfected with connexin43 cDNA. Exp. Cell Res. *206*, 72-84.

Neuhaus,I.M., Dahl,G., and Werner,R. (1995). Use of alternate promoters for tissue specific expression of the gene coding for connexin32. Gene *158*, 257-262.

Nicholson,B., Dermietzel,R., Teplow,D., Traub,O., Willecke,K., and Revel,J.P. (1987). Two homologous protein components of hepatic gap junctions. Nature *329*, 732-734.

Nicholson,B.J., Gros,D.B., Kent,S.B.H., Hood,L.E., and Revel,J.P. (1985). The Mr 28,000 gap junction proteins from rat heart and liver are different but related. J. Biol. Chem. *260*, 6514-6517.

Paul,D.L. (1986). Molecular cloning of cDNA for rat liver gap junction protein. J. Cell Biol. *103*, 123-134.

Paul,D.L., Ebihara,L., Takemoto,L.J., Swenson,K.I., and Goodenough,D.A. (1991). Connexin46, a novel lens gap junction protein, induces voltage- gated currents in nonjunctional plasma membrane of Xenopus oocytes. J. Cell Biol. *115*, 1077-1089.

Peracchia,C., Sotkis,A., Wang,X.G., Peracchia,L.L., and Persechini,A. (2000). Calmodulin directly gates gap junction channels. J. Biol. Chem. *275*, 26220-26224.

Polacek,D., Lal,R., Volin,M.V., and Davies,P.F. (1993). Gap junctional communication between vascular cells. Induction of connexin43 messenger RNA in macrophage foam cells of atherosclerotic lesions. Am. J. Pathol. *142*, 593-606.

Rahman,S., Carlile,G., and Evans,W.H. (1993). Assembly of hepatic gap junctions. Topography and distribution of connexin 32 in intracellular and plasma membranes determined using sequence-specific antibodies. J. Biol. Chem. *268*, 1260-1265.

Reaume,A.G., Desousa,P.A., Kulkarni,S., Langille,B.L., Zhu,D.G., Davies,T.C., Juneja,S.C., Kidder,G.M., and Rossant,J. (1995). Cardiac malformation in neonatal mice lacking connexin43. Science *267*, 1831-1834.

Reed,K.E., Westphale,E.M., Larson,D.M., Wang,H.Z., Veenstra,R.D., and Beyer,E.C. (1993). Molecular cloning and functional expression of human connexin37, an endothelial cell gap junction protein. J. Clin. Invest. *91*, 997-1004.

Revel,J.P. and Karnovsky,M.J. (1967). Hexagonal array of subunits in intercellular junctions of the mouse heart and liver. J. Cell Biol. *33*, C7-C12.

Robertson,J.D. (1963). The occurrence of a subunit pattern in the unit membranes of club endings in Mauthner cell synapses in goldfish brains. J. Cell Biol. *19*, 201-221.

Rosendaal,M., Green,C.R., Rahman,A., and Morgan,D. (1994). Up-regulation of the connexin43+ gap junction network in haemopoietic tissue before the growth of stem cells. J. Cell Sci. *107*, 29-37.

Saez,J.C., Berthoud,V.M., Moreno,A.P., and Spray,D.C. (1993). Gap junctions: multiplicity of controls in differentiated and undifferentiated cells and possible functional implications. In Advances in Second Messenger and Phosphoprotein Research Vol. 27, S.Shenolikar and A.C.Nairn, eds. (New York: Raven Press, Ltd.), pp. 163-198.

Saez,J.C., Martinez,A.D., Branes,M.C., and Gonzalez,H.E. (1998). Regulation of gap junctions by protein phosphorylation. Braz. J. Med. Biol. Res. *31*, 593-600.

Seul,K.H. and Beyer,E.C. (2000a). Heterogeneous localization of connexin40 in the renal vasculature. Microvasc. Res. *59*, 140-148.

Seul,K.H. and Beyer,E.C. (2000b). Mouse connexin37: gene structure and promoter analysis. Biochim. Biophys. Acta *in press*.

Seul,K.H., Tadros,P.N., and Beyer,E.C. (1997). Mouse connexin40: gene structure and promoter analysis. Genomics *46*, 120-126.

Severs,N.J., Shovel,K.S., Slade,A.M., Powell,T., Twist,V.W., and Green,C.R. (1989). Fate of gap junctions in isolated adult mammalian cardiomyocytes. Circ. Res. *65*, 22-42.

Simon,A.M., Goodenough,D.A., li,E., and Paul,D.L. (1997). Female infertility in mice lacking connexin37. Nature *385*, 525-529.

Simon,A.M., Goodenough,D.A., and Paul,D.L. (1998). Mice lacking connexin40 have cardiac conduction abnormalities characteristic of atrioventricular block and bundle branch block. Curr. Biol. *8*, 295-298.

Sohl,G., Gillen,C., Bosse,F., Gleichmann,M., Muller,H.W., and Willecke,K. (1996). A second alternative transcript of the gap junction gene connexin32 is expressed in murine Schwann cells and modulated in injured sciatic nerve. Eur. J. Cell Biol. *69*, 267-275.

Spagnoli,L.G., Villaschi,S., Neri,L., and Palmieri,G. (1982). Gap junctions in myo-endothelial bridges of rabbit carotid arteries. Experientia *38*, 124.

Spray,D.C., Moreno,A.P., Eghbali,B., Chanson,M., and Fishman,G.I. (1992). Gating of gap junction channels as revealed in cells stably transfected with wild type and mutant connexin cDNAs. Biophys. J. *62*, 48-50.

Su,M., Borke,J.L., Donahue,H.J., Li,Z., Warshawsky,N.M., Russell,C.M., and Lewis,J.E. (1997). Expression of connexin 43 in rat mandibular bone and periodontal ligament (PDL) cells during experimental tooth movement. J. Dent. Res. *76*, 1357-1366.

Sullivan,R., Huang,G.Y., Meyer,R.A., Wessels,A., Linask,K.K., and Lo,C.W. (1998). Heart malformations in transgenic mice exhibiting dominant negative inhibition of gap junctional communication in neural crest cells. Dev. Biol. *204*, 224-234.

Sullivan,R., Ruangvoravat,C., Joo,D., Morgan,J., Wang,B.L., Wang,X.K., and Lo,C.W. (1993). Structure, sequence and expression of the mouse Cx43 gene encoding connexin 43. Gene *130*, 191-199.

Swenson,K.I., Jordan,J.R., Beyer,E.C., and Paul,D.L. (1989). Formation of gap junctions by expression of connexins in Xenopus oocyte pairs. Cell *57*, 145-155.

Swenson,K.I., Piwnica Worms,H., McNamee,H., and Paul,D.L. (1990). Tyrosine phosphorylation of the gap junction protein connexin43 is required for the pp60v-src-induced inhibition of communication. Cell Regul. *1*, 989-1002.

TenBroek,E.M., Lampe,P.D., Solan,J.L., Reynhout,J.K., and Johnson,R.G. (2001). Ser364 of connexin43 and the upregulation of gap junction assembly by cAMP. J Cell Biol. *155*, 1307-1318.

Thomas,S.A., Schuessler,R.B., Berul,C.I., Beardslee,M.A., Beyer,E.C., Mendelsohn,M.E., and Saffitz,J.E. (1998). Disparate effects of deficient expression of connexin43 on atrial and ventricular conduction: evidence for chamber-specific molecular determinants of conduction. Circ. *97*, 686-691.

Toyofuku,T., Yabuki,M., Otsu,K., Kuzuya,T., Hori,M., and Tada,M. (1998). Direct association of the gap junction protein connexin-43 with ZO-1 in cardiac myocytes. J. Biol. Chem. *273*, 12725-12731.

Toyofuku,T., Zhang,H., Akamatsu,Y., Kuzuya,T., Tada,M., and Hori,M. (2000). c-Src regulates the interaction between connexin-43 and ZO-1 in cardiac myocytes. J. Biol. Chem.

Traub,O., Druge,P.M., and Willecke,K. (1983). Degradation and resynthesis of gap junction protein in plasma membranes of regenerating liver after partial hepatectomy or cholestasis. Proc. Natl. Acad. Sci. U. S. A. *80*, 755-759.

Traub,O., Look,J., Dermietzel,R., Brummer,F., Hulser,D., and Willecke,K. (1989). Comparative characterization of the 21-kD and 26-kD gap junction proteins in murine liver and cultured hepatocytes. J. Cell Biol. *108*, 1039-1051.

Unger,V.M., Kumar,N.M., Gilula,N.B., and Yeager,M. (1997). Projection structure of a gap junction membrane channel at 7 A resolution. Nat. Struct. Biol. *4*, 39-43.

Unger,V.M., Kumar,N.M., Gilula,N.B., and Yeager,M. (1999). Three-dimensional structure of a recombinant gap junction membrane channel. Science *283*, 1176-1180.

Unwin,P.N.T. and Zampighi,G. (1980). Structure of the junction between communicating cells. Nature *283*, 545-549.

Valiunas,V., Gemel,J., Brink,P.R., and Beyer,E.C. (2001). Gap junction channels formed by coexpressed connexin40 and connexin43. AJP - Heart and Circulatory Physiology *281*, H1675-H1689.

van Kempen,M.J. and Jongsma,H.J. (1999). Distribution of connexin37, connexin40 and connexin43 in the aorta and coronary artery of several mammals. Histochem. Cell Biol. *112*, 479-486.

Van Kempen,M.J.A., Ten Velde,I., Wessels,A., Oosthoek,P.W., Gros,D., Jongsma,H.J., Moorman,A.F.M., and Lamers,W.H. (1995). Differential connexin distribution accomodates cardiac function in different species. Microscopy Research and Technique *31*, 420-436.

van Rijen,H.V., van Veen,T.A., van Kempen,M.J., Wilms-Schopman,F.J., Potse,M., Krueger,O., Willecke,K., Opthof,T., Jongsma,H.J., and de Bakker,J.M. (2001). Impaired conduction in the bundle branches of mouse hearts lacking the gap junction protein connexin40. Circ. *103*, 1591-1598.

van Veen,T.A., van Rijen,H.V., and Jongsma,H.J. (2000). Electrical conductance of mouse connexin45 gap junction channels is modulated by phosphorylation. Cardiovasc. Res. *46*, 496-510.

Veenstra,R.D., Wang,H.Z., Beblo,D.A., Chilton,M.G., Harris,A.L., Beyer,E.C., and Brink,P. (1995). Selectivity of connexin-specific gap junctions does not correlate with channel conductance. Circ. Res. *77*, 1156-1165.

Veenstra,R.D., Wang,H.Z., Westphale,E.M., and Beyer,E.C. (1992). Multiple connexins confer distinct regulatory and conductance properties of gap junctions in developing heart. Circ. Res. *71*, 1277-1283.

Verselis,V.K., Ginter,C.S., and Bargiello,T.A. (1994). Opposite voltage gating polarities of two closely related connexins. Nature *368*, 348-351.

Wang,Y. and Rose,B. (1997). An inhibition of gap-junctional communication by cadherins. J. Cell Sci. *110*, 301-309.

Warn-Cramer,B.J., Cottrell,G.T., Burt,J.M., and Lau,A.F. (1998). Regulation of connexin-43 gap junctional intercellular communication by mitogen-activated protein kinase. J. Biol. Chem *273*, 9188-9196.

Warn-Cramer,B.J., Kurata,W.E., and Lau,A.F. (2001). Biochemical analysis of connexin phosphorylation. Methods Mol. Biol. *154* , 431-446.

Warn-Cramer,B.J., Lampe,P.D., Kurata,W.E., Kanemitsu,M.Y., Loo,L.M., Eckhart,W., and Lau,A.F. (1996). Characterization of the mitogen-activated protein kinase phosphorylation sites on the connexin-43 gap junction protein. J. Biol. Chem. *271*, 3779-3786.

Weidmann,S. (1952). The electrical constants of Purkinje fibres. J. Physiol. (Lond) *118*, 348-360.

Werner,R., Levine,E., Rabadan Diehl,C., and Dahl,G. (1989). Formation of hybrid cell-cell channels. Proc. Natl. Acad. Sci. U. S. A. *86*, 5380-5384.

White,T.W., Paul,D.L., Goodenough,D.A., and Bruzzone,R. (1995). Functional analysis of selective interactions among rodent connexins. Mol. Biol. Cell *6*, 459-470.

Willecke,K., Heynkes,R., Dahl,E., Stutenkemper,R., Hennemann,H., Jungbluth,S., Suchyna,T., and Nicholson,B.J. (1991). Mouse connexin37: cloning and functional expression of a gap junction gene highly expressed in lung. J. Cell Biol. *114*, 1049-1057.

Xu,X., Li,W.E., Huang,G.Y., Meyer,R., Chen,T., Luo,Y., Thomas,M.P., Radice,G.L., and Lo,C.W. (2001). Modulation of mouse neural crest cell motility by N-cadherin and connexin 43 gap junctions. J Cell Biol. *154*, 217-230.

Yancey,S.B., John,S.A., Lal,R., Austin,B.J., and Revel,J.P. (1989). The 43-kD polypeptide of heart gap junctions: immunolocalization, topology, and functional domains. J. Cell Biol. *108*, 2241-2254.

Yeager,M. and Gilula,N.B. (1992). Membrane topology and quaternary structure of cardiac gap junction ion channels. J. Mol. Biol. *223*, 929-948.

Yeager,M., Unger,V.M., and Falk,M.M. (1998). Synthesis, assembly and structure of gap junction intercellular channels. Curr. Opin. Struct. Biol. *8*, 517-524.

Yeh,H.I., Lai,Y.J., Chang,H.M., Ko,Y.S., Severs,N.J., and Tsai,C.H. (2000). Multiple connexin expression in regenerating arterial endothelial gap junctions. Arterioscler. Thromb. Vasc. Biol. *20*, 1753-1762.

Yu,W., Dahl,G., and Werner,R. (1994). The connexin43 gene is responsive to estrogen. Proc. R. Soc. Lond. *255*, 125-132.

Zhou,L., Kasperek,E.M., and Nicholson,B.J. (1999). Dissection of the molecular basis of pp60(v-src) induced gating of connexin 43 gap junction channels [In Process Citation]. J. Cell Biol. *144*, 1033-1045.

Zimmer,D.B., Green,C.R., Evans,W.H., and Gilula,N.B. (1987). Topological analysis of the major protein in isolated intact rat liver gap junctions and gap junction-derived single membrane structures. J. Biol. Chem. *262*, 7751-7763.

4

HETEROMULTIMERIC GAP JUNCTION CHANNELS: A CONNECTION WITH CARDIAC PHYSIOLOGY AND PATHOLOGY

Alonso P. Moreno, Guoqiang Zhong and Volodya Hayrapetyan

Krannert Inst. of Cardiology. Indiana University School of Medicine. Indianapolis IN, 46202

INTRODUCTION

Growing evidence that heteromultimeric channels are formed *in vivo* suggests that junctional communication is not only governed by the permeability and gating mechanism of gap junctions formed by one type of connexin, but also by the interaction of multiple subunits that form channels (Loewenstein1981; Ramon and Rivera1986). Despite our current limited knowledge about interaction among cardiac connexins, it has become necessary to review and interpret how combinations of connexin subunits participate in the physiology and pathology of electrical and metabolic transmission in the heart.

Direct connection between cardiac cells is established by gap junction channels, which can be formed by one or more of members of a family of proteins called connexins, which share great homology in their sequences (Beyer et al., 1990). These distinct connexins can be co-expressed in one or more regions of cardiac tissue including regions of the conduction system. The particular distribution and spatial arrangement of these connexins enhances their functional relevance.

It has been profusely reported that during distinct pathological conditions, the expression of cardiac connexins becomes modified (For a review see (Jongsma and Wilders2000; Peters1996). Cx43 has been the connexin most widely studied because of its predominance in cardiac musculature, but, depending on the cardiac-related disease, Cx43 can be over or under-expressed. The change of expression of Cx43 in cardiac musculature has been accepted as the source of structural support for persistent arrhythmias. Recent reports that propose a model for action potential propagation, propose that even a reduction of 40% in expression will not impact the velocity of propagation of the action potential, therefore, no sustained arrhythmias are expected. Despite this finding, the reduction or increase in connexin expression in other cardiac regions (e.g. the conduction system) has been demonstrated to cause severe conduction disturbances (Gutstein et al., 2001; Kirchhoff et al., 1998; van Rijen et al., 2001a). Furthermore, until now, most studies of pathological conditions have been correlated with Cx43 expression, and the effects of other connexins, like Cx45 have been ignored, in part because of the lack of consistency in the data produced by cross-reaction between antibodies (Coppen et al., 1999b; Kanter et al., 1995). Notwithstanding these distinct interpretations, it is clear that the there is a change in connexin expression during pathological conditions. The importance of these changes in expression is not only related to variations in the level of expression of one specific connexin, but also to the fact that different connexins, when co-expressed at distinct concentrations, can form heteromultimeric channels with novel permeability and gating properties.

In this chapter we will review some evidence that supports the hypothesis that co-expression of cardiac connexins exists, and that this co-expression can induce distinct levels of communication as well as changes in the gating properties of the hetero-multimeric channels produced. We will also try to relate these alterations to cardiac physiology and pathology.

METHODS

Immunocytochemistry. The use of immunocytochemistry becomes necessary to determine the relative abundance of connexins and, in particular, to determine channel distribution (Thomas et al., 1998; Verheule et al., 2001). One main disadvantage of immunocytochemistry is that it does not permit evaluation of functional coupling between tissues, and therefore necessitates the use of parallel systems that allow us to determine the levels of communication between cells. Several attempts have been made to evaluate these levels of communication, especially using fluorescent dyes. Unfortunately the permeability of these dyes varies not only by the number of channels present, but also by the selectivity of the channels formed by the distinct connexins present in regard to the individual dyes (Veenstra et al., 1995).

Electrophysiology: Direct measurement of coupling in a tissue like the heart is not a simple matter because the presence of large numbers of channels in the musculature represents a methodological problem. It is usual to find hundreds of channels present between cells forming large plaques. In some instances, researchers have tried to determine conduction in isolated cells, but the isolation method disrupts these plaques; therefore quantification is inaccurate. The basic problem resides in the fact that, in a double-whole-cell voltage clamp configuration, the resistance of the measuring electrodes equals the resistive levels of the intercellular plaques. Therefore, substantial miscalculations of junctional conductance are expected between cells from the musculature (van Rijen et al., 2001b).

In terms of functional quantification, so far it has not been possible to determine the number of functional channels between cells of the cardiac muscle in its natural condition. Although multiple studies show that the conduction between cardiocytes is very high, (Wilders et al., 1996) and that it could represent hundreds to thousands of gap junction channels. Therefore, the movement of current will not be restricted across these junctions and the anisotropic properties of the tissue appear to be due to cell/tissue morphology rather than to gap junction channel distribution. Furthermore, it is suspected that even during cardiac remodeling due to fibrillation, where connexins change their expression pattern (van der Velden et al., 2000), the conduction may not change substantially (Jongsma and Wilders2000). This abundance of communication may not be the case between some cells that form part of the conduction system wherein communication appears to be substantially lower (e.g. SA node (Trabka-Janik et al., 1994). There, the co-expression of various distinct connexins is noteworthy and the formation of heteromultimeric channels is likely.

An alternative method for understanding the interaction of connexins in this tissue will be to use cellular systems that co-express connexins (Moore et al., 1991) or to develop cellular systems wherein the expression of connexins can be controlled (Eghbali et al., 1990). These systems have already been designed, (including mammalian cells and Xenopus oocytes) and have been used successfully to study the properties of connexins when co-expressed (Barrio et al., 1991; Moreno et al., 1995; Valiunas et al., 2000; Werner et al., 1991).

In vitro induction of connexin co-expression
Mammalian cell lines. Various cell lines have been used to exogenously express connexins, including Skhep1, HeLa, Ros, and N2a cells (Brink et al., 1997; Hopperstad et al., 2001; Moreno et al., 1991; Valiunas et al., 2000). Specific plasmids containing the genes for each connexin have been transfected into these cells, and the gating behavior of the junctional channels formed after co-expression has been studied. A significant advancement in these cell systems is that cells expressing specific connexins can be tagged with membrane or intracellular dyes that make them appear different from untagged cells, or those tagged with a different dye.

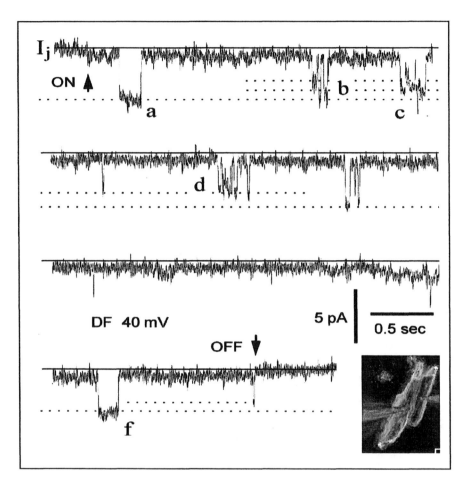

Figure 1. Single channel recordings from murine ventricular isolated cell pairs. Right ventricular cells were isolated by enzymatic micro perfusion through the aorta. The current traces shown correspond to the junctional currents after the cells were under a double whole cell voltage clamp configuration. The presence of multiple current levels (dotted lines) measured from the baseline (solid line) indicates the activity of gap junction channels constituted not only by Cx43. The co-expression of connexin45 is suggested, because the largest size indicated by **a,** corresponds to 120 pS, or the maximal reported for Cx43. The other currents (**b-f)** yield conductance values between 120 pS (homotypic Cx43 channels) and 60 pS (heterotypic Cx43-Cx45 channels).

Xenopus Oocytes. Expression of connexins in Oocytes has also provided substantial knowledge about the behavior of gap junction channels when expression of mRNA for specific connexins is induced. In these cases, the mRNA for each connexin isotype is injected. A great advantage of this method is that the ratios of expression of two distinct isotypes might be partially regulated by the amount of RNA injected, but unfortunately, the expression level of exogenous mRNA might be different for every connexin; with appropriate controls this might be possible to interpret. Another disadvantage compared to mammalian expression systems is that, because of the size of the oocytes, single channel recording from intercellular plaques is not possible, but recordings from hemichannels in cells attached or from excised patch configurations have been successful and substantially informative (Trexler and Verselis2001).

RESULTS

Hetero-multimeric channels in cardiovascular tissue.
Immunocytochemical analysis. This specific-antibody based method has helped to determine that various regions of the cardiovascular system co-express cardiac connexins. In fact, this co-expression has been determined to occur in the same cell (Kwong et al., 1998) and even in the same junction (Yeh et al., 1998). In terms of multiple-expression in selected regions, it is clear that there is spatial/temporal expression of multiple connexins. During development, the expression of cardiac connexins switches according to the tissue, but, in adulthood, segregation becomes major (Delorme et al., 1997). In the conduction regions of the adult mammalian heart, it is also possible to find certain heterogeneity and regionally unbalanced co-expression of connexins. Coppen et al., (1999a) have reported that a clear demarcation of connexins exists between the SA node and the *crista terminalis*. The SA node central regions express mostly Cx40 and Cx43, whereas the escape region co-expresses Cx43 and Cx45. This region is in immediate contact with the *crista*

terminalis, in which Cx43 is mainly expressed. As we will show later, this combination of connexins *in vitro* forms channels of very small conductance, suggesting that the combination of connexins is part of the restriction in communication that prevents atrial musculature hyperpolarization from invading the SA node region, but permits enough communication to allow the pacemaker activity to cross. As we mentioned before, using only immunocytochemistry does not provide exact values for connectivity and the properties of the channels in the tissue. Hence, the formation of heteromultimeric channels can generate new rules for the regulation of metabolic communication and/or gating.

Electrophysiological analysis in vivo. This method requires the performance of more complicated tasks and a more intricate analysis of the data obtained, nonetheless, a growing number of papers have published reliable evidence of functional heteromultimeric channels *in vivo*. In the cases of (Elenes et al., 1999) working with dog ventricular cardiocytes or (Yeh et al., 1998) working with endothelial cells from vascular tissue, the recording of multiple unitary conductances indicates that co-expression of Cx43 and Cx45 induces the formation of multi-heteromeric channels. These manuscripts constitute clear evidence that other channels can be co-expressed besides the dominant Cx43, and what is more important, that this co-expression can definitively affect the properties of the functional channels present. An example of these results is presented in Figure 1.

The *in vivo* data are strongly supported by the formation of heteromultimeric channels *in vitro*. (Brink et al., 1997; He et al., 1999; Hopperstad et al., 2001). When HeLa or N2a cells are induced to express particular pairs of connexins, the electrophysiological data suggest that the new channels formed are heteromultimeric because they produce multiple conductances that cannot be explained by the formation of homomeric connexons alone.

Changes in expression during pathological conditions., Changes in
the expression of Cx43 in various cardiovascular tissues have been
determined during pathological conditions. Although these
changes alone do not completely explain the electrophysiology of
cardiac arrhythmias, not all cardiac connexins have been
extensively explored. Important rigorous work has been done by
(Coppen et al., 1999a) but mostly at the SA node region. We stress
this point, because changes in coupling may not be produced only
through changes in Cx43, but through an increase in Cx45, as we
showed previously during *in vitro* experiments.

Formation of heteromultimeric channels may lead to unpredicted
channel behavior. For every distinct connexin that forms a
functional channel, there has been substantial information
regarding their gating and permeability behavior (White et al.,
1995). So far, it is clear that the characteristics of each connexin
are different, and maintained in different expression systems,
although some differences can be found between mammalian cells
and oocytes (Anumonwo et al., 2001; Moreno et al., 1994a; Revilla
et al., 1999). Most of our fundamental knowledge has been
accumulated for channels formed of only one connexin. Taking
this into consideration, it is natural to conclude that the
combination of subunits, leads to a combination of characteristics.
This conclusion is not necessarily true and the addition of different
subunits may not produce a linear relationship with their gating or
permeability characteristics.

One example is provided by the fact that gating due to
transjunctional voltage might be due to only one connexin in a
connexon, as suggested by (Oh et al., 2000). Other properties such
as the addition or synergism of properties in homo- and
heteromultimeric channels remain to be analyzed. In some
instances, as we will present hereafter, it appears that one plus one
does not always equal two.

Phosphorylation. The regulation of junctional communication has been studied in homotypic cardiac junctions, both in tumor cells

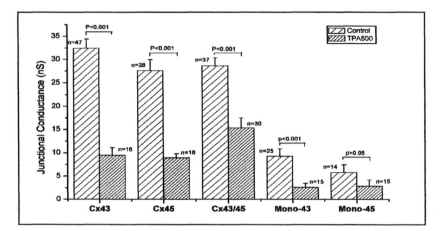

Figure 2. Changes in junctional conductance in channels formed by different combinations of connexins. Mono-43=Cx43-Cx45/Cx43. Mono-45=Cx45-Cx45/Cx43. Cx45 was cloned from chicken and Cx43 from mouse. All connexins were expressed in HeLa cells. Connexin43 homotypic channels are those that communicate best in the cells, whereas Mono-45 channels reduce communication. Note also that Cx45 responds to TPA by uncoupling, contrary to what has been reported for mCx45 by van Rijen et al., 2001b.

expressing connexins, and directly from isolated cardiocytes. It has been consistently shown that the unitary conductance of connexin43 channels decreases after activation of PKC (Moreno et al., 1994b) (Kwak et al., 1995), where serine 368 plays a fundamental role (Lampe et al., 2000). For Cx45, gating by PKC appears to depend on the species. Junctional conductance increases when the mouse isotype is expressed in HeLa cells (van Veen et al., 2000), but not for Chicken Cx45, where gj decreases (see Figure 2). In these experiments, the results indicate that for both Cx43 and chCx45 TPA reduces the conductance of the junction. For heteromeric combinations, according to some of our data, the connexins become less sensitive to gating when phosphorylated (Figure 2).

Unitary conductance and permeability. We have recently detected an unpredicted reduction in unitary conductance from mono-heteromeric channels formed by Cx43-Cx43/Cx45 (unpublished observations). Here, one cell in a pair expresses only Cx43 and the other expresses Cx43 and Cx45 (Mono-43). Our results suggest that the unitary conductance of these Mono-43 channels does not match a predicted sum of conductances, assuming that each subunit contributes identically to the total conductance of the channels. As expected, in the worst scenario, when one cell expresses only Cx43 and the other only Cx45 (very low Cx43), the minimal conductance recorded should be close to 60 pS (Elenes *et al.,* 2001). Surprisingly, our recordings show that, besides the observation that the channels have multiple conductances, some of these channels present conductances as low as 25 pS. This finding is substantiated by the fact that the total conductance of these junctions is much smaller than that of heterotypic junctions, and also by the significant reduction in the permeability of the channel to LY, (Figures 2-3) which indicates the appearance of new smaller conductances.

When the permeability of Lucifer yellow is tested during co-expression of Cx43 and Cx45 in osteoblasts, data indicate that there is also a reduction in permeability (Koval et al., 1995), suggesting again that the newly formed channels are either more

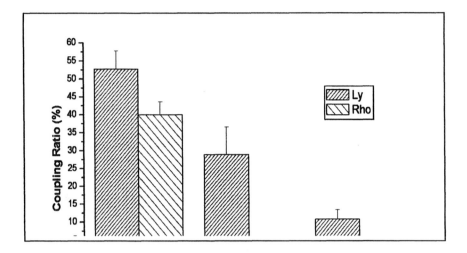

Figure 3. Coupling ratio calculated for homotypic Cx43, Homotypic Cx45 and Mono-45. Microinjecting Lucifer yellow or Rhodamine in groups of HeLa cells we can estimate the coupling ratio of those expressing the same or different combinations of connexins. Cx43 expressing cells are the best coupled, independently of the dye used, whereas those expressing Cx45, whether in the homotypic or the mono-heteromeric configuration are poorly coupled, especially for the positively-charged dye, Rhodamine.

selective or smaller in size. Possibly, the heteromeric connexons formed have a smaller pore, and their selectivity is mainly influenced by the presence of Cx45. Whether other channels with less conductive properties are present, remains to be confirmed. Co-expression of Cx43 and Cx45 in cardiac tissues appears to be non-randomly distributed, but rather, their co-expression may be compartmentalized, and this could generate a distinct scenario in which functional mono-heteromeric channels exist. Again, the localized expression of connexins in the SA node becomes a handy example to suggest that this compartmentalization could be related to the function of the tissue. Our current *in vitro* data suggest that these channels are even more selective than bi-heteromeric channels, indicating that regulation of connexin expression can be used to generate a border zone without the necessity of down-regulating the expression of connexins.

Voltage dependence. Connexons with a heteromeric configuration induce the formation of channels with unpredicted voltage dependence gating. We have recently demonstrated that the interaction between Cx43 and Cx45 as heterotypic channels induces strong impairment of fast gating

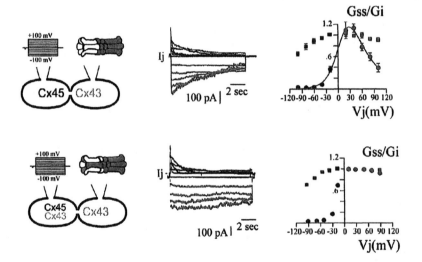

Figure 4. Voltage dependence in heterotypic formation of different combinations of Cx43 and Cx45. The top diagram indicates a pure heterotypic Cx43-Cx45 channel. The current traces indicate that the Cx43 side gates very slowly, although values at steady state are similar to the expected voltage dependence of Cx43. On the bottom, a heteromeric Cx43/Cx45connexon is opposing a homomeric Cx43 connexon. In this case, the gating of Cx43 is completely abolished indicating the importance of heteromeric connexons in the behavior of gap junction plaques.

of Cx43 connexons (See Figure 4). An explanation suggested for this phenomenon is that the carboxyl tail becomes impaired for fast gating after Cx45 docks with Cx43 connexons. As we have previously demonstrated, a similar reduction in fast gating occurs when the tail of Cx43 is removed (Moreno et al., 2002). To our surprise, we have found that the formation of mono-heteromeric channels (Cx43 on one side and Cx43/Cx45 co-expressed in the other) does not recover the voltage dependence of Cx43 (now that more Cx43 subunits are present on the other side) but nullifies completely the voltage dependence gating of connexon43 (Figure 4). These results clearly indicate that interaction between connexins and connexons is complex, and that special consideration must be taken to understand this process.

Intracellular pH gating. This is another type of gating strongly influenced by the interaction of connexins. From recent studies performed in oocytes and reported by (Gu et al., 2000), it has become clear that the presence of two distinct connexins, with different pHi gating sensitivities (pHa of ~6.7) become less sensitive to intracellular acidification when one of the cells expresses both Cx40 and Cx43 (pHa of 7.0). These results intrinsically suggest that co-expression of connexins can be used as a regulatory-defense mechanism to prevent uncoupling during ischemia.

DISCUSSION

In the last three years, it has become evident that many mammalian cells simultaneously express more than one type of connexin, not only in the heart, but also in most tissues of our body. It has also become obvious that this co-expression may induce the appearance of channels with novel characteristics.

We have provided evidence that heteromeric and heterotypic channels can be induced *in vitro*; therefore, it is necessary to consider their impact in the physiology and pathology of mammalian tissues.

For cardiovascular tissue, the presence of multiple connexins in various regions of the heart and smooth muscle has been consistently substantiated by immuno-staining, and there is currently no doubt that co-expression is very important. Of course, electrophysiological data need to be used to support and understand the function of these heteromeric connexons in tissues.

During cardiac development, changes in expression of connexins has been followed and it is clear that the expression of the cardiac connexins, which indeed have different permeability properties occurs, and this could definitively influence the way the tissue differentiate. If, during the co-expression of connexins, there occur heteromeric/heterotypic channels, then the properties of permeation become severely altered, as we have shown in recent publications and from our current data stated above.

Pathological conditions have provided substantial information, mostly immuno-histochemical, specifically about Cx43. It is acquiesced that it is important to know how expression of the "queen of hearts" becomes altered, but it is equally important to characterize and understand the presence of other connexins, like Cx45. As we have shown, the influence of this connexin is substantial to connectivity among cells. The relevance of Cx45 is also substantiated by the fact that hearts from young Cx43 knock out transgenic mice are able to maintain tissue communication (Vaidya et al., 2001). It has been suggested by Wilders et al., (Wilders et al., 1996) that there exists a large safety factor for conductance in cardiocytes in the musculature of the heart, because the cells are amazingly well connected and substantial reduction in expression might not affect conduction. Therefore, changes in the expression of Cx43 might not be involved in cardiac arrhythmias of the musculature. Even when the expression of Cx40, which is suspected to be unable to form functional channels with Cx43, is increased during sustained atrial fibrillation, it is clearly understandable that the effect could be unimportant, but, for the generation of action potentials in ectopic sites, the presence of low conductance junctions is necessary. Therefore, we would like to stress that although the reduction of only connexin43 expression may not cause arrhythmias, it is imperative to understand that an increase in expression of other connexins, like Cx45, and the asymmetric co-expression of connexins can produce a reduction in metabolic or electrical conduction, as has been shown *in vitro*. These heterotypic, or even heteromeric channels are hard to be demonstrated *in vivo*, but it is important to remember that *in vitro*, it has been possible to generate asymmetric multi-heteromeric junctions which lead to the formation of very low conductive junctions, creating a substantial barrier for electrotonic and metabolic coupling.

Moreover, when the heart sustains great damage, the repair of tissue has been shown to modulate the expression of connexins. In these cases, the remodeled tissue is combined with scar tissue, wherein Cx45 is suspected to be abundant. It is important to notice that generation of new activity can only be produced when membrane channels like K+ are highly expressed, and when the input resistance of the cells is high enough to permit a small group of cells to become depolarized, and to trigger an action potential that will propagate across the tissue. This is a clear indication that, close to the scar tissue, low communication levels provided by physical barriers or by the combinations of newly synthesized connexins does not allow strong communication between cardiocytes.

Are these scar-myocyte connections enough to generate small pathways of communication? According to (Rook et al., 1989), the amount of communication is minimal in isolated cells, although their expression and function *in vivo* remain to be quantified. Other questions are still unanswered: Are the surviving cardiocytes sources of new activity and/or low-coupled areas where re-entry is permitted? What is the influence of Cx45 in the generation of ectopic potentials? These questions are expected to be answered in upcoming years, and hopefully the gating properties of gap junction channels between cardiocytes co-expressing multiple connexins will also become understood. In the meantime, we can only speculate on their possible function.

Funding for this research has been provided by the NIH grant HL63969 and cardiology Endowment Funds from the Methodist Research Institute to Alonso P. Moreno. We would also like to thank Patricia Mantel for her accurate technical skills, as well as for the corrections of this manuscript. Thanks also to Dr. Eric C. Beyer and Agustin Martinez from the University of Chicago, USA who provided transfected cells and encouraged numerous discussions.

REFERENCE

Anumonwo J.M., Taffet S., Gu H., Chanson M., Moreno A.P., Delmar M. (2001). The carboxyl terminal domain regulates the unitary conductance and voltage dependence of connexin40 gap junction channels. Circ Res 88, 666-673.

Barrio L.C., Suchyna T., Bargiello T., Xu X., Roginski R., Bennett M.V.L., Nicholson B.J. (1991). Voltage dependence of homo- and hetero-typic Cx26 and Cx32 gap junctions expressed in Xenopus oocytes. Proc Natl Acad Sci USA 88, 8410-8414.

Beyer E.C., Paul D.L., Goodenough D.A. (1990). Connexin family of gap junction proteins. J Membr Biol 116, 187-194.

Brink P.R., Cronin K., Banach K., Peterson E., Westphale E.M., Seul K.H., Ramanan S.V., Beyer E.C. (1997). Evidence for heteromeric gap junction channels formed from rat connexin43 and human connexin37. Am J Physiol 273, C1386-96.

Coppen S.R., Kodama I., Boyett M.R., Dobrzynski H., Takagishi Y., Honjo H., Yeh, HI, Severs N.J. (1999a). Connexin45, a major connexin of the rabbit sinoatrial node, is co-expressed with connexin43 in a restricted zone at the nodal-crista terminalis border. J Histochem Cytochem 47, 907-918.

Coppen S.R., Severs N.J., Gourdie R.G. (1999b). Connexin45 (alpha6) Expression Delineates an Extended Conduction System in the Embryonic and Mature Rodent Heart. Devel Genetics 24, 82-90.

Delorme B., Dahl E., Jarry-Guichard T., Briand J.P., Willecke K., Theveniau-Ruissy M., Gros D. (1997). Expression pattern of connexin gene products at the early developmental stages of the mouse cardiovascular system. Circ Res 81, 423-437.

Eghbali B., Kessler J.A., Spray D.C. (1990). Expression of gap junction channels in communication-incompetent cells after stable transfection with cDNA encoding connexin 32. Proc Natl Acad Sci USA 87, 1328-1331.

Elenes S, Martinez AD, Beyer EC, Moreno AP. Heterotypic docking of Cx43 and Cx45 connexons blocks fast voltage gating of Cx43. Biophys J 81, 1406-1418. 2001.

Elenes S., Rubart M., Moreno A.P. (1999). Junctional communication between isolated pairs of canine atrial cells is mediated by homogeneous and heterogeneous gap junction channels. J Cardiovasc Electrophys 10, 990-1004.

Gu H., Ek-Vitorin J.F., Taffet S.M., Delmar M. (2000). Coexpression of connexins 40 and 43 enhances the pH sensitivity of gap junctions: a model for synergistic interactions among connexins. Circ Res (Online) 86, E98-E103.

Gutstein D.E., Morley G.E., Tamaddon H., Vaidya D., Schneider M.D., Chen J., Chien K.R., Stuhlmann H., Fishman G.I. (2001). Conduction slowing and sudden arrhythmic death in mice with cardiac-restricted inactivation of connexin43. Circ Res 88, 333-339.

He D.S., Jiang J.X., Taffet S.M., Burt J.M. (1999). Formation of heteromeric gap junction channels by connexins 40 and 43 in vascular smooth muscle cells. Proc Natl Acad Sci USA 96, 6495-6500.

Hopperstad M., Srinivas M., Spray D. (2001). Properties of Gap Junction Channels Formed by Cx46 Alone and in Combination with Cx50. Biophys J 79, 1954-1966.

Jongsma H.J., Wilders R. (2000). Gap junctions in cardiovascular disease. Circ Res 86, 1193-1197.

Kanter H.L., Beyer E.C., Saffitz J.E. (1995). Structural and molecular determinants of intercellular coupling in cardiac myocytes. Microscopy Research & Technique 31, 357-363.

Kirchhoff S., Nelles E., Hagendorff A., Kruger O., Traub O., Willecke K. (1998). Reduced cardiac conduction velocity and predisposition to arrhythmias in connexin40-deficient mice. Current Biology 8, 299-302.

Koval M., Geist S.T., Westphale E.M., Kemendy A.E., Civitelli R., Beyer E.C., Steinberg T.H. (1995). Transfected connexin45 alters gap junction permeability in cells expressing endogenous connexin43. J Cell Biol 130, 987-995.

Kwak B.R., Saez J.C., Wilders R., Chanson M., Fishman G.I., Hertzberg E.L., Spray D.C., Jongsma H.J. (1995). Effects of cGMP-dependent phosphorylation on rat and human connexin43 gap junction channels. Pflugers Arch 430, 770-778.

Kwong K.F., Schuessler R.B., Green K.G., Laing J.G., Beyer E.C., Boineau J.P., Saffitz J.E. (1998). Differential expression of gap junction proteins in the canine sinus node. Circ Res 82, 604-612.

Lampe P.D., TenBroek E.M., Burt J.M., Kurata W.E., Johnson R.G. (2000). Phosphorylation of Connexin43 on Serine368 by Protein Kinase C Regulates Gap Junctional Communication. J Cell Biol 149, 1503-1512.

Loewenstein W.R. (1981). Junctional intercellular communication: the cell-to-cell membrane channel. Physiol Rev 61, 829-913.

Moore L.K., Beyer E.C., Burt J.M. (1991). Characterization of gap junction channels in A7r5 vascular smooth muscle cells. Am J Physiol 260, C975-C981.

Moreno A.P., Eghbali B., Spray D.C. (1991). Connexin32 gap junction channels in stably transfected cells. Equilibrium and kinetic properties. Biophys J 60, 1267-1277.

Moreno A.P., Laing J.G., Beyer E.C., Spray D.C. (1995). Properties of gap junction channels formed of connexin 45 endogenously expressed in human hepatoma (SKHep1) cells. Am J Physiol 268, C356-65.

Moreno A.P., Rook M.B., Fishman G.I., Spray D.C. (1994a). Gap junction channels: distinct voltage-sensitive and - insensitive conductance states. Biophys J 67, 113-119.

Moreno A.P., Saez J.C., Fishman G.I., Spray D.C. (1994b). Human connexin43 gap junction channels. Regulation of unitary conductances by phosphorylation. Circ Res 74, 1050-1057.

Moreno A.P., Chanson M., Anumonwo J., Scerri I., Gu H., Taffet S.M., Delmar M. (2002). Role of the Carboxyl Terminal of Connexin43 in Transjunctional Fast Voltage Gating. Circ Res 90, 450-457.

Oh S., Abrams C.K., Verselis V.K., Bargiello T.A. (2000). Stoichiometry of transjunctional voltage-gating polarity reversal by a negative charge substitution in the amino terminus of a Cx32 chimera. J Gen Physiol 116, 13-31.

Peters N.S. (1996). New insights into myocardial arrhythmogenesis: distribution of gap-junctional coupling in normal, ischaemic and hypertrophied human hearts. Clinical Science 90, 447-452.

Ramon F., Rivera A. (1986). Gap junction channel modulation--a physiological viewpoint. Prog Biophys Mol Biol 48, 127-153.

Revilla A., Castro C., Barrio L.C. (1999). Molecular dissection of transjunctional voltage dependence in the connexin-32 and connexin-43 junctions. Biophys J 77, 1374-1383.

Rook M.B., Jongsma H.J., de Jonge B. (1989). Single channel currents of homo- and heterologous gap junctions between cardiac fibroblasts and myocytes. Pflugers Arch 414, 95-98.

Thomas S.A., Schuessler R.B., Berul C.I., Beardslee M.A., Beyer E.C., Mendelsohn M.E., Saffitz J.E. (1998). Disparate effects of deficient expression of connexin43 on atrial and ventricular conduction: evidence for chamber-specific molecular determinants of conduction. Circulation 97, 686-691.

Trabka-Janik E., Coombs W., Lemanski L.F., Delmar M., Jalife, J. (1994). Immunohistochemical localization of gap junction protein channels in hamster sinoatrial node in correlation with electrophysiologic mapping of the pacemaker region. J Cardiovasc Electrophysiol 5, 125-137.

Trexler E.B., Verselis V.K. (2001). The study of connexin hemichannels (connexons) in Xenopus oocytes. Methods in Molecular Biology 154, 341-355.

Vaidya D., Tamaddon H.S., Lo C.W., Taffet S.M., Delmar M., Morley G.E., Jalife J. (2001). Null mutation of connexin43 causes slow propagation of ventricular activation in the late stages of mouse embryonic development. Circ Res 88, 1196-1202.

Valiunas V., Weingart R., Brink P.R. (2000). Formation of heterotypic gap junction channels by connexins 40 and 43. Circ Res (Online) 86, E42-E49.

van der Velden H.M.W., van der Z.L., Wijffels M.C., van Leuven C., Dorland R., Vos M.A., Jongsma H.J., Allessie M.A. (2000). Atrial fibrillation in the goat induces changes in monophasic action potential and mRNA expression of ion channels involved in repolarization. J Cardiovasc Electrophysiol 11, 1262-1269.

van Rijen H.V., van Veen T.A., van Kempen M.J., Wilms-Schopman F.J., Potse M., Krueger O., Willecke K., Opthof T., Jongsma H.J., de Bakker J.M. (2001a). Impaired conduction in the bundle branches of mouse hearts lacking the gap junction protein connexin40. Circulation 103, 1591-1598.

van Rijen H.V., Wilders R., Rook M.B., Jongsma H.J. (2001b). Dual patch clamp. Methods in Molecular Biology 154, 269-292.

van Veen T.A., van Rijen H.V., Jongsma H.J. (2000). Electrical conductance of mouse connexin45 gap junction channels is modulated by phosphorylation. Cardiovasc Res 46, 496-510.

Veenstra R.D., Wang H.Z., Beblo D.A., Chilton M.G., Harris A.L., Beyer E.C., Brink P.R. (1995). Selectivity of connexin-specific gap junctions does not correlate with channel conductance. Circ Res 77, 1156-1165.

Verheule S., van Kempen M.J., Postma S., Rook M.B., Jongsma H.J. (2001). Gap junctions in the rabbit sinoatrial node. Am J Physiol 280, H2103-H2115.

Werner R., Levine E., Rabadan Diehl C., Dahl G. (1991). Gating properties of connexin32 cell-cell channels and their mutants expressed in Xenopus oocytes. Proc R Soc Lond 243, 5-11.

White T.W., Bruzzone R., Paul D.L. (1995). The connexin family of intercellular channel forming proteins. Kidney International 48, 1148-1157.

Wilders R., Kumar R., Joyner R.W., Jongsma H.J., Verheijck E.E., Golod D., van Ginneken A.C., Goolsby W.N. (1996). Action potential conduction between a ventricular cell model and an isolated ventricular cell. Biophys J 70, 281-295.

Yeh H.I., Rothery S., Dupont E., Coppen S.R., Severs N.J. (1998). Individual Gap Junction Plaques Contain Multiple Connexins in Arterial Endothelium. Circ Res 83, 1248-1263.

5

INTERCELLULAR CA^{2+} SIGNALING IN THE CARDIOVASCULAR SYSTEM

Sylvia O. Suadicani and David C. Spray

Department of Neuroscience, Albert Einstein College of Medicine, Bronx, New York 10461

The ability to exchange, integrate and coordinate signals within and between tissues is one of the hallmark features of multicellular organisms. Cells can exchange signals using paracrine, synaptic and endocrine pathways but can also communicate in a more direct way through gap junction channels that provide an intercellular route for cytosol-to-cytosol exchange of small ions and molecules such as metabolites, morphogens and intracellular second messengers. This exchange of diffusible second messengers such as Ca^{2+}- or other messengers with the ability to mobilize Ca^{2+} stores- can trigger the intercellular transmission of Ca^{2+} signals, a wildly used form of cellular communication.

Ca^{2+} ions: ubiquitous cellular messengers

The ubiquity of the Ca^{2+} ion, along with its versatility, contribute to its status as the most widespread cellular messenger. Cells tightly control their intracellular Ca^{2+} levels at around 100 nM whereas local or global transient increases in Ca^{2+} levels can convey information that is essential for cell function. Cell death can be triggered when the amplitude and duration of the Ca^{2+} signal is sustained (Berridge et al., 1998; Clapham, 1995). Cells make broad and diversified use of what has been called the Ca^{2+} "toolkit" (Berridge et al., 2000), composed of a set of channels, pumps, exchangers, intracellular Ca^{2+} buffers and a network of transduction pathways. This Ca^{2+} toolkit equips the cells with the necessary means to promote controlled spatial and temporal changes in intracellular Ca^{2+} levels that will ultimately trigger specific cellular events, depending on the cell type and transduction pathways activated by the Ca^{2+} signal. Sources of intracellular Ca^{2+} include both entry from extracellular space and that mobilized from intracellular Ca^{2+} pools. Influx of Ca^{2+} from the extracellular milieu can occur through voltage-operated Ca^{2+} channels (VOCs) such as the L-type Ca^{2+} channels, receptor-operated Ca^{2+} channels (ROCs), such as the nicotinic, N-methyl-D-aspartate (NMDA) and purinergic P2X-type receptors, stock-operated Ca^{2+} channels (SOCs), transporters such as the Na^{+}/Ca^{2+} exchanger when operating in its reversed mode, and also mechanically activated Ca^{2+} channels (Bootman et al., 2001; Putney and McKay, 1999; Putney et al., 2001; Clapham, 1995). The endoplasmic/ sarcoplasmic reticulum forms the main reservoir for releasable intracellular Ca^{2+}. Mobilization of Ca^{2+} from intracellular stores occurs in a Ca^{2+}-induced Ca^{2+} release (CICR) manner through the activation of ryanodine receptors (RyR) and/or inositol 1,4,5-triphosphate (InsP$_3$) receptors (IP$_3$R) (Berridge, 1993, 1997; Clapham, 1995; Berridge et al., 2000; Bootman et al., 2001). Mechanical distension as well as activation of cell surface metabotropic receptors (including metabotropic glutamate and P2Y type purinergic receptors) can activate phospholipase C (PLC) and lead to the production of InsP$_3$ from the hydrolysis of phosphatidyl inositol, 4,5 biphosphate (PIP2), which readily diffuses within the cell to activate IP$_3$R and modulate the receptor's sensitivity to Ca^{2+}. In the case of the RyRs, those expressed in striated skeletal muscles (RyR "type 1") are activated by conformational changes resultant from their interaction with cell surface voltage-sensors. In cardiac muscle "type 2" RyR are directly activated by Ca^{2+} entering the cell from the extracellular space through VOCs (Berridge, 1997). Besides InsP$_3$ and Ca^{2+} itself, the role of messenger for intracellular Ca^{2+}-release has also been attributed to cyclic ADP-ribose (cADPR), nicotinic acid adenine dinucleotide phosphate (NAADP) and sphingolipids such as sphingosine-1-

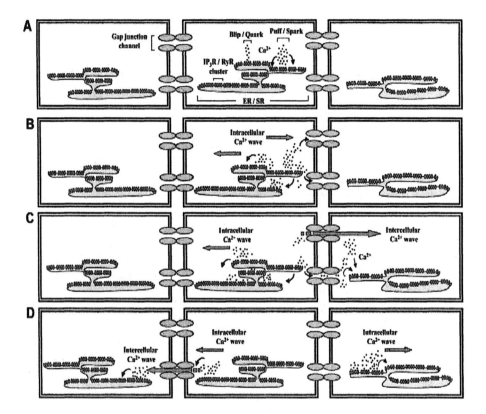

Figure 1 - Elementary and Global Ca2+ events. Blips and quarks, resultant from the individual activation of InP$_3$ receptors (IP$_3$R) and ryanodine receptors (RyR), respectively, contain sufficient Ca2+ to activate adjacent receptors and to amplify the Ca2+ signal in the form of puffs and sparks, resultant from the activation of clusters of IP$_3$R and RyR, respectively (A). The spread of the Ca2+ signal induced by the sequential generation of puffs or sparks results in localized Ca2+ increases that propagate through the cell as intracellular Ca2+ waves (B to D). When cells are coupled by gap junctions, the Ca2+ signal generated in one cell can be communicated to the adjacent coupled cells through the direct cytosol to cytosol diffusion of Ca2+ ions and subsequent activation of the intracellular Ca2+ stores in the adjacent cells, resulting in propagated intercellular Ca2+ waves (C-D).

phosphate (S-1-P) and sphingosylphosphorylcholine (SPC) Berridge et al., 2000; Bootman et al., 2001; Guse, 2000; Genazzani and Gaglione, 1997). Cyclic-ADP ribose (cADPR) has been regarded as an endogenous activator and modulator of RyRs. The identity of the Ca^{2+} stores targeted by NAADP, which is potentially synthesized by the same ribosyl cyclases that produce cADPR, is still not clearly established, but NAADP-mediated Ca^{2+} mobilization apparently involves stores that are resistant to thapsigargin, an inhibitor of the sarco-endoplasmic Ca^{2+}-ATPase pumps (SERCA) (Albrieux et al., 1998). In the case of sphingolipids, the mechanism involved in their Ca^{2+}-mobilizing action is not fully elucidated, but their most probable target seems to be the SCaMPER (sphingolipid Ca^{2+}-release mediating protein of endoplasmic reticulum). The maintenance of Ca^{2+} concentration within manageable levels and its return to basal resting levels is accomplished by the combined action of the intracellular Ca^{2+} buffers, SERCA and plasma membrane Ca^{2+}-ATPase pumps, Na$^+$/Ca^{2+} exchangers and also mitochondrial Ca^{2+} uniporters, which buffer the free Ca^{2+} in the cytoplasm, sequester Ca^{2+} back to the intracellular stores and promote its extrusion to the extracellular space (Berridge et al., 2000; Bootman et al., 2001).

The great diversity of cellular events that can be triggered and modulated by changes in intracellular Ca^{2+} results in great part from the cell's ability to control the rise in Ca^{2+} levels in both time and space, shaping the amplitude and frequency of the signal, and either limiting the signal to a particular region of the cell or allowing it to propagate within and between cells (Berridge, 1997; Berridge et al., 2000; Bootman et al., 2001; Eghbali et al., 1991). Ca^{2+} signals generated by single Ca^{2+} release events, such as the "quarks and blips" that result from activation of an individual RyR or an InsP$_3$R, respectively, are extremely restricted in space and time, but sufficient to trigger the activation of neighboring Ca^{2+}-release channels, thus generating the Ca^{2+} "sparks and puffs" that are amplified but still local Ca^{2+} signals resultant from the activation of clusters of RyR and InsP$_3$R, respectively (Figure 1A).

These elementary Ca^{2+} events, seen as the building blocks of the cellular Ca^{2+} signaling system, can be either individually manipulated or activated as a group, generating a multitude of types of Ca^{2+} signals that can be shaped in space and time. Global Ca^{2+} events that embrace the whole cell can be generated by the coordinated activation of the Ca^{2+}-release channels. One such event is exemplified by the intracellular Ca^{2+} waves that can be observed spreading within a cell and usually propagating throughout its entire length (Figure 1B to D). The initial Ca^{2+} signal that initiates the intracellular wave is usually generated by the activation of clusters of RyR or   InsP$_3$R. The Ca^{2+} released from these channels diffuses and activates the neighboring Ca^{2+}-release receptors, triggering a sequential and regenerative local increase in Ca^{2+} that spreads as a wave within the cell. In some cases, when cells of a same or different cell types are coupled to each other through intercellular channels (gap junction channels), the global increase in Ca^{2+} experienced by one cell can be transmitted to the adjacent cells as an intercellular Ca^{2+} wave (Figure 1C-D) (Rottingen and Iversen, 2000; Sanderson, 1996; Scemes et al., 2000a).

Since it was first reported more than a decade ago (Saez et al., 1989), the phenomenon of intercellular Ca^{2+} signaling has been described in a variety of cell types, and in the majority of the cases the functional presence of gap junction channels has been found to be a primary mechanism for the propagation of the intercellular Ca^{2+} signal (Sanderson et al., 1994; Sanderson, 1996; Scemes et al., 2000a).

Gap junctions: electrical and metabolic couplers of cells and tissues

Gap junctions are clusters of intercellular channels occurring at cell-cell contacts (Figure 2A) (Bennett et al., 1991; Spray et al., 2001a,b; Bruzzone et al., 1996; Kumar and Gilula, 1996). Each intercellular channel is formed by the symmetric pairing and docking of its two halves, the hemichannel or connexon, contributed by each of the juxtaposed cells (Figure 2B). The connexon is composed of six protein subunits, the connexins (Cx), which surround the aqueous pore of the channel. Connexin molecules all possess intracellular amino- and carboxyl-termini, four transmembrane spanning regions, and one cytoplasmic and two extracellular loops (Figure 2C). Despite this uniform membrane topology, connexins can be distinguished from each other by their molecular masses, which are generally used to name the connexins (e.g., Cx43 for the 43kDa connexin). More than twenty different connexin isoforms have been identified in vertebrates and of these, four are expressed at high levels in the mammalian cardiovascular system: Cx37, Cx40, Cx43 and Cx45.

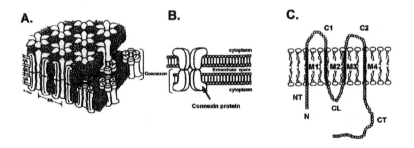

Figure 2 - Gap junctions (**A**) are assemblies of intercellular channels formed by the justaposition of two hemichannels or connexons. The connexons are contributed by each of the apposing cells (**B**) and are composed by six connexin proteins (**C**). The connexin protein contains four transmembrane domains (M1, M2, M3 and M4), two extracellular loops (C1 and C2), one intracellular loop (CL, short in group I or a subfamily and long in group II or b connexin subfamily) and cytoplasmic amino- and carboxyl-terminal domains (NT and CT, respectively).

Cx43 is the most abundantly expressed gap junction protein in the mature heart (see Figure 3) (Spray et al., 2001a). Compared to

Cx43, the spatial distribution and expression level of the other two cardiac connexins, Cx40 and Cx45, change during cardiac development. Cx45 predominates at early stages of heart morphogenesis and is progressively reduced towards maturation, when its expression is mainly confined to the conduction system (Coppen et al., 1999; Coppen et al., 1998). Cx40 is also abundantly expressed during cardiac morphogenesis, but in the mature heart its expression is confined to the atrium, nodal tissue and particularly to the core of the conduction system, where it is enveloped by the predominant expression of Cx45 (Figure 3). In the cardiovascular system the expression of Cx37 is restricted to the endothelial cell lining of the vascular walls, which also expresses Cx40 and Cx43 (Yeh et al., 1998). Compared to Cx37 and Cx40, Cx43 displays a more heterogeneous expression pattern in the endothelial cell lining, showing higher levels of expression in the large arteries (Hong and Hill 1998; van Kempen and Jongsma, 1999; Ko et al., 2001; Little et al., 1995a; van Rijen et al., 1997; Yeh et al., 1997; Ko et al., 1999) and at regions of the vascular tree that are subjected to disturbed blood flow (Gabriels and Paul, 1998). Besides Cx43 and Cx45, Cx40 also forms gap junction plaques in vascular smooth muscle (van Kempen and Jongsma, 1999; Little et al., 1995a; Yeh et al., 1997; Ko et al., 2001).

The intercellular channels formed by each of the connexin isoforms are unique, displaying distinct biophysical properties. However, the functional diversity of the gap junctions is not limited by the properties of individual connexin isoforms. Because most cells express multiple cell specific sets of connexins and because gap junction channels can be formed by oligomers of different connexins, the number of various possible channel

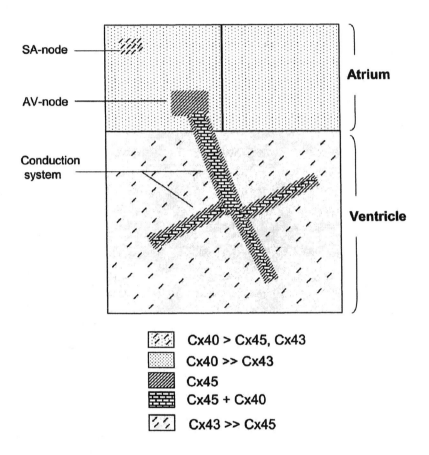

Figure 3 - Schematic drawing representing the cardiac communication compartments and the distribution of the different connexin types that are expressed in the heart (see text).

configurations is greatly expanded and may generate intra- and inter-tissue compartmental boundaries with unusual properties. In the mammalian heart, for instance, differences in the spatial expression of the cardiac connexins, the unique channel properties conferred by each of the connexins, and the fact that Cx43 can form heterotypic channels with Cx45 but not as readily with Cx40, contribute to the functional division of the myocardial tissue in two main compartments, the nodal/His-Purkinje conduction system and the atrial/ventricular contractile myocardium.

In the adult mammalian heart, the high ionic permeability of gap junction channels together with their strategic distribution on the longitudinal ends of the cardiac myocytes in the intercalated discs provide a low resistance intercellular pathway that assures the transmission of signals that are crucial for the propagation of the action potentials and synchronization of contraction (Sanderson et al., 1994; Spray and Burt, 1990; Page and Manjunath, 1996). Functional and morphological changes in cardiac gap junctions, particularly in relation to the arrangement and density of packing of the channels at the junctional membranes, are believed to be responsible for the induction of arrhythmias and for the very slow conduction observed in acutely ischemic myocardium (Peters and Wit, 1998). Disturbances in atrial impulse propagation with A-V block are observed in mice lacking Cx40 (Kirchhoff et al., 2000; Simon et al., 1998; Tamaddon et al., 2000; Verheule et al., 1999) and more profound alterations are observed in Cx43 knockout mice (Eloff et al., 2001; Guerrero et al., 1997; Gutstein et al., 2001; Thomas et al., 1998). Transgenic Cx43-null mice die shortly after birth due to abnormal cardiac formation (Reaume et al., 1995), and the impulse propagation is severely impaired in the neonatal Cx43-null heart, which beats in a completely asynchronous manner.

Besides the role of gap junctions in electrical/ionic coupling, the high permeability to large ions and small molecules (up to 1kDa) confers them the ability to also couple the cells metabolically. Small metabolites, intracellular second messengers (Ca^{2+}, InsP$_3$, cAMP, cGMP, cADPR) and morphogens can be exchanged between coupled cells (Saez et al, 1989; Kumar and Gilula, 1996; Bruzzone et al., 1996) and the "cross talk" between coupled cells can be modulated by changing how many of the channels within a plaque are open and/or the type or level of connexin expression.

The turnover of connexins within gap junctions is a dynamic process, with connexin half-lives being on the order of 1.5 to 3 hours (Beardslee et al., 1998; Spray, 1998; Laird, 1996). The importance of gap junction channels in processes such as embryonic morphogenesis, differentiation, control of cell growth, wound healing, maintenance of intercellular homeostasis and propagation of action potentials have been well documented; the numerous diseases and pathological conditions generated by disruption of connexin expression further emphasizes the functional importance of the intercellular signaling provided by gap junctions (Spray et al., 2000a,b; White and Paul, 1999; Simon and Goodenough, 1998).

Information conveyed by intercellular Ca^{2+} waves

Spatial and temporal alterations in intracellular Ca^{2+} levels are known to mediate and modulate a large number of cellular processes. Increased intracellular Ca^{2+} levels can propagate within the cells as slow intracellular Ca^{2+} waves and can also be communicated between adjacent neighboring cells as intercellular Ca^{2+} waves (see Scemes, 2000). Although the real functional importance of this form of intercellular Ca^{2+} signaling is still a matter of investigation, it is currently believed that the information transmitted by intercellular Ca^{2+} waves is essential to attain the coordination required for certain cooperative cellular activities (Allbritton et al., 1992; Sanderson, 1996; Scemes et al., 2000a).

The initiating signal for the intercellular propagation of Ca^{2+} waves can be generated by electrical, chemical or mechanical stimuli. The increase in intracellular Ca^{2+} level induced in the stimulated cell is promptly transmitted to immediately adjacent cells by diffusion of intracellular second messengers that permeate gap junction channels to release Ca^{2+} from the stores of neighboring cells (see Figure 4).

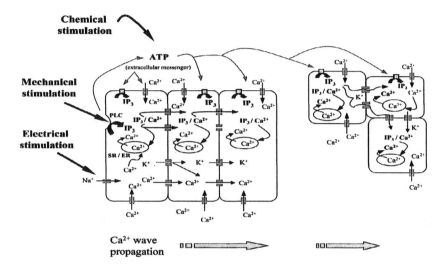

Figure 4 - Model of intercellular Ca2+ signaling. Elevations in the intracellular concentration of second messengers such as InsP$_3$ or Ca^{2+} induced by mechanical, electrical, chemical stimulation or release of active extracellular messengers from the stimulated cell, such as ATP, triggers the release of Ca2+ from the intracellular stores of the stimulated cell and/or influx of Ca2+ from the extracellular milieu. This Ca2+ signal is communicated to adjacent coupled cells when second messengers diffuse through gap junction channels and promote the mobilization of Ca2+ from intra and/or extracellular Ca2+ pools, thus generating propagated intercellular Ca2+ waves. Besides this intracellular pathway provided by gap junction channels, an extracellular pathway mediated through the activation of cell surface membrane receptors by extracellular messengers such as ATP, glutamate or acetylcholine, can also contribute to the transmission of the Ca2+ signal, recruiting cells that are not among those coupled to the primarily stimulated cells.

The diffusion of these messengers thus generates slow waves of Ca^{2+} increase within the adjacent coupled cells that will trail the diffusion of the intercellular messengers, spreading from cell to cell until the threshold for activation of the intracellular stores in no longer achieved (Sanderson, 1996; Scemes et al., 2000a). Besides this intercellular gap junction-mediated pathway, an extracellular pathway can also participate in the communication of intercellular Ca^{2+} signals, working in parallel with the intercellular pathway. This paracrine route involves an extracellular messenger, such as ATP, other adenosine nucleotides, glutamate, or other neurotransmitters or hormones that relay the Ca^{2+} signal through the activation of cell surface membrane receptors. In a few cell types or under certain conditions, the extracellular route is the primary or the sole pathway involved in the transmission of slow intercellular Ca^{2+} signals (Scemes et al., 2000a;(Osipchuk and Cahalan, 1992; Guthrie et al, 1999; Hassinger et al 1996).

Intercellular Ca^{2+} signaling in the heart

In normal working myocardium, this form of slow intercellular Ca^{2+} signaling would presumably be obscured by the fast Ca^{2+} waves associated with action potential propagation and EC coupling, and the duration of sustained Ca^{2+} elevations would be limited by requisite Ca^{2+} buffering and removal. However, although its functional significance is still obscure, this phenomenon has been described in pairs of isolated adult cardiac myocytes (Lopez et al., 1995; Takamatsu et al., 1991) and in primary cultures of neonatal cardiac myocytes (Spray et al., 1998a; Suadicani et al., 2000). Spontaneous intercellular Ca^{2+} waves, which are distinct from the electrically mediated and rapidly transmitted waves of contraction that generate cardiac output, have also been observed propagating on the ventricular surface of the normal working or arrested myocardium of the whole isolated heart (Kaneko et al., 2000; Minamikawa et al., 1997) and in multicellular ventricular trabeculae preparations (Lamont et al., 1998; Miura et al., 1998; Miura et al., 1999). Interestingly, the frequency of these spontaneous waves can be increased by abnormal elevation of extracellular Ca^{2+}, by cellular damage (Kaneko et al., 2000; Lamont et al., 1998; Minamikawa et al., 1997) and by rapid stretch/release of cardiac tissue (Lamont et al., 1998), events that when combined can lead to damage-induced cardiac arrhythmias (ter Keurs and Zhang, 1997). Studies of such triggered arrhythmias in ventricular trabeculae have shown that stretch and release of damaged cardiac tissue during regular twitches induces after-contractions that arise in the damaged region and propagate to the neighboring healthy myocardium as slow waves of contraction accompanied by nearly synchronous delayed after-depolarizations (Daniels et al., 1991; Daniels et al., 1993; Mulder et al., 1989; ter Keurs et al., 1998) (Daniels and ter Keurs, 1990). Such depolarizations may reach threshold for generation of action potentials and thus induce triggered twitches and arrhythmias. These after-contractions seem to result from a chain reaction of Ca^{2+}-induced Ca^{2+} release initiated in the damaged regions by stretch/release-mediated dissociation of Ca^{2+} from the myofilaments followed by Ca^{2+} release from the overloaded sarcoplasmic reticulum (SR) (Daniels et al., 1991; ter Keurs et al., 1998). It has been assumed that the Ca^{2+} transient generated by these events is transmitted to the adjacent cells by a combination of Ca^{2+} diffusion and Ca^{2+}-induced Ca^{2+} release, propagating into the healthy regions as intercellular Ca^{2+} waves (Backx et al., 1989; Daniels et al., 1991; Mulder et al., 1989; ter Keurs et al., 1998) with velocities in the range of about 0.5 to 5 mm/sec (Miura et al., 1998). The transmission of this intercellular Ca^{2+} signal depends on the functional presence of gap junction channels (Daniels et al., 1993; Miura et al., 1998; Zhang et al., 1996). In primary cultures of neonatal mouse cardiac myocytes the presence of gap junctions is also essential for the communication of intercellular Ca^{2+} signals initiated by focal mechanical stimulation of single myocytes Spray et al., 1998a; Suadicani et al., 2000).These intercellular Ca^{2+} waves travel between cardiac myocytes with mean conduction velocities of 14μm/sec, well within the range of velocities measured for the Ca^{2+} signal transmission in other types of cultured cells coupled by gap junction channels (Scemes et al., 2000a) but much slower than the conduction velocities in the ventricular trabeculae preparations (Miura et al., 1998). At least three factors could account for the differences in conduction velocity observed between the adult multicellular preparation and the primary cultures of neonatal cardiac myocytes: the lower degree of SR differentiation in neonatal cardiac myocytes (Husse and Wussling, 1996; Seguchi et al., 1986), the absence in neonatal mycoytes of organized distribution of the gap junction channels in the intercalated discs at the ends of the myocytes (Hoyt et al., 1989; Page and Manjunath, 1996), together with the much longer length of adult myocytes.

Irrespective of the degree of organization displayed by functional gap junctions in non-dissociated and in dissociated cardiac myocytes in culture, gap junction channels would be expected to be the primary transmission route for intercellular Ca^{2+} signal communication between cardiac myocytes. Not only is junctional conductance very high in cardiac tissue Burt and Spray, 1988; Spray et al., 2001a,b; Spray and Burt, 1990), but also the major gap junction protein in cardiac myocytes is Cx43, whose channels are among those with the highest permeability and least selectivity to small ions and molecules. The significant role played by gap junction-mediated metabolic coupling in the communication of intercellular Ca^{2+} signals between cardiac myocytes was suggested from the disruptive effects of gap junction channel blockers such as halothane and heptanol. However, the importance of these intercellular channels was only firmly demonstrated with the generation of Cx43-knockout mice [Cx43(-/-)] (Reaume et al., 1995). The deletion of a single copy of the Cx43 gene did not measurably affect the communication of intercellular Ca^{2+} waves in primary cultures of the heterozygous [Cx43(+/-)] neonatal cardiac myocytes (Suadicani et al., 2000). Although removal of 50% of the functional Cx43 gap junction channels significantly slowed ventricular conduction in the adult Cx43(+/-) mouse heart Eloff et al., 2001; Guerrero et al., 1997; Thomas et al., 1998), the lack of measurable differences in the intercellular Ca^{2+} signaling observed in neonatal cardiac myocytes cultures is consistent with non-measurable difference in dye coupling and junctional conductance between Cx43(+/-) and wild type neonatal cardiac myocytes (Spray et al., 1998b). This presumably reflects the existence of a high safety factor for metabolic coupling in the heart, which is also consistent with the results obtained from optical mapping studies, in which ECG parameters between hearts of heterozygotes did not differ from wild types (Morley et al., 1999). However, a completely different scenario was obtained in the studies with primary cultures of Cx43(-/-) neonatal cardiac myocytes. The complete disruption of Cx43 expression imposed an overall loss of almost 90% in the communication of intercellular Ca^{2+} signals between Cx43(-/-) cardiac myocytes (Suadicani et al., 2000).The few remaining responsive cells in the Cx43(-/-) cultures were those immediately adjacent to the mechanically stimulated cell where the initial Ca^{2+} signal was generated, and the conduction velocity of the Ca^{2+} signal reaching these cells was almost four times slower than that traveling between wild type cardiac myocytes (Suadicani et al., 2000). The persistence of this reduced intercellular communication between Cx43(-/-) cardiac myocytes was attributed to the functional presence of gap junction channels formed by Cx40 and Cx45, and to a minor but relevant participation of an extracellular ATP-mediated route that would contribute to the intercellular gap junction-mediated pathway in the communication of the Ca^{2+} signals (Suadicani et al., 2000).

The participation of ATP as the messenger of an extracellular route that works in parallel with the intercellular gap junction-mediated pathway in the communication of the Ca^{2+} signals has been well described in a variety of cell types (Scemes et al., 2000a). In this paracrine pathway the Ca^{2+} signal is transmitted when ATP released from the stimulated cell diffuses and sequentially activates cell surface membrane P2-receptors that can either induce the influx of Ca^{2+} (ionotropic P2X receptors) or release of Ca^{2+} from intracellular stores via InsP$_3$ (metabotropic P2Y receptors). In primary cultures of neonatal mouse cardiac myocytes the contribution of this paracrine pathway to the actual propagation of the Ca^{2+} signal seems to be minor, assuming only a modulatory role (Suadicani et al., 2000).The ATP released from the stimulated myocyte contributes to the transmission of the Ca^{2+} signal by increasing the number of cells recruited by the signal, but at the same time modulates the communication by controlling and restraining the signal conduction velocity. This dual role played by ATP is attributable to the expression of more than one type of P2-receptor with functionally antagonistic actions that could result in both excitation and inhibition of the neonatal cardiac myocytes in culture. Changes in the population of P2-receptors, in their function and level of expression, could alter the participation of the paracrine pathway in intercellular Ca^{2+} signaling. Furthermore, an interplay between the intercellular and extracellular pathways is also possible and has already been demonstrated in astrocytes, where changes in Cx43 expression seem to alter the population of functional P2-receptors, thus reshaping the participation of ATP in intercellular Ca^{2+} signaling (Scemes et al., 2000b). In the case of cardiac myocytes such an interplay has not yet been demonstrated, but considering the predominance of Cx43 expression and the fact that in Cx43 (-/-) mice the ATP-mediated pathway is still functional and seems even to have been enhanced (Suadicani et al., 2000), it is quite possible that also in the heart a significant change in Cx43 and thus the participation of the gap junction-mediated pathway in the communication of the Ca^{2+} signals will be compensated by an increase in the participation of the paracrine ATP-mediated pathway.

As mentioned previously, the physiological relevance of slow intracellular Ca^{2+} waves is unclear in the normal working myocardium. However, under abnormal conditions such as those imposed by ischemia and cardiac damage, when the release of ATP is increased (Forrester, 1990), the intercellular signaling provided by the paracrine ATP-mediated pathway would be enhanced. In contrast, the contribution of gap junction channels to the communication of the Ca^{2+} signal would be significantly reduced, as the sustained increase in intracellular Ca^{2+} combined with the effects of decrease in pH and accumulation of fatty acid metabolites would result in cellular uncoupling in the damaged region (Kleber et al., 1987; White et al., 1990; Yamada et al., 1994). In such a situation, not only myocytes but also non-myocytes, particularly fibroblasts, would be expected to be recruited into responses mediated by extracellular Ca^{2+} signaling. Such heterocellular myocyte-fibroblast Ca^{2+} signaling has been found in primary cultures of neonatal cardiac cells (Suadicani and Spray, 1999), and the possibility of recruiting fibroblasts in this form of heterocellular ATP-mediated intercellular signaling is intriguing, considering that extracellular ATP can possibly stimulate fibroblast migration (Grierson and Meldolesi, 1995) and that fibroblasts can modulate cardiac myocyte function via secretion of growth factors, such as basic Fibroblast Growth Factor (bFGF or FGF-2), whose expression is increased in the heart in response to injury (Padua and Kardami, 1993).It is thus quite possible, that under normal conditions the information transmitted by slow intercellular Ca^{2+} waves would serve as an internal subthreshold beacon that could be enhanced under abnormal conditions, when the information contained in the intercellular Ca^{2+} signaling would be able to trigger the events that would ultimately lead toward healing and cardiac remodeling.

Intercellular Ca^{2+} signaling in the vascular wall: role in vasomotor response

The main function of the vascular system is to provide an adequate supply of oxygen, nutrients and other factors to meet the short and long-term metabolic requirements of every tissue in the organism and to promote an efficient removal of the toxic end products of this metabolism, achieving tissue homeostasis. The ability of the vascular system to simultaneously attend to a diversity of metabolic demands resides in its capacity to independently and locally control the blood flow in time and space by finely coordinating changes in the diameter of the small arteries and arterioles that supply blood to each organ and tissue of the organism. Vasomotor tone is mainly under the control of the autonomic nervous system but local signals such as those triggered by circulating hormones, other vasoactive substances, shear stress, changes in blood pressure and blood gases also contribute to the regulation of vascular smooth muscle tonus. Ultimately, the response of the vascular wall is dictated by the combined action of both nervous and non-nervous local signals. Precisely how this myriad of signals is integrated and coordinated has not yet been completely unraveled. However, it it clear that the functional coupling between the vascular wall cells, provided by intercellular gap junction channels, plays an essential role in the complex chain of events involved in the vascular wall function and vasomotor regulation (Christ et al., 1996;Dora, 2001;Segal and Duling, 1989).

From a functional point of view, the vascular wall can be regarded as a working unit formed by two parallel compartments, the endothelial cell lining and the enveloping smooth muscle cell layers. A lamina of connective tissue, the elastica interna, separates the endothelial from the smooth muscle compartment, but direct physical contact remains possible through endothelial/smooth muscle cell bridges that transverse the fenestrae of the elastica to form myo-endothelial junctions. These points of heterocellular gap junction contact consummate the functional bond between the endothelial and smooth muscle compartments. This functional coupling and the interplay between the endothelial and smooth muscle compartments form the basis for the local coordination of the vasomotor responses. In this scenario, the endothelial cells would function as the sensors of the changes in the local vascular environment, while the smooth muscle cells would be the effectors, promoting the required alterations in vascular tone and hence vessel diameter.

Endothelial cells can be stimulated by a variety of local vasoactive signals (Furchgott and Vanhoutte, 1989). The response can involve the generation of InsP$_3$ and the subsequent increase in intracellular Ca^{2+} levels that can both mediate the synthesis of endothelium-derived relaxing factors such as NO (nitric oxide), prostacyclin and hyperpolarizing factor(s) (EDHF), and directly induce the opening of Ca^{2+}-activated K^+ channels (K_{Ca2+}) (Chen and Suzuki, 1990; Edwards et al., 1998; Garland et al., 1995; Himmel et al., 1993; Luckhoff and Busse, 1990; Plane et al., 1995). Because endothelial cells are electrically and metabolically coupled by gap junction channels, localized responses can be promptly transmitted to non-stimulated adjacent coupled endothelial cells, leading to coordinated responses up- and downstream from the point of stimulation, recruiting the response of long vascular wall segments. The Ca^{2+} signal triggered locally can be spread to neighboring cells by both the propagation of intercellular Ca^{2+} waves generated by the diffusion of InsP$_3$ and Ca^{2+} and by the electrotonic spread of the electrical signal. This spread of the intercellular signal along the endothelial compartment is rapidly communicated to the smooth muscle compartment that responds with a wave of relaxation that sweeps the vascular wall. Although both forms of endothelial signaling seem to be involved in evoking the overall vasomotor response, the observation that propagated vasodilatation is preceded by the passage of the endothelial wave of hyperpolarization (Dora and Duling, 1997) suggests that the fast electrotonic spread of current rather than the slower intercellular spread of the Ca^{2+} waves is mainly responsible for the fast and long-range recruitment of smooth muscle cells in the vasomotor responses, although opening of K$_{Ca}$+2 channels following the Ca^{2+} wave may sustain the vasorelaxation. An essential and more localized role seems to be reserved for the more slowly propagated endothelial Ca^{2+} waves. This form of intercellular Ca^{2+} communication, generated by an increase in the intracellular Ca^{2+} level of the primarily stimulated endothelial cell(s) (Domenighetti et al., 1998; Demer et al., 1993), would be essential to guarantee the synthesis/release of the endothelium-derived relaxing factors and to attain and sustain the increased intracellular Ca^{2+} levels required to open K$_{Ca2+}$ channels and thus initiate the long-range transmission of the endothelial signal. Since the pioneering work of Furchgott and Zawadski (Furchgott and Zawadski, 1980) much has been learned regarding to the mechanisms involved in endothelial-dependent vasomotor regulation. However, despite compelling evidence for the anatomical and functional presence of myo-endothelial gap junctions Beny and Pacicca, 1994; Emersson and Segal, 2000; Little et al., 1995b; Sandow and Hill, 2000;

Spagnoli et al., 1982; Xia et al., 1995; Yamamoto et al., 1999), the participation of these intercellular channels in endothelium-mediated vasodilatation remains controversial. This can be in part attributed to technical difficulties in distinguishing between the homocellular endothelial-endothelial or smooth muscle-smooth muscle from the heterocellular endothelial-smooth muscle gap junction participation in the complex vasomotor response. However, new evidence for the participation of myo-endothelial junctions in the intercellular signaling from the endothelial to the smooth muscle compartment has been produced by studies conducted to unravel the mechanism of action of EDHF, a Ca^{2+}-dependent endothelium hyperpolarizing factor (Dora et al., 1999; Yamamoto et al., 1998; Chaytor et al., 1998; Brandes et al., 2000; Edwards et al., 1999; Taylor et al., 1998; Yamamoto et al., 1999). Although EDHF may actually be different compounds in different vascular beds, in some of the cases studied the functional presence of myo-endothelial gap junctions has been shown to be required for complete EDHF-mediated vasodilatation. The importance of the gap junction-mediated intercellular pathway for the transmission of the EDHF signal can be even further appreciated from the studies with mice lacking the expression of Cx40, which is normally abundantly expressed in the vascular wall. In the Cx40-knockout mouse the propagation of the endothelium-dependent vasodilatation is severely impaired while the spread of contraction induced by high K^+ solutions is not different from that observed in the wild type animals (de Wit et al., 2000). Interestingly however, the removal of Cx40 significantly attenuated but did not completely prevent the spread of the endothelium-derived signal, suggesting the participation of the other vascular connexins. In fact, the contribution of each of the three endothelial connexins (Cx37, Cx40 and Cx43) to the communication of the EDHF signal was recently claimed using peptides reported to selectively block the channels formed by each of these proteins (Chaytor et al., 2001).

Besides the electrical coupling, myoendothelial junctions should also provide the metabolic coupling of endothelial and smooth muscle cells. Ca^{2+} signals generated in the endothelial compartment would be expected to be transmitted to the smooth muscle compartment by the diffusion of InsP$_3$ and/or Ca^{2+}, leading to an increase in intracellular Ca^{2+} and contraction of the neighboring smooth muscle cells. However, this form of signaling from the endothelial to the smooth muscle cells has not been observed in the vascular wall. It is thus probable that the intercellular Ca^{2+} signal is actually transmitted to the smooth muscle cells but is functionally overridden by the hyperpolarization both induced by the endothelium-derived relaxing factors and opening of K$_{Ca}$2+ channels.

This apparently minor participation of the unidirectional endothelial to smooth muscle cell Ca^{2+} signaling in the regulation of vasomotor responses contrasts with the functional importance that the intercellular Ca^{2+} signaling assumes when it is communicated from the opposite direction, from the smooth muscle to the endothelial cell compartment, as described below. In densely innervated vascular beds the synchronized depolarization and contraction of vascular smooth muscle is mainly dictated by the uniform release of neurotransmitters. However, similar to that described for the endothelial cells, the presence of gap junction channels between smooth muscle cells provides a low resistance pathway for the propagation of the electrical signal and for the diffusion of second messengers (Christ et al., 1996). Thus, the activation of a single or a small group of smooth muscle cells can mediate the activation and contraction of the neighboring non-stimulated cells through the spread of the depolarization and opening of voltage-activated Ca^{2+} channels. Intercellular Ca^{2+} waves initiated by neurotransmitter-mediated generation and diffusion of InsP$_3$ and/or Ca^{2+} through gap junction channels will also contribute to the spread of the contraction, inducing the sequential release of Ca^{2+} from the intracellular Ca^{2+} stores of the neighboring, non-stimulated smooth muscle cells. The contribution of this form of intercellular Ca^{2+} signaling to the activation of smooth muscle cells is restricted to a smaller area of the vascular wall, mainly due to the slower diffusion and intracellular buffering of the intercellular messengers than the electrical spread of the depolarization. However, it seems that the main, if not the most important role that this form of intercellular Ca^{2+} signaling plays in the regulation of vasomotor responses is to keep the endothelial cell compartment informed about the degree of activation of the smooth muscle compartment. When Ca^{2+} signals are transmitted from activated smooth muscle cells to the endothelial cells through the myo-endothelial junctions the increase in endothelial intracellular Ca^{2+} levels triggers the synthesis/release of endothelium-derived relaxing factors that feed back to the smooth muscle cells, reducing the activity in the vascular wall (Budel et al., 2001; Schuster et al., 2001; Dora et al., 1999; Yashiro and Duling, 2000; Dora et al., 2000). This intricate interplay between the endothelial and smooth muscle compartments provides a mechanism through which smooth muscle cells can indirectly control their own level of activation. Such a mechanism may have pathological implications as any impairment of endothelial cell function could result in an abnormal increase in vascular tonus. In this scenario and considering the importance of gap junctions in the conduction of endothelium-derived vasodilatation, it is quite possible that the reported spontaneous hypertension and irregular vasomotion, with cases of local arteriolar vasospasm, observed in the Cx40-knockout mice (de Wit et al., 2000) result from the impairment of the interplay between the endothelial and smooth muscle compartments, the absence of Cx40 gap junction channels resulting in the inability of the endothelium to fully integrate the changes in vascular tonus.

In the vascular wall, the importance of intercellular signals communicated by gap junction channels is not limited to the integration and coordination of vasomotor responses. Regulation of angiogenesis, vascular development and endothelial regeneration, growth and senescence are examples of some other vascular events where gap junction-mediated cell-cell signaling has been shown to participate (de Wit et al., 2000; Kwak et al., 2001; Larson and Haudenschild, 1988; Larson et al., 1996; Pepper et al., 1989; Xie and Hu, 1994). Signals transmitted through Cx45 formed channels seem to be essential for normal vascular development (Kruger et al., 2000). The healing process of the arterial endothelium is accompanied by spatial and temporal changes in the expression pattern of each of the three endothelial connexins, suggesting that successive different intercellular signals participate in the normal endothelial reconstitution (Yeh et al., 2000). Although the nature of the signals and the precise mechanisms involved in these vascular events still remains to be investigated, direct or indirect substantial participation of Ca^{2+} signals can be expected, considering their participation in diverse phenomena such as cellular proliferation, differentiation and migration (Berridge et al., 2000).

Concluding Remarks

The transmission of Ca^{2+} signals is a wide spread form of intercellular communication. In the heart, the functional importance of the slow Ca^{2+} waves in cellular dialogue was initially overlooked. This is in great part due to the overwhelming presence and unquestionable functional importance of the fastest and longer-range form of intercellular signaling provided by the propagation of action potentials and electrotonic spread of current. However, the continuous improvement and advance in Ca^{2+} imaging techniques are providing the tools to document the participation and disclose the importance of intercellular Ca^{2+} signaling in the local integration and coordination of the cellular activities in the cardiovascular system under both normal and pathological conditions.

Acknowledgements: Supported in part by NIH and NIMH grants to DCS. Dr. Suadicani's present address is Institute of Biophysics Carlos Chagas Filho, UFRJ, Rio de Janeiro, BRAZIL. We are grateful for the editorial assistance of Ms. Fran Andrade, and for helpful conversations and collaborations on the subject of this review with Dr. Eliana Scemes (Dept. Neuroscience, AECOM) and Dr. George Christ (Depts. Urology and Physiology, AECOM).

REFERENCE

Albrieux M, Lee HC, Villaz M (1998) Calcium signalling by cyclicADP-ribose, NAADP and inositol trisphosphate are involved in distinct functions in ascidian oocytes. J Biol Chem 273: 14566-14574.

Allbritton NL, Meyer T, Stryer L (1992) Range of messenger action of calcium ion and inositol 1,4,5-trisphosphate. Science 258: 1812-1815.

Backx PH, de Tombe PP, Van Deen JH, Mulder BJ, ter Keurs HE (1989) A model of propagating calcium-induced calcium release mediated by calcium diffusion. J Gen Physiol 93: 963-977.

Beardslee MA, Laing JG, Beyer EC, Saffitz JE (1998) Rapid turnover of connexin43 in the adult rat heart. Circ Res 83: 629-635.

Bennett MV, Barrio LC, Bargiello TA, Spray DC, Hertzberg E, Saez JC (1991) Gap junctions: new tools, new answers, new questions. Neuron 6: 305-320.

Beny J-L, Pacicca C (1994) Bidirectional electrical communication between smooth muscle and endothelial cells in the pig coronary artery. Am J Physiol Heart Circ Physiol 266: H1465-H1472.

Berridge MJ (1993) Inositol trisphosphate and calcium signalling. Nature 361: 315-325.

Berridge MJ (1997) Elementary and global aspects of calcium signalling. J Exp Biol 200: 315-319.

Berridge MJ, Bootman MD, Lipp P (1998) Calcium--a life and death signal. Nature 395: 645-648.

Berridge MJ, Lipp P, Bootman MD (2000) The versatility and universality of calcium signalling. Nat Rev Mol Cell Biol 1: 11-21.

Bootman MD, Collins TJ, Peppiatt CM, Prothero LS, MacKenzie L, De Smet P, Travers M, Tovey SC, Seo JT, Berridge MJ, Ciccolini F, Lipp P (2001) Calcium signalling--an overview. Semin Cell Dev Biol 12: 3-10.

Brandes RP, Schmitz-Winnenthal FH, Feletou M, Godecke A, Huang PL, Vanhoutte PM, Fleming I, Busse R (2000) An endothelium-derived hyperpolarizing factor distinct from NO and prostacyclin is a major endothelium-dependent vasodilator in resistance vessels of wild-type and endothelial NO synthase knockout mice. Proc Natl Acad Sci USA 97: 9747-9752.

Bruzzone R, White TW, Paul DL (1996) Connections with connexins: the molecular basis of direct intercellular signaling. Eur J Biochem 238: 1-27.

Budel S, Schuster A, Stergiopoulos N, Meister JJ, Beny JL (2001) Role of smooth muscle cells on endothelial cell cytosolic free calcium in porcine coronary arteries. Am J Physiol Heart Circ Physiol 281: H1156-H1162.

Burt JM, Spray DC (1988) Single-channel events and gating behavior of the cardiac gap junction channel. Proc Natl Acad Sci U S A 85: 3431-3434.

Chaytor AT, Evans WH, Griffith TM (1998) Central role of heterocellular gap junctional communication in endothelium-dependent relaxations of rabbit arteries. J Physiol 508: 561-573.

Chaytor AT, Martin PE, Edwards DH, Griffith TM (2001) Gap junctional communication underpins EDHF-type relaxations evoked by ACh in the rat hepatic artery. Am J Physiol Heart Circ Physiol 280: H2441-H2450.

Chen G, Suzuki H (1990) Calcium dependency of the endothelium-dependent hyperpolarization in smooth muscle cells of the rabbit carotid artery. J Physiol 421: 521-534.

Christ GJ, Spray DC, el Sabban M, Moore LK, Brink PR (1996) Gap junctions in vascular tissues. Evaluating the role of intercellular communication in the modulation of vasomotor tone. Circ Res 79: 631-646.

Clapham DE (1995) Calcium signaling. Cell 80: 259-268.

Coppen SR, Dupont E, Rothery S, Severs NJ (1998) Connexin45 expression is preferentially associated with the ventricular conduction system in mouse and rat heart. Circ Res 82: 232-243.

Coppen SR, Severs NJ, Gourdie RG (1999) Connexin45 (alpha 6) expression delineates an extended conduction system in the embryonic and mature rodent heart. Dev Genet 24: 82-90.

Daniels MC, Fedida D, Lamont C, ter Keurs HE (1991) Role of the sarcolemma in triggered propagated contractions in rat cardiac trabeculae. Circ Res 68: 1408-1421.

Daniels MC, Kieser T, ter Keurs HE (1993) Triggered propagated contractions in human atrial trabeculae. Cardiovasc Res 27: 1831-1835.

Daniels MC, ter Keurs HE (1990) Spontaneous contractions in rat cardiac trabeculae. Trigger mechanism and propagation velocity. J Gen Physiol 95: 1123-1137.

de Wit C, Roos F, Bolz SS, Kirchhoff S, Kruger O, Willecke K, Pohl U (2000) Impaired conduction of vasodilation along arterioles in connexin40-deficient mice. Circ Res 86: 649-655.

Demer LL, Wortham CM, Dirksen ER, Sanderson MJ (1993) Mechanical stimulation induces intercellular calcium signaling in bovine aortic endothelial cells. Am J Physiol 264: H2094-H2102.

Domenighetti AA, Beny JL, Chabaud F, Frieden M (1998) An intercellular regenerative calcium wave in porcine coronary artery endothelial cells in primary culture. J Physiol 513: 103-116.

Dora KA (2001) Intercellular Ca2+ signalling: the artery wall. Semin Cell Dev Biol 12: 27-35.

Dora KA, Duling BR (1997) Conducted vasodilation: Ca^{2+} is not the intercellular signal. Microcirculation 4: 161.

Dora KA, Hinton JM, Walker SD, Garland CJ (2000) An indirect influence of phenylephrine on the release of endothelium-derived vasodilators in rat small mesenteric artery. Br J Pharmacol 129: 381-387.

Dora KA, Martin PE, Chaytor AT, Evans WH, Garland CJ, Griffith TM (1999) Role of heterocellular Gap junctional communication in endothelium-dependent smooth muscle hyperpolarization: inhibition by a connexin-mimetic peptide. Biochem Biophys Res Commun 254: 27-31.

Edwards G, Dora KA, Gardener MJ, Garland CJ, Weston AH (1998) K$^+$ is an endothelium-derived hyperpolarizing factor in rat arteries. Nature 396: 269-272.

Edwards G, Feletou M, Gardener MJ, Thollon C, Vanhoutte PM, Weston AH (1999) Role of gap junctions in the responses to EDHF in rat and guinea-pig small arteries. Br J Pharmacol 128: 1788-1794.

Eghbali M, Tomek R, Woods C, Bhambi B (1991) Cardiac fibroblasts are predisposed to convert into myocyte phenotype: specific effect of transforming growth factor beta. Proc Natl Acad Sci U S A 88: 795-799.

Eloff BC, Lerner DL, Yamada KA, Schuessler RB, Saffitz JE, Rosenbaum DS (2001) High resolution optical mapping reveals conduction slowing in connexin43 deficient mice. Cardiovasc Res 51: 681-690.

Emersson GG, Segal SS (2000) Electrical coupling between endothelial cells and smooth muscle cells in hamster feed arteries: role in vasomotor control. Circ Res 87: 474-479.

Forrester T (1990) Release of ATP from heart. Presentation of a release model using human erythrocyte. Ann N Y Acad Sci 603:335-51; discussion 351-2.: 335-351.

Furchgott RF, Vanhoutte PM (1989) Endothelium-derived relaxing and contracting factors. FASEB J 3: 2007-2018.

Furchgott RF, Zawadski JV (1980) The obligatory role of endothelial cells in the relaxation of arterial smooth muscle by acetylcholine. Nature 288: 373-376.

Gabriels JE, Paul DL (1998) Connexin43 is highly localized to sites of disturbed flow in rat aortic endothelium but connexin37 and connexin40 are more uniformly distributed. Circ Res 83: 636-643.

Garland CJ, Plane F, Kemp BK, Cocks TM (1995) Endothelium-dependent hyperpolarization: a role in the control of vascular tone. TIPS 16: 23-30.

Genazzani AA, Gaglione A (1997) A Ca^{2+} release mechanism gated by the novel pyridine nucleotide, NAADP. TIPS 18: 108-110.

Grierson JP, Meldolesi J (1995) Shear stress-induced [Ca2+]i transients and oscillations in mouse fibroblasts are mediated by endogenously released ATP. J Biol Chem 270: 4451-4456.

Guerrero PA, Schuessler RB, Davis LM, Beyer EC, Johnson CM, Yamada KA, Saffitz JE (1997) Slow ventricular conduction in mice heterozygous for a connexin43 null mutation. J Clin Invest 99: 1991-1998.

Guse AH (2000) Cyclic ADP-ribose. J Mol Med 78: 26-35.

Guthrie PB, Knappenberger J., Segal M, Bennett MV, Charles AC, Kate SB (1999) ATP release from astrocytes mediates glial calcium waves. J. Neurosci. 19:520-528.

Gutstein DE, Morley GE, Tamaddon H, Vaidya D, Schneider MD, Chen J, Chien KR, Stuhlmann H, Fishman GI (2001) Conduction slowing and sudden arrhythmic death in mice with cardiac-restricted inactivation of connexin43. Circ Res 88: 333-339.

Hassinger TD, Guthrie PB, Atkinson PB, Bennett MV, Kater SB (1996) An extracellular signaling component in propagation of astrocytic calcium waves. Proc. Natl. Acad. Sci USA 93:13268-13273.

Himmel HM, Whorton AR, Strauss HC (1993) Intracellular calcium, currents, and stimulus-response coupling in endothelial cells. Hypertension 21: 112-127.

Hong T, Hill CE (1998) Restricted expression of the gap junctional protein connexin43 in the arterial system of the rat. J Anat 193: 583-593.

Hoyt RH, Cohen ML, Saffitz JE (1989) Distribution and three-dimentional structure of intercellular junctions in canine myocardium. Circ Res 64: 563-574.

Husse B, Wussling M (1996) Developmental changes of calcium transients and contractility during the cultivation of rat neonatal cardiomyocytes. Mol Cell Biochem 163-164:13-21.: 13-21.

Kaneko T, Tanaka H, Oyamada M, Kawata S, Takamatsu T (2000) Three distinct types of Ca(2+) waves in Langendorff-perfused rat heart revealed by real-time confocal microscopy. Circ Res 86: 1093-1099.

Kirchhoff S, Kim JS, Hagendorff A, Thonnissen E, Kruger O, Lamers WH, Willecke K (2000) Abnormal cardiac conduction and morphogenesis in connexin40 and connexin43 double-deficient mice. Circ Res 87: 399-405.

Kleber AG, Riegger CB, Jansen MJ (1987) Electrical uncoupling and increase of extracellular resistance after induction of ischemia in isolated, arterially perfused rabbit papillary muscle. Circ Res 61: 271-279.

Ko YS, Coppen SR, Dupont E, Rothery S, Severs NJ (2001) Regional differentiation of desmin, connexin43, and connexin45 expression patterns in rat aortic smooth muscle. Arterioscler Thromb Vasc Biol 21: 355-364.

Ko YS, Yeh H-I, Rothery S, Dupont E, Coppen S.R., Severs NJ (1999) Connexin make-up of endothelial gap junctions in the rat pulmonary artery as revealed by immunoconfocal microscopy and triple-label immunogold electron microscopy. J Histochem Cytochem 47: 683-692.

Kruger O, Plum A, Kim JS, Winterhager E, Maxeiner S, Hallas G, Kirchhoff S, Traub O, Lamers WH, Willecke K (2000) Defective vascular development in connexin 45-deficient mice. Development 127: 4179-4193.

Kumar NM, Gilula NB (1996) The gap junction communication channel. Cell 84: 381-388.

Kwak BR, Pepper MS, Gros DB, Meda P (2001) Inhibition of endothelial wound repair by dominant negative connexin inhibitors. Mol Biol Cell 12: 831-845.

Laird DW (1996) The life cycle of a connexin: gap junction formation, removal, and degradation. J Bioenerg Biomembr 28: 311-318.

Lamont C, Luther PW, Balke CW, Wier WG (1998) Intercellular Ca2+ waves in rat heart muscle. J Physiol 512: 669-676.

Larson DM, Haudenschild CC (1988) Junctional transfer in wounded cultures of bovine aortic endothelial cells. Lab Invest 59: 373-379.

Larson DM, Wrobleski MJ, Sagar GDV, Westphale EM, Beyer EC (1996) Differential regulation of connexin43 and connexin37 in endothelial cells by cell density, growth, and TGF-β1. Am J Physiol Cell Physiol 272: C405-C415.

Little TL, Beyer EC, Duling BR (1995a) Connexin 43 and connexin 40 gap junctional proteins are present in arteriolar smooth muscle and endothelium in vivo. Am J Physiol 268: H729-H739.

Little TL, Xia J, Duling BR (1995b) Dye tracers define differential endothelial and smooth muscle coupling patterns within the arteriolar wall. Circ Res 76: 498-504.

Lopez JR, Jovanovic A, Terzic A (1995) Spontaneous calcium waves without contraction in cardiac myocytes. Biochem Biophys Res Commun 214: 781-787.

Luckhoff A, Busse R (1990) Calcium influx into endothelial cells and formation of endothelium-derived relaxing factor is controlled by membrane potential. Pflugers Arch 416: 305-311.

Minamikawa T, Cody SH, Williams DA (1997) In situ visualization of spontaneous calcium waves within perfused whole rat heart by confocal imaging. Am J Physiol 272: H236-H243.

Miura M, Boyden PA, ter Keurs HE (1998) Ca2+ waves during triggered propagated contractions in intact trabeculae. Am J Physiol 274: H266-H276.

Miura M, Boyden PA, ter Keurs HE (1999) Ca2+ waves during triggered propagated contractions in intact trabeculae. Determinants of the velocity of propagation. Circ Res 84: 1459-1468.

Morley GE, Vaidya D, Samie FH, Lo C, Delmar M, Jalife J (1999) Characterization of conduction in the ventricles of normal and heterozygous Cx43 knockout mice using optical mapping. J Cardiovasc Electrophysiol 10: 1361-1375.

Mulder BJ, de Tombe PP, ter Keurs HE (1989) Spontaneous and propagated contractions in rat cardiac trabeculae. J Gen Physiol 93: 943-961.

Osipchuk Y, Cahalan M (1992) Cell-to-cell spread of calcium signals mediated by ATP receptors in mast cells. Nature 359: 241-244.

Padua RR, Kardami E (1993) Increased basic fibroblast growth factor (bFGF) accumulation and distinct patterns of localization in isoproterenol-induced cardiomyocyte injury. Growth Factors 8: 291-306.

Page E, Manjunath CK (1996) Communicating junctions between cardiac cells. In: The Heart and Cardiovascular System (Fozzard HA, Haber E, Jennings RB, Katz AM, Morgan HE, eds), pp 573-600. New York: Raven Press.

Pepper MS, Spray D.C., Chanson M, Montesano R, Orci L, Meda P (1989) Junctional communication is induced in migrating capillary endothelial cells. J Cell Biol 109: 3027-3038.

Peters NS, Wit AL (1998) Myocardial architecture and ventricular arrhythmogenesis. Circulation 97: 1746-1754.

Plane F, Pearson T, Garland CJ (1995) Multiple pathways underlying endothelium-dependent relaxation in the rabbit isolated femoral artery. Br J Pharmacol 115: 31-38.

Putney JW, Jr., Broad LM, Braun FJ, Lievremont JP, Bird GS (2001) Mechanisms of capacitative calcium entry. J Cell Sci 114: 2223-2229.

Putney JW, Jr., McKay RR (1999) Capacitative calcium entry channels. Bioessays 21: 38-46.

Reaume AG, de Sousa PA, Kulkarni S, Langille BL, Zhu D, Davies TC, Juneja SC, Kidder GM, Rossant J (1995) Cardiac malformation in neonatal mice lacking connexin43. Science 267: 1831-1834.

Rottingen J, Iversen JG (2000) Ruled by waves? Intracellular and intercellular calcium signalling. Acta Physiol Scand 169: 203-219.

Saez JC, Connor JA, Spray DC, Bennett MV (1989) Hepatocyte gap junctions are permeable to the second messenger, inositol 1,4,5-trisphosphate, and to calcium ions. Proc Natl Acad Sci U S A 86: 2708-2712.

Sanderson MJ (1996) Intercellular waves of communication. News Physiol Sci 11: 262-269.

Sanderson MJ, Charles AC, Boitano S, Dirksen ER (1994) Mechanisms and function of intercellular calcium signaling. Mol Cell Endocrinol 98: 173-187.

Sandow SL, Hill CE (2000) Incidence of myoendothelial gap junctions in the proximal and distal mesentheric arteries of the rat is suggestive of a role in endothelium-derived hyperpolarizing factor-mediated responses. Circ Res 86: 341-346.

Scemes, E. (2000) Components of astrocytic intercellular calcium signaling. Mol. Neurobiol. 22:167-179.

Scemes E, Suadicani SO, Spray DC (2000a) Intercellular calcium wave communication via gap junction dependent and independent mechanisms. In: Gap Junctions: Molecular Basis of Cell Communication in Health and Disease (Peracchia C, ed), pp 145-173. San Diego, CA: Academic Press.

Scemes E, Suadicani SO, Spray DC (2000b) Intercellular communication in spinal cord astrocytes: fine tuning between gap junctions and P2 nucleotide receptors in calcium wave propagation. J Neurosci 20: 1435-1445.

Schuster A, Oishi H, Beny JL, Stergiopulos N, Meister JJ (2001) Simultaneous arterial calcium dynamics and diameter measurements: application to myoendothelial communication. Am J Physiol Heart Circ Physiol 280: H1088-H1096.

Segal SS, Duling BR (1989) Conduction of vasomotor responses in arterioles: a role for cell-to-cell coupling? Am J Physiol 256: H838-H845.

Seguchi M, Harding JA, Jarmakani JM (1986) Developmental changes in the function of sarcoplasmic reticulum. J Mol Cell Cardiol 18: 189-195.

Simon AM, Goodenough DA (1998) Diverse functions of vertebrate gap junctions. Trends Cell Biol 8: 477-483.

Simon AM, Goodenough DA, Paul DL (1998) Mice lacking connexin40 have cardiac conduction abnormalities characteristic of atrioventricular block and bundle branch block. Curr Biol 8: 295-298.

Spagnoli LG, Villaschi S, Neri L, Palmieri G (1982) Gap junctions in myoendothelial bridges of rabbit carotid arteries. Experientia 38: 124-125.

Spray DC (1998) Gap junction proteins: where they live and how they die. Circ Res 83: 679-681.

Spray DC, Burt JM (1990) Structure-activity relations of the cardiac gap junction channel. Am J Physiol 258: C195-C205.

Spray DC, Kojima T, Scemes E, Suadicani SO, Gao Y, Zhao S, Fort A (2000a) Negative physiology: What connexin-deficient mice reveal about the functional roles of individual gap junction proteins. In: Gap Junctions: Molecular Basis of Cell Communication in Health and Disease. (Peracchia C, ed), pp 509-533. San Diego, CA: Academic Press.

Spray DC, Kojima T, Scemes E, Suadicani SO, Gao Y, Zhao S, Fort A (2000b) Negative physiology: What connexin-deficient mice reveal about the functional roles of individual gap junction proteins. In: Gap Junctions: Molecular Basis of Cell Communication in Health and Disease. (Peracchia C, ed), pp 509-533. San Diego, CA: Academic Press.

Spray DC, Suadicani SO, Srinivas M, Gustein, D.E., Fishman GI (2001a) Gap junctions in the cardiovascular system. In: The Heart (Page E, Fozzard HA, Solaro RJ, eds), pp 169-212. Oxford University Press.

Spray DC, Suadicani SO, Vink MJ, Srinivas M (2001b) Gap junction channels and healing-over of injury. In: Heart Physiology and Pathophysiology (Sperelakis N, Kurachi Y, Terzic A, Cohen MV, eds), pp 149-172. San Diego, CA: Academic Press.

Spray DC, Vink MJ, Scemes E, Suadicani SO, Fishman GI, Dermietzel R (1998a) Characteristics of coupling in cardiac myocytes and astrocytes from Cx43(-/-) mice. In: Gap Junctions (Werner R, ed), pp 281-285. New York: ISO.

Spray DC, Vink MJ, Scemes E, Suadicani SO, Fishman GI, Dermietzel R (1998b) Characteristics of coupling in cardiac myocytes and astrocytes from Cx43(-/-) mice. In: Gap Junctions (Werner R, ed), pp 281-285. New York: ISO.

Suadicani SO, Spray DC (1999) Heterocellular Ca^{2+} signaling between cardiac myocytes and fibroblasts. Circulation 100: I-281.

Suadicani SO, Vink MJ, Spray DC (2000) Slow intercellular Ca(2+) signaling in wild-type and Cx43-null neonatal mouse cardiac myocytes. Am J Physiol Heart Circ Physiol 279: H3076-H3088.

Takamatsu T, Minamikawa T, Kawachi H, Fujita S (1991) Imaging of calcium wave propagation in guinea-pig ventricular cell pairs by confocal laser scanning microscopy. Cell Struct Funct 16: 341-346.

Tamaddon HS, Vaidya D, Simon AM, Paul DL, Jalife J, Morley GE (2000) High-resolution optical mapping of the right bundle branch in connexin40 knockout mice reveals slow conduction in the specialized conduction system. Circ Res 87: 929-936.

Taylor HJ, Chaytor AT, Evans WH, Griffith TM (1998) Inhibition of the gap junctional component of endothelium-dependent relaxations in rabbit iliac artery by 18α-glycyrrhetinic acid. Br J Pharmacol 125: 1-4.

ter Keurs HE, Zhang YM, Miura M (1998) Damage-induced arrhythmias: reversal of excitation-contraction coupling. Cardiovasc Res 40: 444-455.

ter Keurs HEDJ, Zhang YM (1997) Triggered propagated contractions and arrhythmias caused by acute damage to cardiac muscle. In: Discontinuous Conduction in the Heart (Spooner PM, Joyner RW, Jalife J, eds), pp 223-239. Armonk, NY: Futura.

Thomas SA, Schuessler RB, Berul CI, Beardslee MA, Beyer EC, Mendelsohn ME, Saffitz JE (1998) Disparate effects of deficient expression of connexin43 on atrial and ventricular conduction: evidence for chamber-specific molecular determinants of conduction. Circulation 97: 686-691.

van Kempen MJ, Jongsma HJ (1999) Distribution of connexin37, connexin40 and connexin43 in the aorta and coronary artery of several mammals. Histochem Cell Biol 112: 479-486.

van Rijen HVM, van Kempen MJA, Analbers LJS, Rook MB, Van Ginneken ACG, Gros D, Jongsma HJ (1997) Gap junctions in human umbilical cord endothelial cells contains multiple connexins. Am J Physiol 272: C117-C130.

Verheule S, van Batenburg CA, Coenjaerts FE, Kirchhoff S, Willecke K, Jongsma HJ (1999) Cardiac conduction abnormalities in mice lacking the gap junction protein connexin40. J Cardiovasc Electrophysiol 10: 1380-1389.

White RL, Doeller JE, Verselis VK, Wittenberg BA (1990) Gap junctional conductance between pairs of ventricular myocytes is modulated synergistically by H$^+$ and Ca^{++}. J Gen Physiol 95: 1061-1075.

White TW, Paul DL (1999) Genetic diseases and gene knockouts reveal diverse connexin functions. Annu Rev Physiol 61: 283-310.

Xia J, Little TL, Duling BR (1995) Cellular pathways of the conducted electrical response in arterioles of hamster cheek pouch in vitro. Am J Physiol Heart Circ Physiol 269: H2031-H2038.

Xie H, Hu VW (1994) Modulation of gap junctions in senescent endothelial cells. Exp Cell Res 214: 172-176.

Yamada KA, McHowat J, Yan GX, Donahue K, Peirick J, Kleber AG, Corr PB (1994) Cellular uncoupling induced by accumulation of long-chain acylcarnitine during ischemia. Circ Res 74: 83-95.

Yamamoto Y, Fukutiz H, Nakahira Y, Suzuki H (1998) Blockade by 18beta-glycyrrhetinic acid of intercelullar electrical coupling in guinea-pig coronary artery. J Physiol 285: 480-489.

Yamamoto Y, Imaeda K, Suzuki H (1999) Endothelium-dependent hyperpolarization and intercellular electrical coupling in guinea-pig mesenteric arterioles. J Physiol 514: 505-513.

Yashiro Y, Duling BR (2000) Integrated Ca^{2+} signaling between smooth muscle and endothelium of resistance vessels. Circ Res 87: 1048-1054.

Yeh H-I, Dupont E, Coppen S, Rothery S, Severs NJ (1997) Gap junction localization and connexin expression in cytochemically identified endothelial cells of arterial tissue. Cytochem 45: 539-550.

Yeh HI, Lai YJ, Chang HM, Ko YS, Severs NJ, Tsai CH (2000) Multiple connexin expression in regenerating arterial endothelial gap junctions. Arterioscler Thromb Vasc Biol 20: 1753-1762.

Yeh HI, Rothery S, Dupont E, Coppen SR, Severs NJ (1998) Individual gap junction plaques contain multiple connexins in arterial endothelium. Circ Res 83: 1248-1263.

Zhang YM, Miura M, ter Keurs HE (1996) Triggered propagated contractions in rat cardiac trabeculae. Inhibition by octanol and heptanol. Circ Res 79: 1077-1085.

6

Biophysics of Gap Junction Channels

Richard D. Veenstra

SUNY Upstate Medical University, Syracuse, NY 13210

INTRODUCTION

All multicellular organisms require a means for long distance intercellular communication for the purpose of tissue homeostasis, coordinated body movements, and receiving sensory input about its environment. Signals are transmitted long distances primarily by electrical impulses through nerve or muscle tissues, whereas chemical signaling is more localized since it is spatially and temporally limited by the constraints of aqueous diffusion within either the extracellular or intracellular fluid compartments of the organism. Signals arising within the cytoplasm of a cell require a mechanism for transmembrane signal transduction if the message is to be received by neighboring cells. The most direct means of intercellular communication between cells is to form cytoplasmic connections with its neighbors thereby permitting the rapid signaling carried by ions and the more specialized chemical signaling provided by intracellular second messengers. The existence of gap junction channels was first proposed in 1964 by Werner Loewenstein (reviewed in Loewenstein, 1981) and are now know to occur by the expression of at least 16 cloned connexin proteins (Beyer and Willecke, 2000). The ability of many of the connexins to facilitate intercellular communication has been clearly demonstrated by electrical coupling assays in a variety of expression systems (White and Bruzzone, 1996; Willecke and Haubrich, 1996). To date, some of the elementary channel properties (e.g. unitary conductance, γ_j) of at least six of these connexins are known (Verselis and Veenstra, 2000). With so many connexin channels in the mammalian body, we must now begin to discern the unique characteristics of each type of gap junction channel in order to determine the physiological consequences of each connexin and their interactions with other connexins. With this in mind, I want to review the essential theories of channel permeability as it pertains to ion channels and relate this body of knowledge to our developing understanding of connexin channel permeability. A more rigorous review of permeability theory and its implications to the study of connexin gap junction channels appears elsewhere (Veenstra, 2000).

1.1 General Description of a Gap Junction Channel

The gap junction channel is commonly portrayed as a weakly selective ion channel capable of passing hydrophilic molecules of nearly 1 kD in molecular mass or 10 to 14 Å in diameter from cell-to-cell. This general description predates present knowledge about the diversity in the molecular composition of gap junction channels and only superficially acknowledges permeability data known since 1980 that demonstrates differential size permeability limits based on the electronegativity of the permeant molecule (Flagg-Newton et al., 1979; Brink and Dewey, 1980). Although the size limitation for permeant molecules decreases with increasing electronegativity, the molecular mass of a molecule is a less accurate indicator of the limiting size of a pore than the abaxial width (second largest dimension) of the molecule (Brink, 1991). Actually the cross sectional area of the largest permeant molecule provides the best estimate of the limiting pore size. In a channel where the molecule remains hydrated for the entire length of the pore, the electrical conductance increases as the square of the pore radius (Hille, 1992). Hence, the larger the channel conductance, the larger the pore radius and the larger the molecular permeability limit should be for a particular channel. This simple interpretation has been directly challenged by experimental evidence from at least four different connexins where the permeability to two anionic fluorescein dye derivatives was not correlated with channel conductance (Veenstra et al., 1995). The generic aqueous pore model serves as a convenient starting point for the discussion of gap junction channel selective permeability (Veenstra, 1996). This is especially true since most published articles still refer to gap junctions as specialized membrane structures that permit the flow of ions and hydrophilic molecules of up to 1 kD in size between mammalian cells. Efforts have already begun to address this issue in a connexin-specific manner.

2 OVERVIEW OF IONIC PERMEABILITY THEORY

No discussion of gap junction channel permeability is complete without considering the initial investigations which provide the existing framework of knowledge of the physical forces that govern ion and nonelectrolyte selective permeability. This subject was extensively reviewed in Diamond and Wright (1969) and Eisenman and Horn (1983) so only the major elements of ionic selectivity theory will be presented here.

2.1 Ionic Selectivity Sequences

In biological systems, the physiologically most relevant ions to consider are the alkali metal cations (Cs^+, Rb^+, K^+, Na^+, Li^+), the halide anions (I^-, Br^-, Cl^-, F^-), and the alkali earth divalent cations (Ba^{++}, Sr^{++}, Ca^{++}, Mg^{++}). Ironically, the origin of the known selectivity sequences for these ions began in nonliving systems (e.g. soils and aluminium silicate glasses). It is now understood that the same finite set of selectivity sequences exists in nature for living and nonliving systems. This is because the same physical forces act to bind these elements in organic materials (e.g. ion channel proteins) or inorganic materials (e.g. glass). To understand how an ordered ionic selectivity sequence arises from intermolecular attractive and repulsive forces, let us begin with the earliest observations of two oppositely ordered sequences and the physical reasons for the sequence inversion.

2.1.1 The Lyotropic Sequence

In an aqueous solution, the measured mobilities of the alkali cations are the exact opposite of their atomic radii. In order of the smallest to the largest monovalent cation, the sequence is $Li^+>Na^+>K^+>Rb^+>Cs^+$. However, the effective radius in water, which can be calculated by the Stokes equation, has the opposite order of $Cs^+ > Rb^+ > K^+ > Na^+ > Li^+$ since the smaller ions are more hydrated (Robinson and Stokes, 1965). This sequence, called the 'lyotropic' or Hofmeister series, was described around the turn of the century. The corresponding sequences for the halide anions and earth divalent cations are $I^- > Br^- > Cl^- > F^-$ and $Ba^{++} > Sr^{++} > Ca^{++} > Mg^{++}$. It was initially thought that the most hydrated ion would be the first to be affected by dehydration, i.e. the first ion to become dehydrated (Jenny, 1932). It is now known that this is not the what occurs for reasons that will become more obvious once we consider the second proposed selectivity sequence.

2.1.2 The Polarizability Sequence

Bungenberg de Jong (1949) forwarded an alternative explanation for ionic selectivity in 1949 that attributed the selectivity to the polarization of water or the binding site by the ion. Since the smallest ion has the highest charge density, ions like Li^+, F^-, and Mg^{++} have the highest relative ability to polarize (orient) the charge on a dipole (e.g. water). Hence, the polarizing sequences are in the exact order of the atomic radii of the monovalent and divalent cations and anions. The result of these two original considerations of how ionic selectivity sequences arise predicts that only Li^+ or Cs^+ would be the most preferred ion under any circumstances. We know this is not the case since K^+ and Ca^{++} channels abound in nature from protozoa to metazoans (Na^+ channels are of metazoan origin). How do these other selectivity sequences arise and what forces are responsible for their occurrence in organic and inorganic matter? The present understanding for the occurrence of a finite set of 'transition' sequences was provided by George Eisenman's investigations using aluminosilicate glass electrodes (reviewed in Eisenman and Horn, 1983).

2.1.3 The Transitional Sequences

Despite the possibility that N! sequences can exist, only a few are commonly observed (seven or eleven). The first sequence always corresponds to the lyotropic sequence and the last sequence in the series for the alkali cations, earth divalent cations, and halide anions always corresponds with the polarizability sequence described above. The intervening sequences, called the 'transitional' sequences, do not have only the smallest or the largest ion of each group as the preferred species. For instance, K^+ channels may correspond to a sequence IV, V or VI while a Na^+ channel may correspond to sequences VII through X. Calcium channels require additional considerations to impart divalent over monovalent selectivity (e.g. two closely spaced cation-binding sites, Diamond and Wright, 1969), but nonetheless correspond to sequences III through VI for the alkaline-earth cations. So what does this have to do with gap junction channels? The same rules will apply and it will depend on the extent to which the permeant ions are hydrated as they pass through the gap junction channel pore. So it follows that we must consider the mechanisms which determine these series of selectivity sequences.

2.2 Mechanisms for Ionic Selectivity

As portrayed in the general definition of a gap junction channel, ions readily pass since they are considerably smaller in diameter than known permeant molecules of 400 to 900 daltons (or 10 to 14 Å in diameter). Hence, the ionic selectivity should be considerably less than the modest charge selectivity observed for large permeant molecules. This is an oversimplification of the interactions that determine the above mentioned selectivity sequences and implies that only lyotropic sequences would be expected to be observed for gap junction channels given their large diameters. There is even more to consider when a channel is permeable to both cations and anions, as gap junction channels are reported to be, and there are only three published models for anion:cation selectivity presently in existence (Borisova et al., 1986; Zambrowicz and Colombini, 1993; Franciolini and Nonner, 1994a,b). Of these three, only one of these models incorporates a central aqueous cylinder within the pore where the ions can electrodiffuse in proportion to their aqueous diffusion coefficients. These models will be considered later in this chapter.

A weak anionic site that selects slightly for cations over anions was suggested by the pioneering gap junction molecular permeability studies (Flagg-Newton et al., 1979; Brink and Dewey, 1980). However, ionic binding sites within gap junction (or more precisely connexin) channel pores were not proposed until the complete alkali cation selectivity sequences for connexin43 and connexin40 were reported by Wang and Veenstra (1997) and Beblo and Veenstra (1997). The first estimates of the physical dimensions of a selectivity filter for a gap junction channel were also obtained from these monovalent cation relative permeability sequences. These findings will be compared to the three existing models for ion permeation through cation and anion permeable channels later in this chapter. Let us first consider further the mechanisms for steric hindrance and binding affinity.

The selection of permeant molecules on the basis of physical size alone we will refer to as 'steric hindrance'. A second mechanism for selectivity involves preferences of related substrates for a specific site or the 'binding affinity' of the ion for the site. Binding sites that result in the observed ionic selectivity of known biological ion channels are more commonly referred to as the 'selectivity filter' of the channel. Selectivity filters for many cation and anion channels have been identified through ionic permeability studies and subsequent structure-function analysis of previously identified pore-forming domains (Galzi et al., 1992; Tomaselli et al., 1993; Ellinor et al., 1995). Definitive structural models depicting the three-dimensional spatial organization of critical amino acid residues that form the selectivity filter of a particular channel are still forthcoming although the conceptual framework for constructing them already exists.

2.2.1 Steric Hindrance

The term steric hindrance implies a physical impediment that separates one molecule from another by its mere presence even though the barrier may not recognize the same locus (pore or site) as the substrate. This is typically less frequent than one might expect, but it forms an essentially insurmountable (absolute) barrier when present. Steric effects involve non-coulomb forces (not involving charge) and are mediated primarily by the relative physical dimensions of, for example, the ion and the pore, and the rigidity of the imposed structure (e.g. the wall of the pore and the crystalline radius of the ion). In the case of two ions where one blocks the other by being impermeant or significantly less permeant, the frequency and order of their occurrence at a common locus is also relevant to the net flux of the ion. For aqueous pores, molecular sieving of the hydrated ion is relevant and results in effectively reducing the mobility of the ion (Levitt, 1991).

2.2.2 Affinity Binding

The term binding affinity implies a mutual attraction between two molecules or a molecule for a site. The primary determinant of the binding affinity is the difference in free energy of the ion for water relative to the site. The difference in free energies largely depends on the electrostatic forces involved in the interactions of the ion with water and the binding site. When these interactions are between two fixed-point charges (non-inducible dipoles), the strength of the coulomb forces decreases as the square of the distance between the ion and the site (Diamond and Wright, 1969). Hence, local concentration of the ion is also important in these intermolecular interactions. Ion selectivity implies the preference of a given site for one ion over another. The selectivity of the site is, therefore, relative in regards to the two competing ions. If ΔG_{ion} = ΔG_{site} - ΔG_{water}, then it follows that $\Delta G_{ion\ A}$ - $\Delta G_{ion\ B}$ provides the difference in free energy between the two ions. At low field strengths, the above equation is dominated by the ΔG_{water} terms and at high electrostatic field strengths the equation is dominated by the ΔG_{site} terms for each ion.

Ionic field strength and the water content of the pore affect the electrostatic forces at distance x from the fixed site. Conventionally, the selectivity of a pore for a series of ions is expressed as the ratio of the ionic permeabilities for two ions calculated from the biionic reversal potential using the Goldman-Hodgkin-Katz (GHK) equation. This form of selectivity measurement is based on the equilibrium established between two ions with oppositely directed electrochemical potentials. Equilibrium selectivity theory has the advantage of not being influenced by kinetic considerations of ion permeation (i.e. channel conductance, Ellinor et al., 1995; Hess et al., 1986). Selectivity can also be modeled as alternating energy barriers and wells that represent the selectivity barriers and binding sites within the pore with which the ion must interact en route (Eisenman and Horn, 1983). The kinetic rate constants for an ion are proportional to the energy difference between the barrier height and the site depth, which vary for different ions.

Alternatively, ions can be modeled to diffuse continuously through a pore rather than by discrete steps using Poisson-Nernst-Planck (PNP) electrodiffusion theory and a mean field approximation of the internal charge within a pore of fixed volume (Nonner and Eisenberg, 1998). All of these approaches are model-dependent and are subject to error (McClesky, 1999). Equilibrium selectivity does not account for ion-ion or ion-site interactions that occur in multi-ion single file (long) pores. Barrier models require more specific information and may be subject to error if the barriers (or sites) vary depending on the state of occupancy for a site. PNP theory integrates all of the channel properties into a single compartment that relies on an average field strength for its calculations. Hence, all ion permeation models require further verification by direct electrophysiological and/or structure-function analysis. The inherent assumption of ionic independence from equilibrium selectivity theory is not likely to be valid for channels that are permeable to both cations and anions since the likelihood of ion-ion interactions is enhanced unless the ions remain fully hydrated. Given the lack of channel conductance and permeability properties and specific structural information about gap junction channels to date, each offers a perspective view of an ion channel that may benefit gap junction electrophysiologists in their research (Veenstra, 2000).

3 GAP JUNCTION CHANNEL PERMEABILITY

Ionic permeability ratios were performed on many plasmalemmal ion channels as early as 1973 on the sodium current from the frog node of Ranvier (Hille, 1973).   The development of the patch clamp recording technique permitted investigators to perform selectivity experiments on single channels, rather than whole cell membrane currents, from native cell membranes or cloned ion channels expressed in *Xenopus* oocytes (Hamill et at., 1981; Mishina et al., 1985; Stühmer et al., 1987). Alternatively, intracellular ion channels can be studied using artificial lipid bilayer reconstitution techniques (Miller, 1978).   Similar conductance and permeability experiments performed on native gap junction channels or connexin-specific channels have been less forthcoming owing mostly to the technical difficulties of either recording from the double membrane gap junction channel using the patch clamp technique or attempting to reconstitute the channels into planar lipid bilayers.   Hence, knowledge about the ionic permeabilities of gap junction channels and their subsequent structure-function relationships is comparatively sparse.   There exist only two published accounts of ionic permeability ratios from native gap junction channels. How this limited experimental data correlates with previous interpretations of the 'generic' gap junction channel based on molecular permeability investigations will now be considered.

3.1 Ionic Permeability Ratios

Bionic reversal potential experiments are more difficult to perform on gap junction channels since they are intercellular channels and are, therefore, not accessible from the extracellular surface of the plasmamembrane.   Indeed, the first accounts of gap junction channel recordings required intracellular recordings from two electrically coupled cells (Neyton and Trautmann, 1985; Veenstra and DeHaan, 1986). Two cell voltage clamp approaches to the recording of net junctional currents existed prior to these dual whole cell patch clamp recordings, but both approaches suffer from the need to modify the intracellular ionic composition of both cells in order to perform the necessary reversal potential experiments. Junctional reversal potential measurements are further hindered by the present knowledge that cells typically express more than one type of gap junction channel and selective blockers necessary to isolate the current of interest were not yet known for gap junction channels. Nonetheless, there are two accounts of ionic permeability ratios from native gap junction channels.

Membrane potential is measured relative to the external ground reference that is taken as 0 mV and assumed to be invariant. Junctional current flows between the interior of two cells and is, by definition, isolated from ground by the input resistance of each cell. Therefore, the measurement of ionic reversal potentials imposed across the junction within a cell pair becomes more difficult to ascertain (Veenstra, 2001). Typically, one side of the channel-containing membrane is exposed to the bath and the bath ground is maintained essentially constant by the use of a chloride salt bridge that minimizes the junction potentials between the bath and the recording reference electrode. Still, the measurement of net junctional current in coupled cell pairs is determined from the baseline whole cell currents obtained when there is no net transjunctional voltage. The zero junctional current ($I_j = 0$) level is readily ascertained under symmetrical ionic conditions, but is not readily defined under biionic conditions (asymmetric pipette solutions, Veenstra 2001). Neyton and Trautmann (1985) reported relative potassium to sodium and potassium to chloride permeability ratios (P_K/P_{Na} and P_K/P_{Cl}) of 1.23 and 1.45 respectively for the rat lacrimal gland gap junction channels. The junctional biionic reversal potential was measured as the voltage applied to the prejunctional cell (cell 1) that was required to make the current in the post-junctional cell (cell 2) equal to zero. This measurement requires knowing the holding current value required to clamp cell 2 to -50 mV in the absence of the biionic- or differential voltage-clamp amplifier-induced transjunctional voltage gradient. Their reported P_K, P_{Na}, and P_{Cl} values of 1.0, 0.81, and 0.69 were consistent with the interpretation of a modest

(<2:1) cation:anion selectivity for a mammalian gap junction channel. This investigation remains the only quantitative estimate of the ionic permeabilities for native mammalian gap junction channels to date.

Brink and Fan (1989) developed a more novel approach to the patch clamp analysis of gap junction channel currents by directly patching onto the septal membrane of the earthworm axon, a large surface area junctional membrane not typically found between mammalian cells. Using a cocktail of ionic blockers to limit nonjunctional membrane currents, a 100 pS monovalent permeant ion channel was isolated. This junctional membrane channel had ionic conductance ratios of $K^+ = 1.0$, $Cs^+ = 1.0$, $Na^+ = 0.84$, $TMA^+ = 0.64$, $Cl^- = 0.52$, and $TEA^+ = 0.20$. These conductance ratios can be equated to ionic permeability ratios if the assumption that $P_{ion} = G_{ion}(RT/F^2[K])$ is valid. This expression is derived from the GHK current equation where G is the conductance of the ion and [K] is the ion (K^+) concentration. The similarity of the relative P_K, P_{Na}, and P_{Cl} values to the previous interpretation of gap junction channels was again consistent with the conventional interpretation of the gap junction channel. In either case, the molecular composition of the junctional channels was not known.

3.2 Molecular (Dye) Permeability Limits

The often stated upper size limit of approximately 1 kD is derived from fluorescent tracer studies performed on native gap junction channels performed during the late 1970's until 1980. Of the numerous investigations performed, only a few provide significant information about the selectivity of gap junction channels. To be precise, the largest molecular tracers known to permeate a mammalian gap junction channel are the multiple glycine conjugates of lissamine rhodamine B-200 (LRB, Flagg-Newton et al., 1979). LRB(glycine)$_6$OH ($M_r = 901$) was permeable in all cultured mammalian cells investigated and LRB(glycine)$_4$OH ($M_r = 859$) was shown to diffuse through mammalian ventricular myocyte gap junctions (Imanaga et al., 1987). It should be noted that the permeability limit decreased with increasing negative charge on the rhodamine or fluorescein dye conjugates (e.g. FITC(glutamate)$_2$OH, M_r = 665 and 6-carboxyfluorescein, M_r = 376), suggestive of fixed negative charge within the gap junction channel pore (Flagg-Newton et al., 1979; Brink and Dewey, 1980; Veenstra et al., 1995). Precise information about the limiting cross sectional area of the gap junction channel pore and its charge selectivity cannot be determined without knowing the cross-sectional area of the tracer molecule and its permeability coefficient relative to other permeant molecules. Furthermore, most published accounts of fluorescent tracer studies were performed independently of junctional conductance measurements in the observed cell pairs or clusters (Veenstra et al., 1995; Veenstra, 1996). Suitable tracer molecules should be membrane impermeant and have little or no cytoplasmic binding, which would falsely increase or decrease the dyes observed junctional permeability (Brink and Ramanan, 1985; Safranyos et al., 1987).

What are the physiological consequences of this molecular permeability to cellular function? Activation of membrane-bound receptors by ligand binding triggers a cytoplasmic cascade of events culminating in modulation of protein kinases or phosphatases and transcription regulatory binding proteins to give only a few general examples. Membrane signal transduction by the generation of physiologically relevant second messengers (e.g. Ca^{++}, cAMP, 1,4,5-inositoltrisphosphate (IP$_3$)) is vital to cellular function and the integration of neurohumoral signals within a tissue is provided by intercellular chemical signaling via gap junctions. There are reports of cell-to-cell transfer of all of these second messengers in the present gap junction literature (Tsien and Weingart, 1976; Saez et al., 1989), although there is increasing evidence that IP$_3$, and not Ca^{++}, is responsible for the propagation of intercellular calcium waves (Sanderson, 1995). Some of these second messengers are also believed to regulate junctional conductance (e.g. cAMP, DeMello, 1991), which is another related area of investigation that has been reviewed elsewhere (Brink, 1991; Veenstra, 1991). The reported acute increase in junctional communication via cAMP-dependent pathways has recently been disputed in mammalian heart preparations and various serine and tyrosine protein kinases regulate gap junction communication in a connexin- and species-specific manner (Jongsma et al., 2000; Lau et al., 2000). Without the spatial and temporal signal averaging that occurs via gap junctions, all cells in a tissue would have to receive identical neurohumoral signals in order to coordinate their functional activity. Hence, direct coupling via gap junctions provide for functional homogeneity and tissue homeostasis. The loss of junctional communication is often associated with developmental defects and cellular transformation (Loewenstein, 1981; Guthrie and Gilula, 1989, Swenson et al., 1990; Réaume et al., 1995). The host of potential permeable molecules could also include a variety of metabolites and enzyme products provided that the molecular permeability limit is in excess of 10 Å and ≈ 1 kD (Hobbie et al., 1989).

4 CONNEXIN-SPECIFIC CHANNEL PERMEABILITY

All of the above investigations were performed on native gap junction channels from mammalian or invertebrate cells. In 1986, the first gap junction channel protein, connexin32 (Cx32; Paul, 1986), was cloned and electrophysiological methodologies for recording unitary gap junction channel currents were developed (Neyton and Trautmann, 1985; Veenstra and DeHaan, 1986; Veenstra, 2001). With sixteen mammalian connexins identified thus far (Beyer and Willecke, 2000), the discussion of ionic and molecular permeabilities of gap junctions now must be considered in the context of the specific proteins expressed rather than the conceptualized version of a generic gap junction channel. The use of expression systems for connexins has contributed new evidence that has begun to advance our understanding of gap junction channels from the cellular to the molecular level (Dahl et al., 1987; Eghbali et al., 1990; Veenstra et al., 1992; Elfgang et al., 1995). Let us reconsider the previous interpretations about gap junction channels in the context of these most recent findings.

4.1 Ionic Permeability

The first approach taken regarding the relative ionic permeabilities of connexin-specific channels was to assess the relative cation:anion selectivity of several connexin channels by substituting glutamate⁻ for Cl⁻ in both patch pipettes and determining the change in unitary channel conductance (γ_j) for four different connexin channels (Veenstra et al., 1995). Given the measured aqueous diffusion coefficient for glutamate⁻, a 33% decrease in γ_j was predicted (Veenstra, 1996). All four cardiovascular connexins examined exhibited decreases in γ_j in excess of the predicted value, indicative of a modest cation:anion selectivity of 2:1 or higher. Hence, hCx37, rCx40, rCx43, cCx43, and rCx45 (r = rat, h = human, c = chicken) all fit this one general interpretation of a gap junction channel. However, the predicted inverse correlation of increasing conductance (i.e. pore diameter) and decreasing ionic selectivity expected for an aqueous pore was not observed. In fact, no correlation between channel conductance and cation:anion selectivity was evident at all. This simply implies that conductance and pore diameter need not be directly correlated, as was already known to be true for ion-selective channels (Hille, 1992), and/or that the connexin γ_j may not be limited by restricted aqueous diffusion alone.

4.2 Differential Dye Permeability

These observations were echoed at the molecular level by the differential dye permeability of these five connexin channels to 2,7-dichlorofluorescein (diCl-F) and 6-carboxyfluorescein (6-CF) (Veenstra et al., 1995). It was striking to note that the highest γ_j channel, hCx37, exhibited only sporadic dye passage while rCx43 (1/3 the γ_j of hCx37) was the only connexin channel to be 100% permeable to both dyes. It should be noted that only the presence or absence of dye transfer was determined following a 10 min recording period to assess the junctional conductance of the cell pair. Still, this was the first investigation that directly determined the junctional conductance of cells in which dye transfer was assayed. Another key advantage of this investigation was the use of two dyes that were structurally similar except for side-chain substitutions to the fluorescein molecule that minimize the physical constraints (i.e. diameter) and maximize the effect of net surface charge (i.e. valence) on the permeability through a connexin channel.

Evidence in support of the differential permeability of connexin-specific channels also came from Hela-transfected cells expressing Cx26, Cx31, Cx32, Cx37, Cx40, Cx43, and Cx45 (Elfgang et al., 1995). Although all connexins were permeable to Lucifer Yellow, a known fluorescent tracer with properties suitable for assaying gap junction permeability (M_r = 443, valence = -2, ≈10 Å diameter), differential dye transfer was noted for the less conventional dyes ethidium bromide, propridium iodide, and DAPI. All of these dyes are cationic and are known to bind to DNA, which may limit their junctional permeability. It is also true that the dye transfer assays were performed by dye microinjection into clusters of connexin-transfected Hela cells so the junctional conductances of the dye-coupled or uncoupled cells were not known. Nonetheless, the data are consistent with a reduced dye permeability of Cx31 and, to a lesser extent, Cx32 to propridium iodide and ethidium bromide relative to the other connexins. There are experimental discrepancies between the above two investigations, particularly regarding the dye permeability of Cx45 to anionic dyes such as Lucifer Yellow that should be investigated further under more closely correlated experimental conditions.

Connexin-specific molecular permeability has likely physiological implications. The intercellular transfer of ^{14}C-labeled metabolites in C6 glioma cells transfected with either Cx43 or Cx32 reportedly differ by 40- to 160-fold in their permeability to ^{14}C-labeled glutamate, glutathione, and ATP or ADP (Goldberg et al., 1999). Glucose was reportedly not permeable through Cx32 gap junctions, in contrast to Cx43 and past gap junction literature on molecular permeability (Brink, 1991; Wang and Veenstra, 1997). Another steady state molecular permeability assay elegantly demonstrated reduced molecular permeability to cAMP, cGMP, and uncharged tri- and tetra-maltose polysaccharides of mouse and rat liver liposomes that correlated with increasing Cx26 content in the presence of Cx32 (Bevans et al., 1998). This study suggests that glucose is readily permeable through Cx32 gap junctions and further demonstrates the possible role of heteromeric gap junction channels in regulating molecular permeability limits. Although these methods are not as quantitative as direct molecular permeability measurements using fluorescent techniques in combination with electrical measurements of junctional conductance, these results are consistent with the hypothesis of connexin-specific gap junction permeability limits (Veenstra et al., 1995).

4.3 Hemichannel Permeability

Although most connexins appear to form functional channels only when paired with connexins from a partner cell, a few cloned connexins are capable of forming hemichannels where the extracellular domain of the connexin opens to the extracellular space. This allows the investigator to study the voltage gating and permeability of the connexin hemichannel. The lens fiber cell connexins, Cx46, Cx50, and Cx56 are capable of forming functional hemichannels. While their physiological function is not known, hemichannels provide a unique opportunity to investigate the ionic permeability of half a gap junction channel. This information will also be useful when considering heterotypic gap junction channels where each hemichannel is formed from a different connexin. These results will also be considered in the context of the homotypic gap junction channel formed from a single connexin.

There are only two such reports of connexin hemichannel permeability ratios. Subsequent to the ionic permeability experiments performed on rCx43, rCx40, and others as mentioned above and to be presented in more detail later in this chapter, biionic reversal potential measurements were performed on Cx46 hemichannels expressed in *Xenopus* oocytes (Trexler et al., 1996). They found the monovalent cation sequence to follow the aqueous mobility sequence for the alkali cations (minus Rb^+) and the tetraalkylammonium ions tetramethylammonium (TMA) and tetraethylammonium (TEA). This corresponds to a selectivity sequence I or II. The P_X/P_K ratios were: Cs^+, 1.19; K^+, 1.00; Na^+, 0.80; Li^+, 0.64; TMA^+, 0.34; and TEA^+, 0.20. The two-fold lower permeability ratios for TMA^+ and TEA^+ relative to Li^+ suggest additional factors (i.e. pore diameter) may be involved in reducing their permeability, although an estimate of pore diameter was not made from these data (see Figure 1). These values were based on a P_K/P_{Cl} value of 10.3 and a P_{TEA}/P_{Cl} value of 2.8 as determined from asymmetric KCl and KCl:TEACl salt gradients. Anionic reversal potentials for Cl^-, Br^-, NO_3^-, and acetate$^-$ were not reported. The inherent difficulty of measuring relative permeability ratios of a channel that is permeable to monovalent anions and cations will be discussed later in this chapter.

The *Xenopus* oocyte possesses an endogenous connexin38 (Cx38) that also forms a functional hemichannel (Zhang et al., 1998). The P_X/P_K ratios were: Na^+, 0.99; TEA^+, 0.35; $NMDG^+$, 0.45; TPA^+, 0.20; and TBA^+, 0.20. The P_{Cl}/P_K ratio was 0.24 and the $P_{gluconate}/P_K$ was 0.20. The higher Na^+, TEA^+, and Cl^- permeability ratios suggest that the Cx38 hemichannel is larger and/or less selective than Cx46. Hydrodynamic estimates of the pore sizes based on the measured P_X/P_K ratios and hydrated radii of the monovalent cations were 8.1 ± 1.0 Å for Cx38 and 5.5 ± 0.6 Å for Cx46 (Veenstra, 2000 and Figure 1).

4.4 Heterotypic Connexin Channel Permeability

Every connexin cloned to date is capable of forming heterotypic junctions with at least one other connexin (White and Bruzzone, 1996). It is not known if heterotypic junctions occur naturally in native cell types, but expression systems permit the investigator to determine if two connexins can couple when brought into contact with one another. This also provides insight into how two connexins interact to form a functional channel, namely, whether each connexin maintains its intrinsic properties or not. Cx26/Cx32

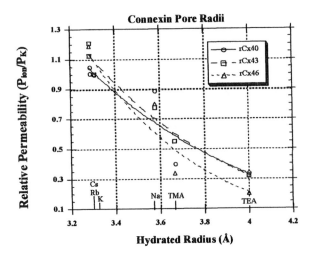

Figure 1. Relative ionic permeability ratios for rCx40, rCx43, and rCx46 (Trexler et al., 1996; Wang and Veenstra, 1997; Beblo and Veenstra, 1997). Curved lines are the theoretical fit of the permeability data by the hydrodynamic equation (Dwyer et al., 1980). Estimates of pore radii in Å are: Cx40, 6.6±0.9; Cx43, 6.3±0.4, and Cx46, 5.5±0.6. Hydrated ionic radii as reported by Nightingale (1959).

heterotypic pairs were one of the first combinations tested and produced some unique conductance properties not found in the homotypic channels of Cx26 or Cx32. While the voltage gating properties of the heterotypic pair were attributed to the opposite polarity of their transjunctional gating mechanisms, the channel conductance and permeability properties are less well understood. The Cx26/Cx32 channel has a nonlinear conductance with respect to transjunctional voltage similar to the instantaneous junctional current-voltage relationship observed in *Xenopus* oocytes (Barrio et al., 1991; Bukauskas et al., 1995). Mutation of a single amino acid residue in the N-terminal cytoplasmic domain (Cx32N2D or Cx26D2N) appeared to alter transjunctional voltage-gating polarity (- to + or + to -, respectively) as evidenced by the current-voltage relationships (Verselis et al., 1994). The voltage sensor was thought to be formed by two residues at the M1-E1 border on the opposite side of the membrane (ES in most connexins, KE in Cx26) since the reciprocal mutations alter the kinetics and sensitivity of the transjunctional voltage-dependent inactivation of current (and conductance). The opposite polarity of the voltage gate for Cx26 and Cx32 (D2 or N2) can explain the rectifying instantaneous junctional current-voltage relationship for the Cx26/Cx32 channel. The similarity of the single channel Cx26/Cx32 I-V relationship lead Bukauskas et al. (1995) to propose that the rectifying I-V is due to the asymmetric voltage-sensitivity of the channel open state that are not predicted from the homotypic connexin channels.

In what began as a collaborative effort to investigate the channel properties of the Cx26P87L mutant gap junction, we also investigated the properties of the heterotypic Cx26/Cx32 gap junction channels (Suchyna et al., 1993). Our homotypic Cx26 and Cx32 γ_j values were nearly identical to those reported by Bukauskas et al. (1995) and the heterotypic single channel I-V curve also rectified in the same manner (Suchyna et al., 1999). In addition to the above experiments, however, we performed the glutamate$^-$ for Cl$^-$ substitutions described above for Cx43, etc. and estimated their relative cation:anion selectivity (Veenstra et al., 1995; Veenstra, 1996). From these results, we concluded that Cx26 and Cx32 also have opposite ionic selectivities (Suchyna et al., 1999). Cx26 favors cations by $\approx$2:1 while Cx32 is slightly anionic ($\approx$1.0:1.1). Specific ionic conductances were calculated for Cx26 and Cx32 from the homotypic γ_j values and the estimated cation:anion selectivities for each connexin. I-V relations for the heterotypic Cx26/Cx32 channel were calculated using the unidirectional flux equations and by equating ionic conductance and permeability according to the assumption $P_{ion} = G_{ion}(RT/F^2(z_{ion})^2[ion])$. The results are summarized in Figure 2 where the homotypic Cx26, homotypic Cx32, and heterotypic Cx26/Cx32 channel I-V relations are plotted in 115 mM Kglutamate pipette solutions.

It is apparent upon visual inspection that the conductance of the hybrid channel asymptotes towards the conductance of one connexin hemichannel or another depending on the voltage polarity (negative transjunctional voltage = Cx26 cell negative for Figure 2).   The results illustrate one model that describes the asymmetric rectification of a heterotypic gap junction channel based on the intrinsic ionic permeability properties of each connexin to one hemichannel of the junction.   While there are further experimental tests of the model that should be performed, this experimental evidence provides an alternative explanation to the asymmetry of the instantaneous   I-V of the Cx26/Cx32 channel. It should be noted that channel activity was altered in an asymmetric manner across the junction (Suchyna et al., 1999). Figure 2 represents the simplest approach to modeling heterotypic gap junction channels, but it presents the essential concept that rectification results from asymmetric conductance and permeability properties of an asymmetric channel even under symmetrical ionic conditions.   It also illustrates that ion-ion interactions, such as the flux coupling modeled here, further increase the rectification. It should also be noted that modeling each hemichannel is not necessarily valid since all experimental measurements were made on homotypic or heterotypic Cx26 and Cx32 gap junctions.

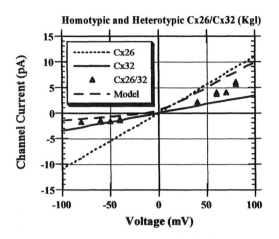

Figure 2. Single channel current-voltage relationships for homotypic Cx26/26, homotypic Cx32/32, and heterotypic Cx26/32 channels in 115 mM Kglutamate (Kgl). Conductance of the Cx26 channel was 110 pS and 35 pS for Cx32. The heterotypic channel has a nonlinear I-V as illustrated by the data points (▲). The dashed line is a theoretical fit of the data derived by calculating the unidirectional fluxes for the homotypic Cx26/26 and Cx32/32 channels according to the following equations for each

$$\overrightarrow{I_{ion}} = P_{ion}\frac{z_{ion}F^2}{RT}E\frac{[ion]_1}{1-\exp\left(-z_{ion}FEn\big/_{RT}\right)} \quad \text{and} \quad \overleftarrow{I}_{ion} = P_{ion}\frac{z_{ion}F^2}{RT}E\frac{[ion]_2}{1-\exp\left(z_{ion}FEn\big/_{RT}\right)}$$

ion where 1 = cell 1, 2 = cell 2, and n = flux coupling coefficient (= 4 for the fitted line). The ionic permeability (P_{ion}) was determined from the channel conductance using the GHK current equation and the relation $P_{ion} = g_{ion} \times RT/F^2$. The cation:anion selectivities of the Cx26/26 and Cx32/32 channel were assumed to be 2.6:1.0 and 0.94:1.0 respectively (Veenstra, 1996; Suchyna et al., 1999). For the heterotypic channel the P_{ion} values of Cx26 were assigned to one unidirectional flux ($\overrightarrow{I}_{ion}$) and the P_{ion} values of Cx32 were assigned to the opposite unidirectional flux ($\overleftarrow{I}_{ion}$). $P_{ion} = (D_{ion} \bullet \beta_{ion})/l$ by thermodynamic definition and β_{ion}/l was assumed to equal one since the channel was assumed to be aqueous and the partition coefficient (β) into the membrane will equal the energy required to travel the length (l) of the channel pore.

Two new observations regarding the Cx46 hemichannel also suggest that charges on opposite sides of the membrane alter the rectification of a connexin channel (Trexler et al., 2000). Replacing the first extracellular loop of Cx46 with that from Cx32 replaces two acidic (D51 and E62) with neutral (S50 and N61) amino acids at these loci and converts the channel rectification from inward to outward under symmetrical 100 mM KCl conditions. As expected for a symmetrical channel, the Cx46 homotypic gap junction channel does not rectify since the charges on both sides of the channel are identical. These wild type and chimeric Cx46 hemichannels demonstrate that asymmetric charge profiles indeed produce rectification in the expected direction with a decrease in negative charge on the extracellular side of the membrane. From Teorell (1953), the rectification ratio under symmetrical ionic conditions is equal to the Donnan ratio for the two sides of the membrane (= 1 for a gap junction channel). This was modeled for the heterotypic Cx26/Cx32 channel where the Donnan ratio was estimated for a homotypic channel by comparing the ohmic conductances of each homotypic channel under symmetrical KCl and Kglutamate conditions (Veenstra, 1996; Suchyna et al., 1999). A native hemichannel provides the unique opportunity to compare the Donnan ratio from the cytoplasmic side to the central extracellular compartment of a homotypic gap junction channel, although this was not conducted on the Cx46 hemi- and gap junction channel preparation. This approach could lead to a more complete model for homotypic and heterotypic gap junction channels as was attempted with Cx26 and Cx32 and outlined in more detail in Veenstra (2000). Trexler et al. (2000) also observed that the reversal potential of the wild-type Cx46 hemichannel continued to increase with increasing intracellular [KCl] but not extracellular [KCl] above 400 mM, indicative of a selectivity filter between the cytoplasmic and extracellular sides of the Cx46 channel. The extracellular site would appear to be saturated near 400 mM KCl, an observation that would be readily altered by altering the Donnan potential on the extracellular side of the channel.

5 MECHANISMS OF ION PERMEATION

The details of ion permeation through ion-selective channels are being elucidated by site-directed mutagenesis of pore-forming residues and critical sites for ion binding within the pore are being identified. Already, key residues involved in determining whether two highly homologous proteins form a Na^+ or Ca^{++} channel are known. Furthermore, recent models directly impact on a previous two-site model developed from important Ca^{++} channel conductance and permeability data from the previous decade (Hess et al., 1986). The originally proposed two-site, three-barrier model relied on electrostatic repulsion between two Ca^{++} ions separated by ≈ 10 Å to produce high rates of Ca^{++} flux. Present models now suggest that four glutamate residues form a single high affinity site and the increased divalent current is due to competition between like ligands for a single site (Ellinor et al., 1995; Dang and McClesky 1998; Nonner and Eisenberg, 1998). The high divalent ion affinity effectively blocks any monovalent cation current and the apparent low affinity of the conducting divalent channel can be due either to repulsion (increased energy) or steps in potential energy (lower energy). This model is consistent with all previous permeability and conductance data on the L-type calcium channel and is supported by data from other divalent cation-binding proteins (Matthews and Weaver, 1974). Permeation models developed from other ion channels may assist us as we continue our investigations into the permeability properties of connexin-mediated gap junction channels.

5.1 Independent Electrodiffusion

The GHK current and voltage equations all assume that ions move through the pore independently of other ions. For long, single-file (narrow multi-ion) pores, this assumption does not hold (Hille, 1992). Electrodiffusion theory has accounted for ion-ion interactions within the pore by introducing a flux-coupling coefficient to the flux-ratio equation. To experimentally test this theory, one must perform tracer flux experiments measuring both efflux and influx independently, a difficult task (Stampe and Begenisich, 1996). Conventionally, equilibrium selectivity theory is applied to biionic permeability ratios and mole-fraction effects on conductance are employed to determine ion-ion interactions within the pore. If two different ions are competing for a single site within the pore, the reversal potential can accurately reflect the relative affinity of the site for the two ions under biionic conditions. On other occasions, ionic permeability ratios cannot be determined using the GHK voltage equation. This is frequently the case for channels that are permeable to both cations and anions since electrostatic attraction within a restricted space is favored and the binding energies for a fixed electrostatic site will be oppositely-directed. This adds another dimension of complexity to the measurement of ionic permeabilities unless impermeant counterions can be used. There are three examples in the literature that explores the cation:anion selectivity of three different ion channels. In all cases, non-compliance with constant field theory occurred due to ion-dependent permeabilities.

5.2 Ion-dependent Counterion Permeability

Ionic permeability ratios that are dependent on the concentration of a different ion can are consistent with ion-ion interactions within a pore. I would like to summarize three examples of ion channels that exhibit ionic permeabilities that cannot be accounted for by the GHK equation and the models presented to account for these results. In some cases, the cation:anion reversal potential does not follow the GHK relationship with varying ionic gradients and in other cases the cation:anion permeability ratio cannot be calculated using the GHK equation.

5.2.1 Large Channel Theory

VDAC is a voltage-dependent anion channel found in the outer mitochondrial membrane (Zambrowicz and Colombini, 1993). It is estimated to form an aqueous pore approximately 3 nm in diameter and 5 nm in length. As is expected for a large diameter aqueous pore, any ionic selectivity was not presumed to be due to specific binding sites but rather electrostatic interactions between (partially) hydrated ions and the wall of the channel. It is widely accepted that electrostatic interactions are concentration-dependent and are strongest at low ionic strength. Hence, measuring the concentration-dependence of the cation:anion reversal potential provides a direct test of this facet of the Large Channel Theory (LCT, Zambrowicz and Colombini, 1993). The two essential features of the VDAC permeability are that (i) the cation:anion reversal potential deviates from linearity as the KCl gradient increases above 5-fold and (ii) the KCl reversal potential decreases with increasing concentration (constant KCl gradient of 2.0). Neither of these observations fit with GHK theory and was indicative of concentration-dependent permeability ratios. A third test is to measure the cation:anion reversal potential using salts with different aqueous mobilities. Whereas GHK theory predicts changes in the reversal potential, LCT predicts less change in the biionic reversal potential than expected from the mobility difference between the cations and anions.

The essential feature of the LCT theory is that the pore forms two compartments (Figure 3A). An outer compartment lining the wall of the channel where electrostatic interactions attract permeant ions and reduce their permeability through the channel. This screening of electrostatic charge along the pore wall creates a central aqueous compartment where ions can electrodiffuse through the channel without interacting with the wall of the channel. This screening is more effective at higher ionic strength, thus reducing the cation:anion reversal potential of the channel. The pore diameter and amount of electrostatic charge is critical to this theory since the diameter must be sufficient to allow ions to screen the pore wall and create a central cylinder still sufficient in diameter to allow other ions to electrodiffuse with minimal interaction. Concentration-dependent anion:cation reversal potentials using salts with similar or different aqueous mobilities provide an experimental test of this hypothesis.

5.2.2 Counterion-dependent Bidirectional Flux

A different observation was made on the model channel formed by the polyene antibiotic, amphotericin B (Borisova et al., 1986). This compound aligns in an end-to-end fashion between the inner and outer membrane leaflets to form a continuous pore of ≈ 8 Å in diameter across the membrane. Again, the cation:anion selectivity is less than an order of magnitude (<1:10). A striking difference between this anion channel and VDAC is that the cation permeability was not observed to be concentration-dependent, but rather dependent on the sum of the monovalent permeant anions on both sides of the membrane. The anion permeability, however, is independent of the monovalent cation concentration. The key experimental test of their hypothesis involved the use of impermeant divalent ions (Mg^{++}, SO_4^{2-}) in combination with permeant monovalent cations and anions. They derived an equation resembling the GHK voltage equation where the cation:anion permeability ratio, $r_{ca} = L_{ca}([A_1] + [A_2])$, thus replacing P_c/P_a in the normal GHK equation. In the above modified relative permeability coefficient expression, a = anion, c = cation, [A] is the concentration of anions 1 and 2 respectively, and L_{ca} = the cation:anion selectivity coefficient as determined by the expression $L = \alpha_c/\beta_a[(\beta_c/v)+2]$. The terms α, β, and v are model-dependent rate constants for the entry rate (α) of an ion to an electrostatic site, release rate (β) of the same ion from the site, and the rate of cation c and anion a trading places at the same site.

The essential feature of the permeation model for the amphotericin B channel is that there is a site that selects highly for anions and does not allow a cation to pass unless a permeant anion is also present (Figure 3B). In other words, the cation permeability of the channel is observed only in the presence of a permeant anion. An anion may occupy this site alone and binds to or dissociates from this site with rate constants α_a and β_a. A cation can bind to and dissociate from the anion-bound site with rate constants α_c and β_c. The cation:anion pair can also exchange places at the site in an electroneutral manner with rate constant v. If the site is anion-selective, α_c is rate limited by α_a and β_a is rate limited by β_c since a cation cannot occupy the site alone. Hence, $L = \alpha_c/\beta_a[(\beta_c/v)+2]$. This model can be tested experimentally by examining the counterion-dependent or -independent permeability ratios using the modified GHK equation. These permeability coefficients will also be constant for a given cation-anion pair, in sharp contrast to the LCT theory. It is possible that the permeability ratios could be concentration-dependent if α_a is concentration-dependent, which is only likely if the site is accessible to the bulk solution. The distinguishing characteristic of this model is that the permeability of one ion is dependent on the presence of a permeant counterion whereas the reciprocal relationship is not true.

5.2.3 Counterion-dependent Unidirectional Flux

The data for the third permeation model comes from a background Cl⁻ channel found in nerve and skeletal muscle (Franciolini and Nonner, 1994a, b). This channel had been previously found to be permeable to Na^+ and even large organic cations (Franciolini and Nonner, 1987). Again, the cation permeability was < 1:10 relative to Cl⁻ (0.1-0.35). Originally thought to be a cation-dependent anion channel, this channel exhibited some uniquely interesting characteristics. First, substitution of Na^+ with a large organic cation had a minimal effect on channel conductance (Franciolini and Nonner, 1994a). Biionic cation:Cl⁻ reversal potentials demonstrated that even a large divalent cation, bis-tris-propane (BTP), was permeable through this channel. Second, substitution of Cl⁻ or Br⁻ with the larger and less permeable propionate produced smaller changes in the Na^+:anion reversal potential than expected from GHK, and the shift was in the opposite direction, indicating a reduced cation permeability in the presence of less permeable anions. Third, the channel was blocked by large hydrophobic cations (benzyltrimethylammonium, BTMA) and anions (9-anthracene carboxylic acid, 9-ACA), but not by the small hydrophobic anion benzoate. Again the anion channel was not permeable to divalent anions (SO_4^{2-}). So the data suggests a lyotropic sequence for the permeant monovalent anions and a hydrophobic moiety as well. Furthermore, the cation permeability sequence ($Li^+ \approx Cs^+ > K^+ \approx Na^+$) does not correspond to any of the transitional selectivity sequences. Franciolini and Nonner (1994b) interpreted these results as suggestive of a large diameter aqueous pore with only weak electrostatic groups and a strong hydrophobic site. This molecular model for ion permeation is similar to the previous model in so far as they propose that a single permeable anion may bind to a site while transiting through the pore while the permeable cation must associate with the bound anion at the site. The difference is that the cation can only dissociate from the site and pass on through the pore by associating with a permeant anion (Figure 3C). This can explain the anion-dependence of the cation permeability and the minimal effect of cation substitution on the channel conductance for a common anion. Hence, the two models involving ion-pairing at a site within the pore are mutually exclusive and can be distinguished by the direction of the cation:anion reversal potential measurements (Borisova et al., 1986; Franciolini and Nonner, 1994a). In their permeation model, they predicted the pore to be ≈7 Å in diameter and 15 Å in length with an anion-binding site that senses 56% of the transmembrane voltage.

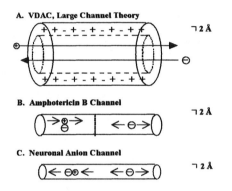

Figure 3. Illustrations of three different mechanisms for cation and anion permeation through a common pore. **A,** Diagrammatic representation of the 30 Å by 50 Å mitochondrial voltage-dependent anion channel (VDAC) channel and the Large Channel Theory for ion permeation (Zambrowicz and Colombini, 1993). Electrostatic charge associated with the wall of the pore attracts ions of opposite charge creating an outer shell of ions within the pore. This alters the electrostatic profile of the central pore compartment whereby ions (K$^+$ and Cl$^-$ drawn to scale) can diffuse down their electrochemical gradient. **B,** Channels formed by polyene antibiotics are 8 Å in diameter and do not possess fixed charges. Nonetheless, anions are readily permeable while cations can produce a counter flux only when a permeant anion is present (Borisova et al., 1986). **C,** A similar mechanism is proposed for the 7 Å diameter neuronal Cl$^-$ channel except that the cation reversal potentials shift in the opposite direction of their mobilities and are correlated with the anion permeability (Franciolini and Nonner, 1994a, b). The anion-dependent cation permeability is consistent with an occasional cation-anion pair transiting through the pore.

5.3 Connexin Channel Cation/Anion Permeability

The observation that most connexin channels were slightly cationic (2:1 - 10:1 cation:anion selectivity) prompted us to examine the ionic permeabilities of homotypic connexin channels in more detail in order to elucidate the selectivity sequence for the monovalent cations and anions. For this purpose, we chose two related connexins that varied in their relative cation:anion selectivity by a factor of two, rat Cx43 and Cx40. Cx43 was of primary interest since it is expressed in a greater variety of tissues than any other cloned connexin and because it appears to be less selective as demonstrated by its low relative cation:anion permeability ratio and highest permeability to fluorescent dyes (Veenstra et al., 1995; Veenstra, 1996). These two connexins are also of interest since they are coexpressed in the mammalian heart and vasculature (Gros and Jongsma, 1996). Cx43 and Cx40 were previously thought to be atypical of other coexpressed connexins due to their inability to form heterotypic gap junctions when expressed in *Xenopus* oocytes (White and Bruzzone, 1996). However, Cx43 and Cx40 were recently observed to form heterotypic gap junctions between pairs of mammalian cells expressing homomeric Cx40 and Cx43 hemichannels (Valiunas et al., 2000). Our approach has been to characterize the conductance and permeability properties of the homotypic Cx43 and Cx40 gap junctions prior to attempting to understand the heterotypic conformation. The results of our ionic permeability investigations are summarized below and presented in the context of the favored model for cation and anion permeation based on our observations and the above previous three examples of distinct cation and anion permeable channels.

5.3.1 Connexin43

Previously we had estimated the rCx43 cation:anion selectivity ratio to be 0.77 based on equimolar substitution of Cl⁻ by glutamate⁻ (Veenstra, 1996). To further elucidate the mechanism for this modest selectivity, we performed conductance and permeability ratio experiments on the rCx43 channel using the alkali metal cations and the tetraalkylammonium organic cations

(Wang and Veenstra, 1997). The monovalent cationic γ_j and permeability ratios were in close agreement both in the magnitude of the ratios and the order of the selectivity sequence. For the alkali cations, the equilibrium selectivity sequence was $Rb^+ \geq Cs^+ > K^+ > Na^+ \geq Li^+ > TMA^+ > TEA^+$. This corresponded to a series II sequence and was not indicative of a high affinity cation binding site within the pore. The most significant deviation from the aqueous mobility sequence occurred with Li^+, whose aqueous mobility in bulk solution is lower than that of Na^+ and TMA^+. This discrepancy in the ionic γ_j ratios was modeled using the Levitt approximation for the relative reduction (D_x) in the aqueous diffusion coefficient (D_o) based on frictional drag of water molecules associated with the permeant ion within a pore of limited diameter (Levitt, 1991). This effect was most pronounced for Li^+ since it is the most hydrated ion (Wang and Veenstra, 1997).

More importantly, a direct measure of the cation:anion permeability ratio was obtained using an asymmetric LiCl salt gradient using impermeant sugars (e.g. raffinose) to maintain osmotic balance between the two cells (Wang and Veenstra, 1997). Surprizingly, this yielded a P_{Cl}/P_K value of 0.13, or a cation:anion selectivity of $\approx$ 8:1. Hence, estimation of relative permeabilities based on aqueous diffusion theory appears to underestimate the selectivity of the rCx43 channel. This could be true if stronger ion-site and cation-anion interactions are occurring within the pore (i.e. ionic independence principal is violated). Ionic conductance ratio and permeability ratios should be performed on a homotypic and subsequent heterotypic gap junction channel to estimate the potential contributions of Donnan potentials and internal pore chemical potentials to the net permeation of cations and anions through a connexin gap junction channel (Veenstra, 2000).

Opposing viewpoints suggest that that there may not be separate sites for both partitioning and binding, as in the mean field approximations inherent to PNP theory that others have used to model the rectification of Cx46 hemichannels (Nonner and Eisenberg 1998; Trexler et al., 2000). These same authors also dispute the Cx43 P_{Cl}/P_K ratio of 0.13, but used different methods for maintaining osmotic balance and determining the reversal potential between the two cells. A comparison of the methods used to obtain these measurements is needed to resolve this reported discrepancy. Our own observations of a nearly neutral chloride/glutamate conductance ratio originally lead us to believe that Cx43 was essentially electroneutral. Under similar ionic conditions, another report of an identical 17 mV reversal potential value for Cx43 gap junctions substantiates our original measurements, although the calculated P_{Cl}/P_K ratio of 0.25 differs by a factor of 2 from our own estimate (Sokolova et al., 2001). The contributions of the other monovalent ions were only estimated in the most recent calculation rather than individually calculated as previously reported.

Even more surprising were the relative anionic permeability measurements. Asymmetric KCl:Kanion equilibrium reversal potential experiments produced anionic reversal potentials of the same magnitude as those observed for the monovalent cations. This is not expected, according to the GHK voltage equation, if the anionic flux is less than 1/8th that of K^+. The anionic reversal potential and permeability ratios are listed in Table 1.

Calculation of the relative P_{anion}/P_{Cl} permeability ratios, while taking into account all of the permeant ions and their relative permeability coefficients, required dividing all of the cationic concentration terms by 135 mM, which is equivalent to the total monovalent cation concentration of the IPS. The exact equation

$$E_{rev} = \frac{RT}{zF} \ln \left| \frac{P_K([K]_1/135) + P_{Cs}([Cs]_1/135) + P_{Na}([Na]_1/135) + P_{TEA}([TEA]_1/135) + P_{Cl}[Cl]_2 + P_Y[Y]_2}{P_K([K]_2/135) + P_{Cs}([Cs]_2/135) + P_{Na}([Na]_2/135) + P_{TEA}([TEA]_2/135) + P_{Cl}[Cl]_1 + P_Y[Y]_1} \right|$$

used was:
where 1= cell 1, 2 = cell 2, Y = substitute anion, $P_K = 1.35$, $P_{Na} = 1.05$, $P_{Cs} = 1.53$, and $P_{TEA} = 0.43$ (relative to $P_{Li} = 1.0$; Wang and Veenstra, 1997). Although empirically derived for the ionic conditions used on the rCx43 channel, this equation is analogous to the one derived by Borisova et al. (1986) where $L_{ac} = 1$ and P_{Cl} and P_Y are multiplied by ($[K^+] + [Na^+] + [Cs^+] + [TEA^+] = 135$). Hence, our solution to the anionic reversal potential measurements

requires the same assumption made for the amphotericin B channel except that it is the anion that must pair with one bound cation at the site in order to permeate through the rCx43 pore. This hypothesis for cation:anion selective permeability in the rCx43 channel can be examined experimentally to distinguish between this model and the other two alternative models for cation:anion permeability.

Table 1. Cx43 Relative Anion Reversal Potential and Permeability Measurements

Ion	N	Mean E_{rev} (mV)	Measured E_{rev} (mV)	P_{ion}	Calculated E_{rev} (mV)	γ_j Ratio
Br⁻	4	-0.9 ± 1.2	-1.5	1.08	-1.5	1.08
Cl⁻	--	-----	-----	1.00	-----	1.00
Acetate⁻	4	+3.8 ± 0.5	+3.6	0.85	+3.6	0.79
Glutamate⁻	3	+13.2 ± 1.2	+13.1	0.52	+13.1	0.63

N = number of cell pairs.
Mean E_{rev} = statistical mean from N experiments ± S.D.
Measured E_{rev} = value obtained from pooled data from N experiments.
Calculated E_{rev} = value from modified GHK voltage equation.
γ_j ratio = unitary channel conductance ratios obtained using symmetrical solutions.

The rCx43 γ_j was observed to increase nonlinearly when increasing KCl from 115 mM to 140 mM in subsequent experiments. Based on the above hypothesis of a cation-binding site within the pore, γ_j was determined for varying KCl concentrations in the absence of other monovalent cations. The results are summarized graphically in Figure 4 and, although saturating concentrations of KCl were not achieved, extrapolation of the data from the theoretical fit provided by the Hill equation estimates a saturating KCl γ_j of 253 pS and a half-maximal γ_j at a concentration (K_d) of 143 mM. This is slightly higher than the intracellular $[K^+]$ in mammalian cells, consistent with the hypothesis that K^+ ions are largely responsible for the electrical coupling between mammalian cells *in situ*.

5.3.2 Connexin40

Similar experiments were performed on the rCx40 channel and

revealed some quantitative differences between these two connexin channels (Beblo and Veenstra, 1997). Although the quantitative differences in the cation γ_j and permeability ratios are small relative to rCx43 (series I sequence and $P_{Cl}/P_K = 0.14$), some notable differences were observed when using impermeant sugars for the asymmetric LiCl reversal potential experiments and the monovalent anion γ_j and permeability experiments. Although raffinose produced similar results with both channels, mannitol produced the same result in the rCx40 channel, but not in the rCx43 channel. The reduction in γ_j and the 115:30 mM LiCl reversal potential in the presence of mannitol with rCx43, but not rCx40, is consistent with mannitol being permeable through the rCx43 pore and impermeant through the rCx40 channel (Wang and Veenstra, 1997; Beblo and Veenstra, 1997). The concept that the rCx40 pore may be smaller than the rCx43 pore, despite the similarities illustrated in Figure 1, were further substantiated by the observed blocking effect of TBA^+ on the rCx40 channel. Even more startling was the observation that the rCx40 γ_j did not decrease when Cl^- was replaced with less mobile anions. Furthermore, the asymmetric anion reversal potentials shifted in the opposite direction than expected, which prompted us to examine the effects of even more anions (e.g.aspartate$^-$,nitrate$^-$, F$^-$).

Equilibrium reversal potentials for the monovalent cations and anions were determined using the conventional GHK equation provided that glutamate$^-$ was assumed to be more permeable than Cl^-. This contrast to the anion results on the rCx43 channel suggests a different mechanism for anion permeation. Again, by analogy to a previously examined model, we hypothesize that the rCx40 channel exhibits the ion-pair permeation scheme forwarded by Franciolini and Nonner (1994a, 1994b; Fig. 3C). The oppositely shifted reversal potentials and the lack of a change in γ_j when less mobile anions were used are consistent with this hypothesis. If this is the case, then the anion permeabilities are the reciprocal of the values presented in Table V of Beblo and Veenstra (1997). These model-dependent values for $P_{glutamate}/P_{Cl}$ and $P_{nitrate}/P_{Cl}$ are 0.17 and 0.76 respectively. This hypothesis for cation:anion selective permeability of the rCx40 channel should also be examined experimentally to distinguish between the three alternative models for cation:anion permeability. The permeability studies of the rCx40 and rCx43 channels are hampered by the lack of a known nonblocking impermeant cation and/or anion for the connexin channels to date.

The rCx40 γ_j – [KCl] curve was examined using the same methods employed to examine the rCx43 channel. The results are illustrated in Figure 4 and again indicate that γ_j approaches saturation with increasing KCl concentrations saturation with increasing KCl concentrations in the absence of other monovalent cations. The theoretical fit provided by the Hill equation estimates a saturating KCl γ_j of 233 pS and a half-maximal γ_j at a concentration (K_d) of 127 mM. This is again slightly higher than the equivalent intracellular [K^+] in mammalian cells, but still consistent with the hypothesis that K^+ ions are primarily responsible for the electrical coupling between mammalian cells *in situ*.

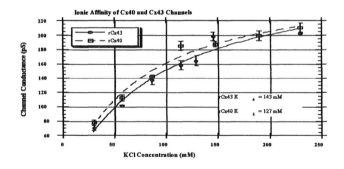

Figure 4. Channel conductance-KCl concentration curves for rCx40 and rCx43. The curved lines are the theoretical fits according to the Hill equation with Hill coefficients of 1.14 and 1.11, K_d values of 127 and 143 mM, and limiting conductances of 233 and 253 pS for rCx40 and rCx40 respectively. Data points are mean ± S.D. of two to six experiments. All conductances were determined from the slope of a single channel current-voltage relationship (Wang and Veenstra, unpublished results).

6 IONIC BLOCK OF CONNEXIN CHANNELS

All known blockers of gap junctions were amphipathic lipophilic compounds until the recent observation of organic cations that disproportionately reduce junctional currents. Among the tetraalkylammonium (TAA) series of monovalent cations, tetrabutylammonium (TBA) was the first to exhibit properties of ionic block in rCx40 gap junctions (Beblo and Veenstra, 1997). Larger TAA ions block rCx40 gap junctions in a voltage-dependent manner with K_d values in the mM range (Musa et al., 2001). Preliminary data indicates that tetrapentylammonium (TPeA) ions also partially block rCx43 gap junction currents (Veenstra, 2000). In this study, we were not able to definitively identify the site of block because TPeA and tetrahexylammonium (THxA) ions appeared to be poorly permeant through the rCx40 channel. This was confirmed from the observations of prolonged (gating-type) channel block in the presence of unilateral concentrations of TPeA and rapid flicker block (open channel permeation) block under bilateral conditions. The polyamines, such as spermine, are naturally present organic polyvalent cations that cause rectification of several types of ion channels (Williams, 1997). Spermine was observed to completely block rCx40 gap junctions while having no effect on rCx43 gap junctions. It appeared to act as an impermeant blocking molecule of the rCx40 gap junction channel and continued analysis of the voltage-dependent block by spermine may provide a more definitive identification of a site of cationic block of the rCx40 gap junction channel (Musa and Veenstra, unpublished results).

7 FUTURE DIRECTIONS

It is apparent from existing permeability theories that simple aqueous diffusion models are inadequate to explain channel permeability to both cations and anions. Even in large diameter pores, ionic permeabilities are not predicted by constant field (GHK) theory. Channel diameters approximating a single KCl ion pair ($\approx 7\text{Å}$) develop complex cation-anion interactions within the pore. Connexin pore diameters are estimated to be 11 - 13 Å from ionic permeability ratios, or only about 2 to 3 water molecules greater than the diameter of the passing ions. Preliminary comparisons to other cation:anion channels are consistent with a cation-dependent anion permeability, indicative of specific cation-anion interactions occurring within the connexin pores. The relative cation:anion selectivity of the rat Cx40, Cx43, and Cx46 channels are $\approx$ 10:1. What remains to be determined are the exact mechanisms for cation and anion permeation through connexin pores and the identity of the pore forming domains and specific residues involved in these interactions. Ionic block provides another approach towards identifying sites of ionic interactions within the permeation pathway of connexin pores.

REFERENCE

Barrio, LC, Suchyna, T, Bargiello, TA, Xu, LX, Roginsk,i R, Bennett, MVL, and Nicholson B. (1991). Gap junctions formed by connexin 26 and 32 alone and in combination are differently affected by applied voltage. Proc Natl Acad Sci USA 88, 8410-8414.

Beblo, DA, and Veenstra, RD. (1997). Monovalent cation permeation through the connexin40 gap junction channel. Cs, Rb, K, Na, Li, TEA, TMA, TBA, and effects of anions Br, Cl, F, acetate, aspartate, glutamate, and NO₃. J Gen Physiol 109, 509-522.

Bevans, CG, Kordel, M, Rhee, SK, and Harris, AL. (1998). Isoform composition of connexin channels determines selectivity among second messengers and uncharged molecules. J Biol Chem 272, 2808-2816.

Beyer, EC, and Willecke K. (2000). Gap junction genes and their regulation. In Gap Junctions, Advances in Molecular and Cell Biology, Vol. 30, EL Hertzberg (ed.), JAI Press, Stamford, CT, pp. 1-30.

Borisova, MP, Brutyan, RA, and Ermishkin, LN. (1986). Mechanism of anion-cation selectivity of amphotericin B channels. J Membr Biol 90, 13-20.

Brink, PR. (1991). Gap junction channels and cell-to-cell messengers in myocardium. J Cardiovasc Electrophysiol 2, 360-366.

Brink, PR, and Dewey, MM. (1980). Evidence for fixed charge in the nexus. Nature 285, 101-102.

Brink, PR, and Fan, S-F. (1989). Patch clamp recordings from membranes which contain gap junction channels. Biophys J 56, 579-593.

Brink, PR, and Ramanan, SV. (1985). A model for the diffusion of fluorescent probes in the septate giant axon of earthworm. Biophys J 48, 299-309.

Bukauskas, FF, Elfgang, C, Willecke, K, and Weingart R. (1995). Heterotypic gap junction channels (connexin26-connexin32) violate the paradigm of unitary conductance. Pflügers Arch - Eur J Physiol 429, 870-872.

Bungenberg de Jong, HG. (1949). In Kruyt HR (ed.): Colloid Science, II, New York, NY, Elsevier, pp. 259-334.

Dahl, G, Miller, T, Paul, D, Voellmy, R, and Werner, R. (1987). Expression of functional cell-cell channels from cloned rat liver gap junction complementary cDNA. Science 236, 1290-1293.

Dang, TX, and McClesky, EW. (1998). Ion channel selectivity through stepwise changes in binding affinity. J Gen Physiol 111, 185-193.

DeMello WC. Further studies on the influence of cAMP-dependent protein kinase on junctional conductance in isolated heart cell pairs. J Molec Cell Cardiol 1991;23:371-379.

Diamond, JM, and Wright, EM. (1969). Biological membranes: the physical basis of ion and nonelectrolyte selectivity. Annu Rev Physiol 31, 581-646.

Dwyer, TM, Adams, DJ, and Hille, B. (1980). The permeability of the endplate channel to orgainc cations in frog muscle. J Gen Physiol 75, 469-492.

Eghbali, B, Kessler, JA, and Spray, DC. (1990). Expression of gap junction channels in communication-incompetent cells after stable transfection with cDNA encoding connexin32. Proc Natl Acad Sci USA 1990;87:1328-1331.

Eisenman, G, and Horn, R. (1983). Ionic selectivity revisited: The role of kinetic and equilibrium processes in ion permeation through ion channels. J Membr Biol 76, 197-225.

Elfgang, C, Eckert, R, Lichtenberg-Frate, H, Butterweck, A, Traub, O, Klein, RA, Hülser, D, and Willecke, K. (1995). Specific permeability and selective formation of gap junction channels in connexin-transfected HeLa cells. J Cell Biol 129, 805-817.

Ellinor, PT, Yang, J, Sather, WA, Zhang, J-F, and Tsien, RW. (1995). Ca^{2+} channel selectivity at a single locus for high-affinity Ca^{2+} interactions. Neuron 15, 1121-1132.

Flagg-Newton, J, Simpson, I, and Loewenstein, WR. (1979). Permeability of the cell-to-cell membrane channels in mammalian cell junction. Science 205, 404-407.

Franciolini, F, and Nonner, W. (1987). Anion and cation permeability of a chloride channel in rat hippocampal neurons. J Gen Physiol 90, 453-478.

Franciolini, F, and Nonner, W. (1994a). Anion-cation interactions in the pore of neuronal background chloride channels. J Gen Physiol 104, 711-723.

Franciolini, F, and Nonner W. (1994b). A multi-ion mechanism in neuronal background chloride channels. J Gen Physiol 104, 725-746.

Galzi, J-L, Devillers-Thiery, A, Hussy, N, Bertrand, S, Changeux, J-P, and Bertrand, D. (1992). Mutations in the channel domain of a neuronal nicotinic receptor convert ion selectivity from cationic to anionic. Nature 359, 500-505.

Gros, DB, and Jongsma, HJ.   (1996).   Connexins in mammalian heart. Bioessays 18, 719-730.

Goldberg, G, Lampe, PD, and Nicholson, BJ. (1999). Selective transfer of endogenous metabolites through gap junctions composed of different connexins. Nature Cell Biology 1, 457-459.

Guthrie, SC, and Gilula, NB. (1989). Gap junctional communication and development. Trends Neurosci 12, 12-16.

Hamill, OP, Marty, A, Neher, E, Sakmann, B, and Sigworth, FJ. (1981). Improved patch-clamp techniques for high-resolution current recording from cells and cell-free membrane patches. Pflügers Arch - Eur J Physiol 391, 85-100.

Hess, P, Lansman, JB, and Tsien, RW. (1986). Calcium channel selectivity sequence for divalent and monovalent cations. Voltage and concentration dependence of single channel current in ventricular heart cells. J Gen Physiol 88, 293-319.

Hille B. (1973).   Potassium channels in myelinated nerve.   Selective permeability to small cations. J Gen Physiol 61, 669-686.

Hille, B. (1992).   Ionic Channels of Excitable Membranes, 2nd edition, Sunderland, MA, Sinauer Associates Inc., 607 pp.

Hobbie, L, Kingsley, DM, Kozarsky, KF, Jackman, RW, Krieger, M. (1989). Restoration of LDL receptor activity in mutant cells by intercellular junctional communication. Science 235, 69-73.

Imanaga, I, Kameyama, M, and Irisawa, H. (1987). Cell-to-cell diffusion of fluorescent dyes in paired ventricular cells. Am J Physiol 252, H223-H232.

Jenny H. (1932).   Studies on the mechanism of ionic exchange in colloidal aluminum silicates. J Physiol Chem 36, 2217-2258.

Jongsma, HJ, van Rijen, HVM, Kwak, BR, and Chanson, M.   (2000). Phosphorylation of connexins: consequences for permeability, conductance, and kinetics of gap junction channels. In Gap Junctions. Molecular Basis of Cell Communication in Health and Disease, Current Topics in Membranes, Vol. 49, C Peracchia (ed.), Academic Press, San Diego, CA, pp. 131-144.

Lau, AF, Warn-Cramer, B, and Lin, R. (2000). Regulation of connexin43 by tyrosine protein kinases. In Gap Junctions. Molecular Basis of Cell Communication in Health and Disease, Current Topics in Membranes, Vol. 49, C Peracchia (ed.), Academic Press, San Diego, CA, pp. 315-341.

Levitt, DG. (1991).   General continuum theory for multiion channel. II. Application to acetylcholine channel. Biophys J 59, 278-288.

Loewenstein, WR. (1981). Junctional intercellular communication: the cell-to-cell membrane channel. Physiol Rev 61, 829-913.

Matthews, BW, and Weaver, LH. (1974). Binding of lanthanide ions to thermolysin. Biochemistry 13, 1719-1725.

McClesky, EW. (1999). Calcium channel permeation: A field in flux. J Gen Physiol 113, 765-772.

Miller C. (1978). Voltage-gated cation conductance channel from fragmented sarcoplasmic reticulum. Steady-state electrical properties. J Membr Biol 40, 1-23.

Mishina, M, Tobimatsu, T, Imoto K, Tanaka, K-i, Fujita, Y, Fukuda, K, Kurasaki, M, Takahashi, H, Morimoto, Y, Hirose, T, Inayama, S, Takahashi, T, Kuno M, and Numa, S. (1985). Location of functional regions of acetylcholine receptor □-subunit by site-directed mutagenesis. Nature 313, 364-369.

Musa, H., Gough, JD, Lees, WJ, and Veenstra, RD. (2001). Ionic blockade of the rat connexin40 gap junction channel by large tetraalkylammonium ions. Biophys. J. 81, 3253-3274.

Neyton, J, and Trautmann, A. (1985). Single channel currents of an intercellular junction. Nature 317:331-335.

Nightingale, ER. (1959). Phenomenological theory of ion solvation. Effective radii of hydrated ions. J Phys Chem 63, 1381-1387.

Nonner, W, and Eisenberg, B. (1998). Ion permeation and glutamate residues linked by Poisson-Nernst-Planck theory in L-type calcium channels. Biophys J 75, 1287-1305.

Paul, DL. (1986). Molecular cloning of cDNA for rat liver gap junction protein. J Cell Biol 103, 123-134.

Réaume, AG, de Sousa, PA, Kulkarni, S, Langille, BL, Zhu, D, Davies, TC, Juneja, SC, Kidder, GM, and Rossant, J. (1995). Cardiac malformation in mice lacking connexin43. Science 267, 1831-1834.

Robinson, RA, and Stokes, RH. (1965). Electrolyte Solutions, 2nd edition, London, UK, Butterworths, 571 pp.

Saez JC, Conner JA, Spray DC, Bennett MVL. (1989). Hepatocyte gap junctions are permeable to the second messenger, inositol 1,4,5-trisphosphate and to calcium ions. Proc Natl Acad Sci USA 86, 2708-2712.

Safranyos, RGA, Caveney, S, Miller, JG, and Petersen, NO. (1987) Relative roles of gap junction channels and cytoplasm in cell-to-cell diffusion of fluorescent tracers. Proc Natl Acad Sci USA 84, 2272-2276.

Sanderson, MJ. (1995). Intercellular calcium waves mediated by inositol trisphosphate. Ciba Found Symp 188, 175-194.

Sokolova, IV, Hessinger, DA, and Fletcher, WH. (2001). Ionic selectivity of gap junctions formed by mouse Cx43. Biophys J 80, 174a.

Stampe, P, and Begenisich, T. (1996). Unidirectional K^+ fluxes through recombinant Shaker potassium channels expressed in single *Xenopus* oocytes. J Gen Physiol 107, 49-457.

Stühmer, W, Methfessel, C, Sakmann, B, Noda, M, and Numa, S. (1987). Patch clamp characterization of sodium channels expressed from rat brain cDNA. Eur Biophys J 14, 131-138.

Suchyna, TM, Nitsche, JM, Chilton, M, Harris, AL, Veenstra, RD, and Nicholson, BJ. (1999). Different ionic selectivities for connexins 26 and 32 produce rectifying gap junction channels. Biophys J 77, 2968-2987.

Suchyna, T, Xu, LX, Gao, F, Fourtner, CR, and Nicholson, BJ. (1993). Identification of a proline residue as a transduction element involved in voltage gating of gap junction channels. Nature 365, 847-849.

Swenson, KI, Piwnica-Worms, H, McNamee, H, and Paul, DL. (1990). Tyrosine phosphorylation of the gap junction protein connexin43 is required for the pp60vsrc-induced inhibition of communication. Cell Regulation 1, 989-1002.

Teorell, T. (1953). Transport processes and electrical phenomena in ionic membranes. Prog Biophys Mol Biol 3, 305-369.

Tomaselli, GF, Backx, PH, and Marban, E. (1993). Molecular basis of ion permeation in voltage-gated ion channels. Circ Res 72, 491-496.

Trexler, EB, Bennett, MVL, Bargiello, TA, and Verselis, VK. (1996). Voltage gating and permeation in a gap junction hemichannel. Proc Natl Acad Sci USA 93, 5836-5841.

Trexler, EB, Bukauskas, FF, Kronengold, J, Bargiello, TA, and Verselis, VK. (2000). The first extracellular loop domain is a major determinant of charge selectivity in connexin46 channels. Biophys J 79, 3036-3051.

Tsien, RW, and Weingart, R. (1976). Inotropic effect of cAMP in calf ventricular muscle studied by a cut end method. J Physiol 260, 117-141.

Valiunas, V, Weingart, R, and Brink, PR. (2000). Formation of heterotypic gap junction channels by connexins 40 and 43. Circ Res 86, e42-e49.

Veenstra RD. (1991). Physiological modulation of cardiac gap junction channels. J Cardiovasc Electrophysiol 2, 168-189.

Veenstra, RD. (1996). Size and selectivity of gap junction channels formed from different connexins. J Bioener Biomembr 28, 327-337.

Veenstra, RD. (2000). Ion permeation through connexin gap junction channels: effects on conductance and selectivity. In Gap Junctions. Molecular Basis of Cell Communication in Health and Disease, Current Topics in Membranes, Vol. 49, C Peracchia (ed.), Academic Press, San Diego, CA, pp. 95-129.

Veenstra, RD. (2001). Voltage clamp limitations of dual whole-cell gap junction current and voltage recordings. I. Conductance measurements. Biophys J 80, 2231-2247.

Veenstra, RD, and DeHaan, RL. (1986). Measurement of single channel currents from cardiac gap junctions. Science 233:972-974.

Veenstra, RD, Wang, H-Z, Westphale, EM, and Beyer, EC. (1992). Multiple connexins confer distinct regulatory and conductance properties of gap junctions in developing heart. Circ Res 75, 1277-1283.

Veenstra, RD, Wang, H-Z, Beblo, DA, Chilton, MG, Harris, AL, Beyer, EC, and Brink, PR. (1995). Selectivity of connexin-specific gap junctions does not correlate with channel conductance. Circ Res 77, 1156-1165.

Verselis, VK, Ginter, CS, and Bargiello, TA (1994). Opposite voltage gating polarities of two closely related connexins. Nature 368, 348-351.

Verselis, VK, and Veenstra R. (2000). Gap junction channels. Permeability and voltage gating. In Gap Junctions, Advances in Molecular and Cell Biology, Vol. 30, EL Hertzberg (ed.), JAI Press, Stamford, CT, pp. 129-192.

Wang, H-Z, and Veenstra, RD. (1997). Monovalent ion selectivity sequences of the rat connexin43 gap junction channel. J Gen Physiol 109, 491-507.

White, TW, and Bruzzone R. (1996). Multiple connexin proteins in single intercellular channels: Connexin compatibility and functional consequences. J Bioener Biomembr 28, 339-350.

Willecke, K, and Haubrich, S. (1996). Connexin expression systems: To what extent do they reflect the situation in the animal? J Bioener Biomembr 28, 319-326.

Williams, K. (1997). Interaction of polyamines with ion channels. Biochem J 325, 289-297.

Zambrowicz EB and Colombini M. (1993). Zero-current potentials in a large membrane channel: A simple theory accounts for complex behavior. Biophys J 65, 1093-1100.

Zhang, Y, McBride, DW, and Hamill, OP. (1998). The ion selectivity of a membrane conductance inactivated by extracellular calcium in *Xenopus* oocytes. J Physiol 508, 763-776.

7

PHOSPHORYLATION OF CONNEXIN43 AND REGULATION OF CARDIAC GAP JUNCTION

Issei Imanaga, Nobue Hirosawa, Hai Lin, Yasuji Sakamoto, Takashi Matsumura & Ken Mayama

Department of Physiology, School of Medicine, Fukuoka University, Fukuoka, 814-0180, Japan

Introduction

In the cardiac muscle, the gap junctions make it possible the cell-to-cell coupling and the intercellular impulse conduction. This physiological function of the gap junction depends on the open or close state of the intercellular channels which depends on the phosphorylation of the connexins which are phosphoproteins.

It is generally accepted that cyclic AMP increases the gap junction conductance (gj) and enhances the electrical cell-to cell coupling in the heart (Burt, Spray 1988; De Mello,1991) through PKA-dependent phosphorylation of the connexins since the effects of cAMP were abolished by PKA inhibitor (Burt, Spray, 1988; De Mello,1988).On the other hand, Ca (Burt et al, 1982; Burt,1987; Maurer, Weingart 1987; Noma, Tsuboi 1987; Toyama et al,1994; Firek, Weingart 1995) and proton (Burt 1097; Noma,Tsuboi,1987; Firek, Weingart 1995) ions decrease gj and the electrical cell-to-cell coupling with consequent changes in impulse conduction and generation of cardiac arrhythmias. Therefore, hypoxia-or ischemia -induced arrhythmias are possibly caused by cell-to-cell decoupling, since progressive increase in intracellular Ca (overload) and progressive intracellular acidosis are brought about during hypoxia or ischemia (Kléber et al,1987; Streenbergen et al 1987;Dekker et al 1996). Previously we reported that cyclic AMP and satolol (d-sotalol) which elevates intracellular cAMP level) prevented and restored hypoxia-induced electrical cell-to-cell decoupling (Manoach et al 1996). However, these effects of cyclic AMP were not observed when hypoxia lasted for a long time (more than one hour) (Imanaga et al 1997). This finding rises the question whether phosphorylation of gap junction connexin is affected by ionic strength of Ca and protons. In this study, the effect of intracellular Ca overload and acidosis as well as activation of PKC on PKA-dependent phosphorylation of connexin43 were investigated on the ventricular muscle of the adult guinea-pig heart.

Methods

Material

Adult male guinea-pigs weighing 385±15.5g were sacrificed by a blow of the head, being approved by the Institutional Animal Care and Use Committees of Fukuoka University. The animals were heparinized 30 minutes before sacrifice.

Evaluation of electrical cell-to-cell coupling

The longitudinal internal resistance was evaluated as the functional cell-to-cell coupling. Measurement of the longitudinal internal resistance was based on the principle described by Tuganowski (Tuganowsky et al 1986). Briefly, thin endocardial muscle strips (less than 1 mm in thickness,10~15 mm in length, 2~3 mm in width) were isolated from right ventricular wall after rapid removal of the heart, and fixed in the three-compartment chamber separated with thin silicon membranes being superfused with well oxygenated normal Krebs solution (in mmol/L: NaCl,130; KCl,5.4; NaHCO3, 11.9; NaH2PO4, 1.2; MgCl2, 1.2; CaCl2, 2.5; glucose, 5.5; saturated with mixture gasses of 97% oxygen and 3% carbon dioxide; pH7.4) at constant flow (5 ml/min) and at constant temperature (37° C). The middle part was 0.8 mm wide and 0.1 ml in volume. The preparation in the middle part was superfused with reagents and test solutions. Transmembrane action potential was recorded at one of both sides of the preparation with conventional glass microelectrode and extracellular action potential was recorded at both sides of the preparation with suction electrodes. The preparation was electrically stimulated with a suction electrode at 0.5 Hz at one of both sides. Shunt resistance in the electrical circuit was 50 K ohom.ri = rs×Eo (1/E2 - 1/E1)where ri is the longitudinal internal resistance, rs is the shunt resistance in the electrical circuit, Eo is the transmembrane action potential, and E1 and E2 are the extracellular action potentials before and after shunting with rs.

Immunoblot and evaluation of phosphoryation of Cx43

Hearts removed rapidly from the animal were perfused with oxygenated Krebs solution at constant pressure (60 mmHg) and at constant flow (18 ml/min) on a Langendorff apparatus. Sixty to 90 minutes after perfusion of control and test solutions, ventricular tissues were frozen in liquid nitrogen and used for Western blot analysis.

Tissue samples were homogenized in the Tris-buffer containing PMSF and centrifuged. The supernatants were mixed with 10% Triton X-100 and centrifuged again at 30,000 rpm for 30 minutes. The pellets were proposed to Western blot analysis. Twenty five microgram of total protein was run on a 10% SDS polyacrylamide gel (SDS-PAGE) and the separated protein was electrophoretically transferred to PVDF membranes. After blocking with 5% skimmed milk in T-PBS phosphate buffer saline containing 0.1% Tween-20), membranes were incubated with the primary antibody (specific mouse anti-Cx43 monoclonal antibodies, Chemicon Int.Inc. Lot.No.19100924) at dilutions of 1:4000 for an hour at room temperature. Secondary antibody (anti-mouse IgG,

Amersham Pharmacia biotech, U.K., Lot.NO.145660) were used at dilutions of 1:5000. Cx43 protein-antibody complexes was transcribed on chemiluminescence film. Molecular weight was calibrated using Low Molecular Weight Calibration Kit for SDS Electrophoresis (Amersham Pharmacia Biotech, U.K.)

Two isoforms were observed near 43Kda (Fig.2). Mean density of Cx43 complex bands was analyzed by NIH Image. Mean density of the higher molecular isoform was remarkably reduced by a treatment of alkaline phosphatase (Fig.3) and then this isoform was decided as hosphorylated isoform (P1). The lower molecular isoform was not affected by alkaline phosphatase (Fig.3) and decided as non-phosphorylated isoform (P0). The density ratio of P1 to P0, P1/P0 was evaluated as a magnitude of phosphorylation of the connexin. Alkaline phosphatase (from bovine intestinal mucosa, Sigma, Lot.No.109H7045) was added in the first homogenizing procedure at a dose of 20 u/ml.

Test solutions

Intracellular Ca overload was induced by reduction of sodium ions in the external perfusing solution substituted with N-methyl-d-glucamine adjusting pH.7.4 with HCl. Intracelluar Ca level was measured by Fura-2 on ventricular myocyte isolated by collagenase. When external Na ions were reduced from standard concentration, 141.9 mM to 80 mM, 60 mM,30 mM and 10 mM, intracellular Ca level was raised exponentially (Table 1).

Table 1

Emission ratio of 340/360

External Na concentration (mM)	143.1	80	30	20	10
Relative value	1	1.083± 0.033	1.34±0.05	1.49±0.08	1.84 ± 0.06

Intracellular Ca concentration was calculated by experimental results to be 1.04 ± 0.06 μM at an extracellular Na concentration of 20mM.

Intracellular acidosis was induced by increasing the partial pressure of carbon dioxide. The pH of the perfusing solution was changed from 7.4 (standard) to 7.1-6.9 and 6.1-5.9 by altering of proportion of oxygen and carbon dioxide while checking the in a pH meter (Protable Clinical Analyser, i-STAT, i-STT Cooperation, U.S.A.). In low pH solution, external Ca ions were excluded.

Other chemical reagents

8Bromo-cAMP (8bromoadenosine 3':5'-cyclic monophosphate sodium salt; Sigma, Lot.No.85H7808) as cyclic AMP (cAMP), PKA activator (Spadenosine 3',5'-cyclic monophosphothioate triethylamine salt, Sigma, Lot.No.97H4681), PKA inhibitor (Rp-adenosine 3',5'-cyclic monophosphothioate triethylamine salt, RBI (Research Biochemicals Internatinonal), Lot. No. 087H4643), PKC activator (12-o-tetradecanoyl phorbol-13-acetate, TPA, Sigma, Lot.No.38F0179), PKC inhibitor (Calphostin C, RBI, Lot. No.087H4652) were used.

Perfusion of test solution and reagents

The hearts were perfused with 8Bromo cyclic AMP, PKA activator, PKA inhibitor, low Na and low pH solution for at least 60 min, and perfused with TPA and PKC inhibitor for at least 90 min on Langendorff, before measurements were performed. Tissue samples for Western blot were extracted after treatment with the test solutions and reagents.

Statistical analysis

Data were expressed as mean±SEM (standard error of means). A paired or un-paired Student's t-test was used to analyze the statistical significance ($p < 0.001$) between means.

Results

Effects of cyclic AMP

Cyclic AMP (1 μM) applied for 60 min decreased the longitudinal internal resistance by about 30%. This effect of cAMP was abolished by PKA inhibitor (10 μM) (Fig.1). Effects of cAMP and PKA activator (1μM) on phosphorylation of the Cx43 were

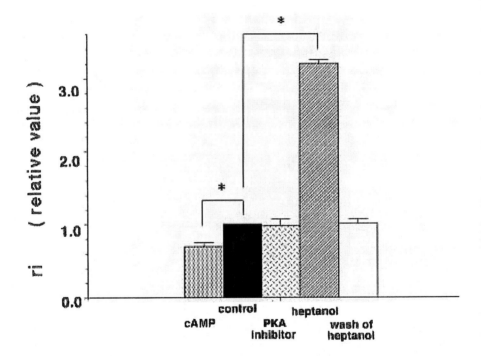

Fig.1 Effects of 8Bromo cyclic AMP on the longitudinal internal resistance (ri). ri (ordinate) represents relative value. 1 and control mean value before treatment of reagents. A dose of 8Bromo cyclic AMP, PKA inhibitor and heptanol were 1.M, 10.M and 1mM, respectively. Bars correspond to means ± SEM. Stars represent statistical significance (p<0.001).

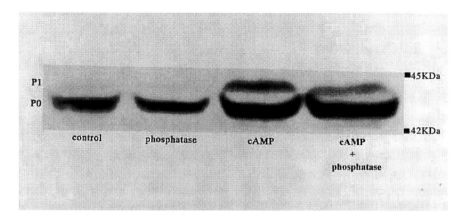

Fig.2 Representative of Western blot for Cx43 showing effects of cAMP and phosphatase. Control is value without treatment of reagents. 8Bronmo cyclic AMP (1.M) was applied for 60 min on Langendorff. Phosphatase at dose of 20 u/ml was treated at first homogenizing procedure (see methods).

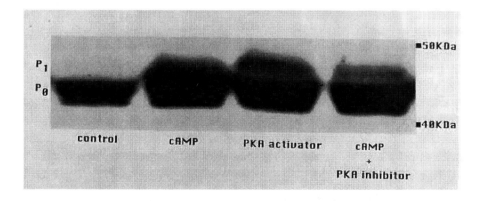

Fig.3 Representative of Western blot for C43 showing effects of cAMP and PKA activator. 8Bromo cyclic AMP (1.M), PKA activator (1.M) and PKA inhibitor (10.M) were perfused for 60 min on Langendorff.

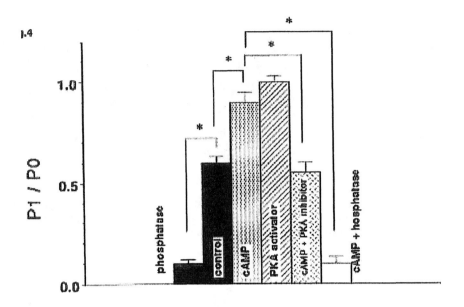

Fig.4 Effects of 8Bromo cyclic AMP, PKA activator, PKA inhibitor and phosphatase on mean density ratio of two isoforms of Cx43, P1/P0. Treatments and dose of reagents are the same as those shown in Fig.2 and Fig.3. Control means absence of reagents. Bars correspond to menas±SEM. Stars mean statistical significance, p<0.001.

analyzed with Western blot (Fig.2, 3).P1/P0 ratio was significantly increased by treatment with cAMP and PKA activator (Fig.4). These effects of cAMP and PKA activator on P1/P0 ratio 10 were inhibited by the presence of PKA inhibitor (10 μM) and treatment of alkaline phosphatase (20ug/ ml) (Fig.4).

Effects of cAMP on intracellular Ca-overload

Intracellular Ca overload was induced by a reducing the external Na concentration, as mentioned above. When the external Na concentration was reduced from standard concentration 143.1 mM to 78.1mM and 13.1 mM, the longitudinal internal resistance was increased depending on reduction of Na concentration. In the presence of cAMP(1 μ.M), the increment of the internal resistance at 78.1 mM of Na concentration was reduced. The effect cAMP was abolished by PKA inhibitor (10 μ.M) (Fig.5). However, when

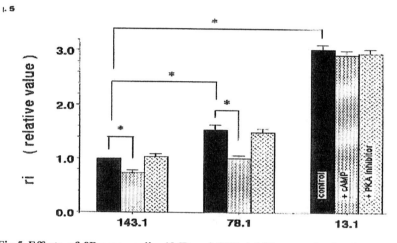

Fig.5 Effects of 8Bromo cyclic AMP and PKA inhibitor on the longitudinal internal resistance (ri) at low external Na concentration. External concentration of Na ions were reduced from 143.1 to 78.1 and 13.1 mM. Doses of 8Bormo cAMP and PKA inhibitor were 1.M and 10.M, respectively. ri (ordinate) represents relative value. 1 means value at the standard concentration of Na ions without any reagents. Black, shadow and dotted column represent control (before treatment of reagents), cAMPand PKA inhibitor, respectively. Bars correspond to means±SEM. Stars mean statistical significance, p<0.001.

external Na concentration was reduced to 13.1 mM, cAMP was not able to change the resistance (Fig.5). Phosphorylation of Cx43 in the presence or absence of cAMP (1 μ.M) was analyzed with Western folt at 143.1, 78.1 and 13.1 mM external Na concentration (Fig.6) and the P1/P0 ratio was compared between each Na concentration in several examples (Fig.7). At 13.1 mM of external Na concentration, phosphprylation of cx43 was significantly reduced. cAMP (1 μM) augmented P1/P0 at 143.1 and 78.1 mM of external Na concentrations but not at 13.1mM.

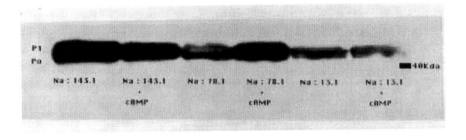

Fig.6 Representative of Western blot for Cx43 showing effects of cAMP at low concentration of external Na ions. Low Na solutions and 8Bromo cyclic AMP (1.M) were perfused for 60 min on Langendorff.

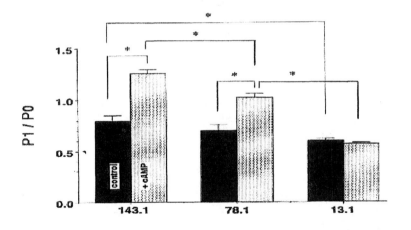

Fig.7 Effects of 8Bromo cyclic AMP at low external concentration of Na ions on P1/P0 ratio. Treatment and dose of solution and reagents are the same as those in Fig.6. Control (black column) means absence of cAMP.

Effects of cAMP on intracellular acidosis

The longitudinal internal resistance was increased as the external pH was decreased from standard, 7.4 to 7.1- 6.9 and 6.1-5.9. The increase of the resistance was reduced at pH 7.1- 6.9 by cAMP (1 µM). The effects of cAMP were abolished by PKA inhibitor (10 µM). When pH was in the range of 6.1-5.9, the effect of cAMP on the increasd resistance was not observed at all (Fig.8). Phosphorylation of Cx43 in presence or absence of cAMP (1 µ.M) was analyzed at pH of 7.4, 7.1-6.9 and 6.1-5.9 with Western blot

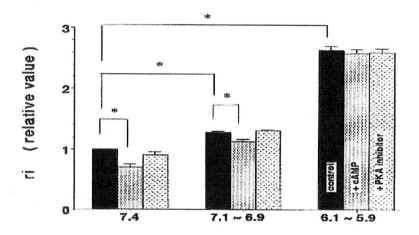

Fig. 8 Effects of 8Bromo cyclic AMP and PKA inhibitor on the longitudinal internal resistance (ri) at low pH. The pH was reduced from 7.4 to 7.1~6.9 and 6.1~5.9. Doses of 8Bormo cAMP and PKA inhibitor were 1.M and 10.M, respectively. ri (ordinate) represents relative value.1 means value at 7.4 of pH without any reagents. Black, shadow and dotted column represent control (before treatment of reagents), cAMP and PKA inhibitor, respectively. Bars correspond to means ± SEM. Stars mean statistical significance, p<0.001.

(Fig.9). P1/P0 ratio was compared between each pH in several examples (Fig.10). At pH 6.1-5.9 , phosphorylation of Cx43 was significantly reduced. cAMP augmented P1/P0 ratio at pH 7.4 and 7.1-6.9 of pH, but not at pH 6.1-5.9 .

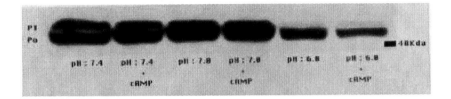

Fig. 9 Representative of Western blot for Cx43 showing effects of cAMP at low pH.
Low pH solutions and 8Bromo cyclic AMP 1.M) was perfused for 60 min
on Langendorff

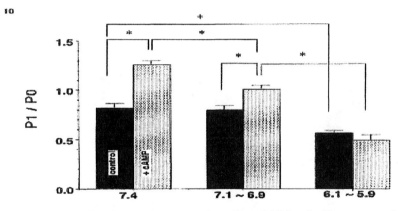

Fig.10 Effects of 8Bromo cyclic AMP at low pH on P1/P0 ratio. Treatment and dose of
solution and reagents are the same as those in Fig.9. Control (black column) means
absence of cAMP. Bars correspond to means± SEM. Stars represent statistical
significance, p<0.001.

Effects of cAMP at the presence of TPA

The longitudinal internal resistance was increased by a long period
exposure (for about 90 min) to TPA (0.1 μM). This event was
abolished by Calphostin C (1 μM) (Fig.11). Western blot for Cx43
in the presence of cAMP (1 μM) and TPA (0.1 μM) was shown in
Fig.12. TPA raised slightly but significantly the P1/P0 ratio

(Fig.13). However, cAMP did not augment P1/P0 ratio in the presence of TPA.

11

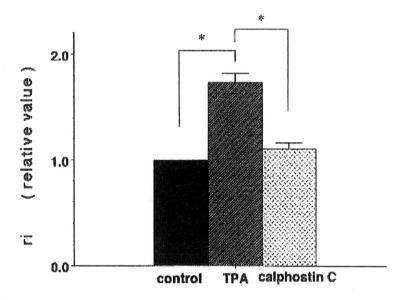

Fig.11 Effects of TPA and Calphostin C on the longitudinal internal resistance (ri). TPA and Calphostin C were superfused for 90 min at a dose of 0.1μ M and 1μM, respectively. Ordinate (ri) represents relative value, and 1 and control mean value without reagents. Bars correspond to means ± SEM. Stars represent statistical significance, p<0.001.

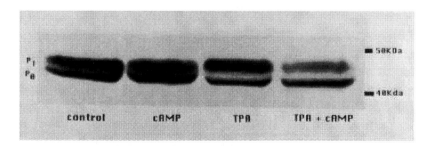

Fig.12 Representative of Western blot for cx43 showing effects of cAMP and TPA. 8Bromo cyclic AMP (1μM) and TPA (0.1μM) were perfused for 90 min on langendorff.

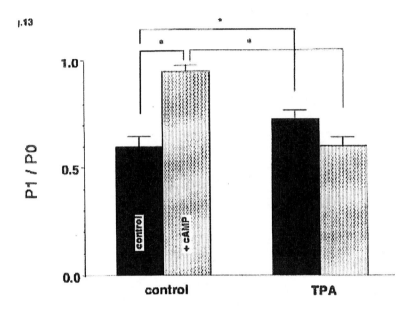

Fig.13 Effects of 8Bromo cyclic AMP and TPA on P1/P0 ratio. Treatment and dose of reagents are the same as those in Fig.12. Bars correspond to means ± SEM. Stars represent statistical significance, p<0.001.

Discussion

Two isoforms of Cx43 were distinctly detected in the Western blot. It is mentioned in Method that the ratio of mean density of the higher molecular isoform (P1) to the lower molecular isoform (P0), P1/P0 is available for evaluation of phosphorylation of Cx43. We used mouse monoclonal anti-Cx43 antibody. It was reported in the rat heart that monoclonal anti-Cx43 antibody could not detect phosphorylated isoform but polyclonal anti-Cx43antibody was available for evaluation of phosphorylation (Beard et al,2000). However, there is a report that some phosphorylated isoforms of Cx43 near 41 KDa can be detected with monoclonal antibody (Cruciani, Mikalsen 1999). We could not observe definite difference between phosphorylated and non-phosphorylated isoform of Cx43 on trial use of polyclonal anti-Cx43 antibody (not shown in figure). It is concluded that monoclonal anti-Cx43 antibody is useful for the detection of phosphoryalted isoform of Cx43 in the adult guinea-pig heart.

It is generally accepted that cAMP increases macroscopic conductance of the cardiac gap junction (gj) (Burt,Spray 1988; De Mello 1991). This effect of cAMP is inhibited by PKA inhibitor (Burt,Spray 1988; De Mello 1988). It was also shown in this study that cAMP decreases the longitudinal internal resistance - an effect suppressed by PKA inhibitor.Therefore, there is no doubt that the action of cAMP on the gap junction conductance is mediated by activation of PKA. In this study it was shown by analysis of Western blot that cAMP and PKA activator augmented phosphorylation of Cx43. These findings suggest that the effect of cAMP on the junctional conductance is attributed to phosphoryation of Cx43 by PKA. Phosphorylation of Cx43 by PKA up-regulates the connexin, that is, increases open probability of the gap junction channel, maintains the channel at open-state or prevents the degradation of the connexin.

In ischemic or hypoxic cardiac muscle, arrhythmias due to abnormalities of intercellular impulse conductivity are often observed. When cardiac muscle is exposed to hypoxia, intracellular Ca overload and intracellular acidosis are induced (Kleber et al,1987; Strenbergen et al 1987; Dekker et al 1996)(see also Chpater 10).Because Ca and protons reduced gj (Burt et al 1982; Burt 1987; Maurer,Weingart 1987;Noma,Tsuboi 1987; Toyama et al,1994; Firek,Weingart 1995) it is possible to conclude that hypoxia-induced cell-to-cell decoupling is explainable by the increase of intracellular Ca or proton ions (see Chaper 10).

In the present study it was shown that the electrical cell-to-cell coupling was impaired by Ca overload induced by the reduction of external Na concentration. When intracellular Ca overload was moderate (at 78.1mM of external Na concentration) the Ca-induced cell-to-cell decoupling was reduced by cAMP and the effect of cAMP was suppressed by PKA inhibitor. However, when the Ca overloaded was high (such as that achieved at 13.1 mM Na),the effect of cAMP was not observed. Phosphorylation of Cx43 by PKA was slightly impaired at 78.1mM Na and remarkably impaired at an external Na concentration of 13.1 mM. During Ca overload, the effect of cAMP on the electrical cell coupling is consistent with that found on phosphorylation of Cx43. These findings suggest that PKA dependent phosphoryation of Cx43 is affected by the ionic strength of Ca and it is inhibited by higher ionic strength of Ca.

Intracellular acidosis (pH) is equivalent to extracellular acidosis induced by elevation of pCO2 (Reber,Weingart 1982; Pressler 1987). Intracellular acidosis possibly promotes inflow of Ca into the cell through activation of Na-Ca exchange following Na-H exchange. In this study the effect of increase in intracellular Ca was prevented by nominative deletion of extracellular Ca ions and the electrical intercellular communication was decreased depending on the decrease of pH. The raise of longitudinal internal resistance at pH 7.1-6.9 was reduced by cAMP but not that at a pH range of 6.1-5.9. Phosphorylation of Cx43 by PKA was suppressed depending on the fall in pH. cAMP augmented phosphorylation at a pH range of 7.1- 6.9 but not at the range of 6.1~5.9. The effect of cAMP on the electrical cell coupling is consistent with that seen on the phosphorylation of Cx43. These findings suggest that PKA- dependent phosphorylation of Cx43 is affected by ionic strength of protons. In our experiments,the effect of cAMP on the electrical cell communication and phosphorylation of Cx43 were not observed at a pH below 6.5 .

The effect of activation of PKC on the electrical cell-to-cell coupling is a controversial issue. According to some authors the activation of PKC increases gj (Kwak et al 1995; Kwak,Jongsma 1996; Saez et al,1997) but other author reported a decrease of gj (Munster,Weingart 1993; De Mello 1997; Husoy et al,2000). This discrepancy may be caused by the different state of phosphorylation of Cx43, phosphorylated or non-phosphorylated form, before the activation of PKC (Saez et al,1997; Brissete et al 1991;Oh et al 1991;Berhoud et al 1992; Reynout et al 1992; Berthoud et al 1993). In the present study it was found that the activation of PKC by TPA enhanced the cell-to-cell decoupling. TPA was applied for about 90 min because the half-time of cardiac Cx43 has been reported to be about 1.3 hours (Beardslee et al 1998). The activation of PKC increased slightly but significantly the phosphorylation of Cx43. It is interesting that phosphorylation of Cx43 by PKC may lead of the protein to subsequent degradation (Saez et al 1997;Musil,Goodenough 1991). In rat liver epithelial cells,for instance, degradation of Cx43 due to activation of proteolysis pathway was observed after phosphorylation of Cx43 by PKC (Matesic et al 1994; Houssain, Boynton 1998).

Moreover, in the mouse embryo, assembly of Cx43 into the gap junction plaque was suppressed by phosphorylation of the connexin due to PKC activation (Ogawa et al 2000). Confocal image analysis and immunohistochemical studies of Cx43, 90 min after treatment with TPA (0.1 μM), revealed a remarkable reduction of immunoreactive particle area at the intercalated disk of the ventricular myocardial cells,in spite of the increased phosphorylation of the connexin (Imanaga et al, not shown here). It was shown in this study that Cx43 isoform phosphorylated by PKC was fairly resistive to PKA. These evidences suggest that PKC dependent phosphorylation of cardiac Cx43 may be lead to degradation of connexin.

It is reported that angiotensin II (Ang II) induced cell-to-cell decoupling in heart muscle (De Mello,Altieri 1992; De Mello 1994; De Mello 1996) an effect probably due to the phosphorylation of junctional proteins by PKC.

Conclusions

Cyclic AMP promotes electical cell-to-cell coupling and junctional communication in the ventricular muscle cells of the heart. This effect of cyclic AMP is attributed to the phosphorylation of connexin43 by activation of PKA. PKA dependent phoshorylation of Cx43 is downward affected by intracellular ionic strength of Ca and protons and by activation of PKC. Isoform of Cx43 phosphorylated by PKC may be target of subsequent degradation.

Abstracts of this study were previously reported (Imanaga et al 1998; Imanaga et al 2000; Imanaga et al 2001).

Acknowledgements

This study was supported by a Grant from The Vehicle Racing Commemorative Foundation, and a Grant (No.016010) from The Central Research Institute of Fukuoka University.

REFERENCE

Beardslee MA, Laing JG, Beyer EC, Saffitz JE. 1998 Rapid turnover of connexin43 in the adult rat heart. Circ Res; 83: 629–635.

Beardslee MA, Lerner DL, Tadros PN, Laing JG, Beyer EC, Yamada KA, Kleber AG, Schuessler RB, Saffitz JE. 2000 Dephosphorylation and intracellular redistribution of ventricular connexin43 during electrical uncoupling induced by ischemia. Circ Res 87: 656-662..

Berthoud VM, Ledbetter MLS, Hertzberg EL, Saez JC. 1992 Connexin43 in MDCK cells: regulation by a tumor-promoting phorbol ester and Ca2+. Eur J Cell Biol 57:40-50.

Berthoud VM, Rook M, Hertzberg EL, Sáez JC. 1993 On the mechanism of cell uncoupling induced by a tumor promoter phorbol ester in clone 9 cells, a rat liver epithelial cell line. Eur J Cell Biol; 62: 384–396.

Brissette JK, Kumar NM, Gilula NB, Dotto GP. 1991 The tumor promoter 12-o-teradecanoylphorbol-13-acetate and the ras oncogene modulate expression and phosphorylation of gap junction proteins. Mol Cell Biol 11: 5364-5371.

Burt JM, Frank JS, Berns MW. 1982 Permeability and structural studies of heart cell gap junctions under normal and altered ionic conditions. J Membr Biol 68: 227-238.

Burt JM, Spray DC.1988 Inotropic agents modulate gap junctional conductance between cardiac myocytes. Am J Physiol 254 (Heart Circ. Physiol. 25): H1206-H1210.

Burt JM. 1987 Block of intercellular communication: interaction of intracellular H+ and Ca2+. Am J Physiol 253 (Cell Physiol 22): C607-C612.

Cruciani V, Mikalsen SO. 1999 Stimulated phosphorylation of intracellular connexin43. Exp Cell Res; 251: 285-298.

De Mello WC, Altieri P. 1992 The role of the renin-angiotensin system in the control of cell communication in the heart; effects of enalapril and angiotensin II. J Cardiovac Pharmacol 20: 643-651.

De Mello WC. 1991 Further studies on the influence of c-AMP-dependent protein kinase on junctional conductance in isolated heart cell pairs. J Mol Cell Cardiol 23: 371-379.

De Mello WC. 1988 Increase in junctional conductance caused by 20 isoproterenol in heart cell pairs is suppressed by c-AMP dependent protein kinase inhibitor. Biochem Biophys Res Commun 154: 509-514.

De Mello WC. 1994 Is an intracellular renin-angiotensin system involved in control of cell communication in heart? J Cadiovac Pharmacol 23: 640-646.

De Mello WC. 1996 Renin-angiotensin system and cell communication in failing heart. Hypertension 27: 1267-1272.

De Mello WC. 1997 Influence of α-adrenergic –receptor activation of junctional conductance in heart cells: interaction with β –adrenergic agonists. J Cardiovasc Pharmacol 29: 273-277.

Dekker LR, Fiolet JW, van Bavel E, Coronel R, Opthof T, Spaan JA, Janse MJ. 1996 Intracellular Ca2+, intercellular electrical coupling, and mechanical activity in ischemic rabbit papillary muscle. Effects of preconditioning and metabolic blockade. Circ Res 79; 237-246.

Firek L, Weingart R. 1995 Modification of gap junction conductance by divalent cations and protons in neonatal rat heart cells. J Mol Cell Cardiol 27: 1633-1643.

Hossain MZ, AO P, Boynton AL. 1998 Rapid disruption of gap junctional communication and phosphorylation of connexin43 by platelet-derived growth factor in T51B rat liver epithelial cells expressing platelet derived growth factor receptor. J Cell Physiol 174: 66-77.

Husφy T, Cruciani V, Sanner T, Mikalsen SO. 2001 Phosphorylation of connexin43 and inhibition of gap junctional communication in 12-otetradecanoylphorbol-13-acetate-exposed R6 fibroblasts: minor role of protein kinase CβI andμ. Carcinogenesis 22: 221-231.

Imanaga I, Hirosawa n, HiLin, Matumura K, Mayama T. 2001 Factors influencing phosphorylation of connexin of the cardiac gap junction-with special reference to intercellular impulse conductivity. (Abstract) J Mol Cell Cardiol 33: A50.

Imanaga I, Hirosawa N, Matsumura K, Mayama T. 2000 Effects of Ca ions and acidosis on phosphorylation of cardiac gap junction connexin434 in adult guinea pig heart. (Abstract) J Mol Cell Cardiol 32: A119.

Imanaga I, Matsumura K. 1997 Effects of C-AMP on disturbance of impulse propagation during hypoxia in myocardium. (Abstract) J Mol Cell Cardiol29: A6.

Imanaga I, Mayama T. 1998 Effects of C-AMP on intercellular electrical decoupling induced by intracellular Ca2+-overload and acidosis in myocardium. (Abstract) J Mol Cell Cardiol 30: A306.

Kléber AG, Riegger CB, Janse MJ. 1987 Electrical uncoupling and increase of extracellular resistance after induction of ischemia in isolated, arterially perfused rabbit papillary muscle. Circ Res 61: 271-279.

Kwak BR, Jongsma, HJ. 1996 Regulation of cardiac gap junction channel permeability and conductance by several phosphorylating conditions. Mol Cell Biochem 157: 93-99.

Kwak BR, van Veen TBA, Analbers LJS, Jongsma HJ. 1995 TPA increases conductance but decreases permeability in neonatal rat cardiomyocyte gap junction channels. Exp Cell Res 220: 456–463.

Manoach M, Tribulová N, Imanaga I. 1996 The protective effect d-sotalol against hypoxia-induced myocardial uncoupling. Heart Vessels 11;281-288.

Matesic DF, Rupp HL, Bonney WJ, Ruch RJ, Trosko JE. 1994 Changes in gap junction permeability, phosphorylation, and number mediated by phorbol ester and non-phorbol-ester tumor promoters in rat liver epithelial cells. Mol Carcinog 10: 226-236.

Maurer P, Weingart R. 1987 Cell pairs isolated from adult guinea pig and rat hearts: effects of [Ca2+]i, on nexal membrane resistance. Pflügers Arch-Eur J Physiol 409: 394-402.

Münster PN, Weingart R. 1993 Effects of phorbol ester on gap junctions of neonatal rat heart cells. Pflügers Arch-Eur J Physiol 423: 181-188.

Musil LS, Goodenough DA. 1991 Biochemical analysis of connexin43 intracellular transport, phosphorylation, and assembly into gap junctional plaques. J Cell Biol; 115: 1357–1374.

Noma A, Tsuboi N. 1987 Dependence of junctional conductance on proton, calcium and magnesium ions in cardiac paired cells of guinea pig. J Physiol 382: 193-211.

Ogawa h, Oyamada M, Mori T, Mori M, Shimizu H. 2000 Relationship of gap junction to phosphorylation of connexin43 in mouse preimplantation embryos. Mol.Reprod Dev 55: 393–398.

Oh SY, Grupen CG, Murry AW. 1991 Phorbol ester induces phosphorylation and down-regulation of connexin43 in WB cells. Biochemica Biophysica Acta (BBA); 1094: 243–245.

Pressler M. Effects of pCa and pHi on cell-to-cell coupling. Experientia 1987; 43:1084-1091.

Reber WR, Weingart P. 1982 Ungulate cardiac Purkinje fibres: the influence of intracellular pH on the electrical cell-to-cell coupling. J Physiol 328: 87-104.

Reynout JK. 1992 Lampe PD, Johnson RG. An activation of protein kinase C inhibits gap junctional communication between cultured bovine lens cells. Exp Cell Res 198: 337-342.

Strenbergen C, Murphy E, Levy L, London RE. 1987 Elevation in cytosolic free calcium concentration early in myocardial ischemia in perfused rat heart. Circ Res 60: 700-707.

Toyama J, Sugiura H, Kamiya K, Kodama I, Terasawa M, Hidaka H. 1994 Ca2+-calmodulin mediated modulation of the electrical coupling of ventricular myocytes isolated from guinea pig heart. J Mol Cell Cardiol 26: 1007-1015.

Tuganowski W, Bukowski M, Korczynska I, Wójcik B, Wasik K. 1986 A method of measurement of longitudinal resistances in an isolated cardiacand smooth muscle preparation. Pflügers Arch-Eur J Physiol 406:232-233.

Záez JC, Narin AC, Czernik AJ, Fishman GI, Spray DC, Hertzberg EL. 1997 Phosphorylation of connexin 43 and the regulation of neonatal rat cardiac myocyte gap junction. J Mol Cell Cardiol 29: 2131-2145.

8

THE SINOATRIAL NODE GAP JUNCTION DISTRIBUTION AND IMPULSE PROPAGATION

Mark R. Boyett, Haruo Honjo, Henggui Zhang, Yoshiko Takagishi and Itsuo Kodama

Reseach Institute of Environmental Medicine, Nagoya University, Nagoya 464-8601, Japan and School of Biomedical Sciences, University of Leeds, Leeds LS2 9JT, UK

INTRODUCTION

The function of the sinoatrial (SA) node is to act as the heart's pacemaker and for this the cells of the SA node have to be electrically connected both to one another and also the atrial cells surrounding them. This chapter is concerned with the electrical coupling between cells in and around the SA node – it is shown that this is special, perhaps in order for the SA node to carry out its normal function. This chapter is written to complement our recent review of the functional and morphological organisation of the SA node (Boyett et al., 2000).

Fig. 1 shows the activation sequence of the rabbit SA node. SA node tissue lies almost throughout the intercaval region between the two venae cavae (SVC and IVC) and the SA node is bounded by the atrial muscle of the crista terminalis (CT) on one side and the atrial muscle of the interatrial septum (SEP) on the other. As shown by the 0 ms isochrone in Fig. 1, the action potential is first initiated in the centre of the SA node (distant from the crista terminalis). From here, the action potential preferentially propagates in an oblique cranial direction. The action potential first propagates to the periphery of the SA node (where the SA node meets the atrial muscle) and then into the atrial muscle of the crista terminalis. Towards the interatrial septum, conduction is blocked (extent of the block zone is shown by the shaded area in Fig. 1) and the action potential must propagate around the block zone to reach the interatrial septum. A movie of the activation sequence in Fig. 1 is available at http://www.leeds.ac.uk/bms/staff/boyett.

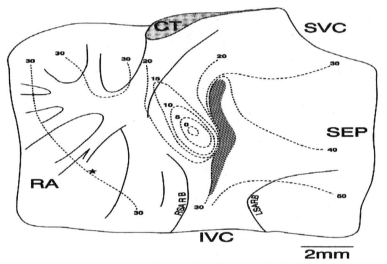

Figure 1. Activation sequence of the rabbit SA node. Dashed lines, isochrones showing activation times in ms. Hashed area, block zone. CT, crista terminalis. SVC, superior vena cava. SEP, interatrial septum. LSARB, left branch of SA ring bundle. IVC, inferior vena cava. RSARB, right branch of SA ring bundle. RA, right atrial appendage.

THE REQUIREMENTS OF THE SA NODE

In order for the SA node to drive the surrounding atrial muscle, it must be electrically coupled to it and yet, because of the resulting electrotonic interaction, the atrial muscle (which is more hyperpolarized than the SA node) tends to suppress the activity of the SA node. This is known from various lines of evidence: cutting off the atrial muscle surrounding the SA node results in an acceleration of the pacemaker activity of the SA node (Fig. 2A; Kodama and Boyett, 1985; Kirchhof et al., 1987; Boyett et al.,

1995) and coupling of an atrial cell to a SA node cell can cause the pacemaker activity of the SA node cell to slow and perhaps cease (Boyett et al., 1995; Toyama et al., 1995; Watanabe et al., 1995a, 1995b; Joyner et al., 1998). We have even argued that ACh, by increasing the K^+ conductance of the atrial muscle surrounding the SA node, may increase the suppressive effect of the atrial muscle on the SA node and thereby slow the pacemaker activity of the SA node (Boyett et al., 1995; Kodama et al., 1996).

It is likely that the SA node is organized in a way such that the suppressive effect of the atrial muscle on the SA node is minimised and yet the SA node is still able to drive the atrial muscle. This is probably achieved in various ways (Boyett et al., 2000). Using mathematical modelling, Joyner and van Capelle (1986) were the first to address this issue. They suggested that the SA node should be a minimum size. Fig. 2B summarises simulations in which a simple model was used – a group of isopotential SA node cells was connected to a group of isopotential atrial cells (isopotential means that all cells within a group have the same membrane potential, i.e. the coupling resistance and distance between cells in a group are ignored). Three types of behaviour were observed depending on the coupling resistance (reciprocal of conductance) between the two cell groups and the size of the group of SA node cells (size of group of atrial cells fixed): 1) the SA node cells did not show pacemaking; 2) the SA node cells did show pacemaking but failed to drive the atrial cells; and 3) the SA node cells showed pacemaking and did drive the atrial cells (normal physiological situation) (Fig. 2B). The group of SA node cells showed pacemaking and was able to drive the atrial cells only when it exceeded a minimum size (Fig. 2B). The reason for this is that the SA node must have sufficient capacity to withstand the hyperpolarizing influence of the atrial muscle (which causes the SA node to cease pacemaking) and to provide sufficient depolarizing current to drive the atrial muscle.

These results were obtained using a simple model (see above). In the case of the real SA node, these effects of size will be influenced by the space constant of the SA node (the SA node is not isopotential). The space constant of rabbit SA node is 465-828 μm parallel to the crista terminalis and 205-310 μm perpendicular to it (see Boyett et al., 2000, for references). The suppressive effect of atrial muscle on SA node tissue, as the result of electrotonic interaction, will diminish the greater the distance of the SA node tissue from the atrial muscle, and the suppressive effect will be small when the SA node tissue is more than say two space constants from the atrial muscle. Furthermore, an increase in the size of the SA node up to a radius of say two space constants will provide more and more depolarizing current to drive the atrial muscle (however, an increase in size beyond this will not provide more, because the SA node tissue will be too distant from the atrial muscle to be able to influence it). On this basis, it can be argued that the distance between the leading pacemaker site within the SA node and the atrial muscle should be at least several space constants. Fig. 1 suggests that in the rabbit the leading pacemaker site is located more than several space constants from the atrial muscle of the crista terminalis.

Joyner and van Capelle (1986) also suggested that some degree of electrical uncoupling of the cells within the SA node might be an essential design feature of the normal SA node-atrial muscle system. Fig. 2B shows that, in order for the SA node cells to show pacemaker activity, the coupling resistance must exceed (i.e. the coupling conductance must be less than) a critical value that depends on the size of the group of SA node cells. For the SA node cells to show pacemaker activity and drive the atrial cells, the group of SA node cells must be of sufficient size and the coupling resistance must lie within a small range (the coupling resistance

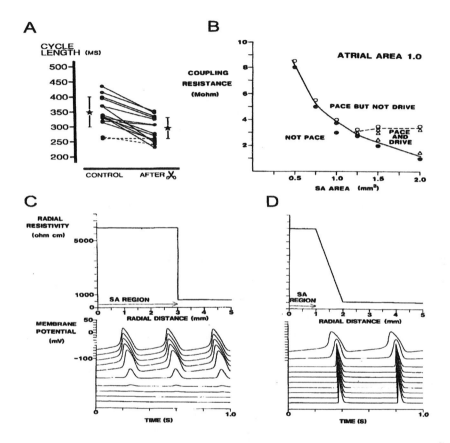

Figure 2. The suppressive effect of the atrial muscle on the SA node. A, effect of cutting off the atrial muscle surrounding the SA node on the spontaneous cycle length of the rabbit SA node. Values for individual preparations shown as well as the mean ± SEM for all prep-arations. From Kirchhof et al. (1987). B, importance of the coupling resistance between SA node and atrium and the size of the SA node on the function of the SA node as shown by mathematical modelling. Three types of behaviour were observed depending on the coupling resistance and the size (area) of the SA node. See text for further details. C, D, importance of a gradual decrease in coupling resistance at the border of the SA node with the atrial muscle as shown by mathematical modelling. Action potentials are shown at different radial distances (from 0 to 5 mm in 0.5 mm increments) within a circular SA node and surrounding ring of atrial muscle when, from the atrial muscle to the SA node, the coupling resistance was decreased in a step-like manner (C) or in a gradual manner (D). B-D from Joyner and van Capelle (1986).

must be sufficiently low so that the SA node cells are protected from the suppressive effect of the atrial cells, but sufficiently high so that the SA node cells can drive the atrial cells).

Finally, Joyner and van Capelle (1986) suggested that there should be a gradual increase in electrical coupling at the border of the SA node and atrial muscle. The results in Fig. 2C, D (also from Joyner and van Capelle, 1986) were obtained using a more realistic model of a circular SA node surrounded by a ring of atrial tissue. In this model, the membrane potential could vary in each group of cells (SA node and atrial), i.e. the coupling resistance and distance between cells in a group were taken into account. In the first case (Fig. 2C), connectivity was low (i.e. radial resistivity was high) in the SA node and connectivity was high (i.e. radial resistivity was low) in the atrial muscle. The low connectivity within the SA node protects the SA node from the hyperpolarizing influence of the atrial muscle, but does not allow it drive the atrial muscle – the action potential failed to exit from the SA node (Fig. 2C, bottom panel). In this case, increasing the size of the SA node may not allow the SA node to drive the atrial muscle (because the radius of SA node was already large, the space constant consideration above means that increasing the radius further may not assist). A possible solution is suggested by Fig. 2D: here, there was a progressive increase in connectivity (decrease in radial resistivity) at the junction of SA node and atrial muscle – now the action potential exited from the SA node (Fig. 2D, bottom panel). Evidence for such a transitional connectivity at the junction of the two tissues is considered below by action potentials from outside of the SA node, from either a reentrant arrhythmia or one of the many latent pacemakers in the atria. This could lead to a resetting of the SA node or perhaps even overdrive suppression of the SA node. It appears that the SA node is well protected: Kirchhof and Allessie (1992) have shown that during atrial fibrillation, normal pacemaker activity is still present in the centre of the SA node and hardly overdrive suppressed due to a high degree of SA node entrance block. This protection is probably achieved in various ways (Boyett et al., 2000), but one way could again be some degree of electrical uncoupling of the cells within the SA node.

THERE IS SOME DEGREE OF ELECTRICAL UNCOUPLING OF CELLS WITHIN THE SA NODE

Many lines of evidence show that there is weak electrical coupling within the SA node. Intercellular coupling is a major determinant of the conduction velocity. The conduction velocity is low in the centre of the SA node. In rabbit heart, the conduction velocity in the centre of the SA node is 4.5 cm/s parallel to and 3.0 cm/s perpendicular to the crista terminalis (Yamamoto et al., 1998). The conduction velocity from the periphery of the SA node to the surrounding atrial muscle is higher at 49.7 cm/s parallel to and 36.3 cm/s perpendicular to the crista terminalis (Yamamoto et al, 1998). This is in accord with the hypothesis of Joyner and van Capelle (1986) of a transitional connectivity at the junction of the SA node and atrial muscle.

The space constant is another measure of electrical coupling and the space constant of SA node is lower than that of atrial muscle (Bonke, 1973a, 1973b; Seyama, 1976; Bleeker et al., 1982; Bukauskas et al., 1982; Bouman et al., 1989). Finally, gap junction conductance measurements between pairs of cells have confirmed that electrical coupling in the SA node is weak. Verheule et al. (2001) measured the gap junction conductance between pairs of rabbit SA node cells to be 7.5 ± 6.4 nS, whereas for rabbit atrial and ventricular cells the same group measured it to be 169 ± 146 and 175 ± 147 nS, respectively (Verheule et al., 1997). Anumonwo et al. (1992) measured the gap junction conductance between pairs of rabbit SA node cells to be on average 2.6 nS, in keeping with the low value above. By experiment or mathematical modeling, various investigators have estimated the minimal coupling

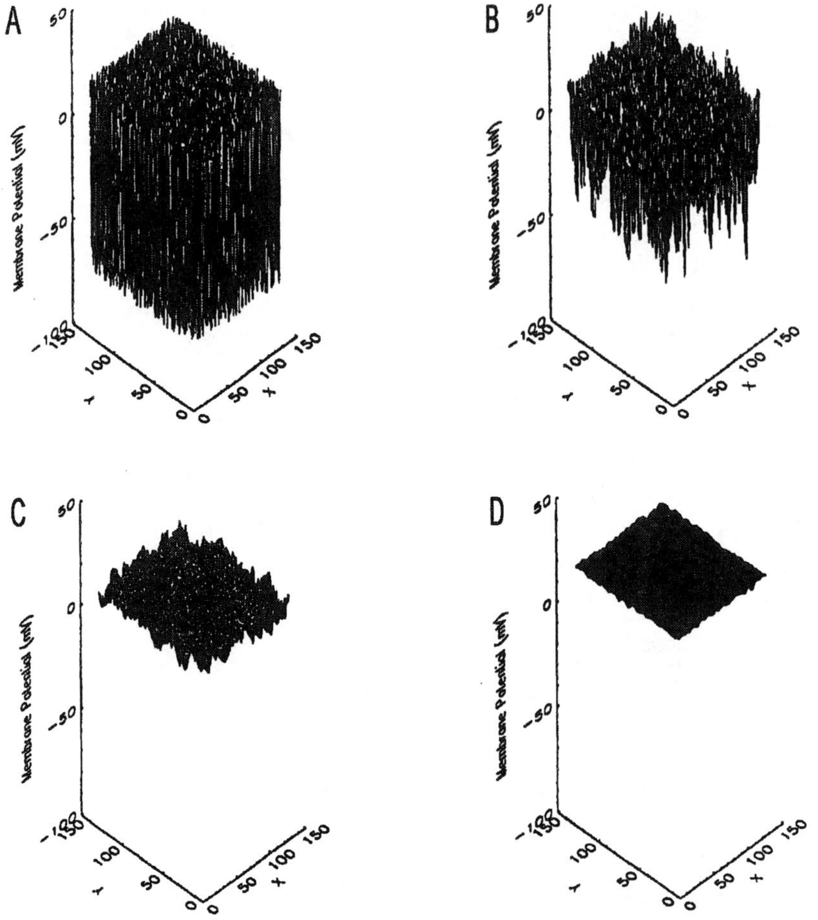

Figure 3. The effect of the coupling conductance on the synchronisation of SA node cells as shown by mathematical modelling. Membrane potential is shown at a given moment in time in each cell of a 128×128 mesh of SA node cells with different intrinsic frequencies (randomly distributed). The coupling conductance was 0 (A), 0.2 (B), 1 (C) and 50 (D) nS. From Cai et al. (1994).

conductance between SA node cells in order to achieve a synchronisation of electrical activity within the SA node to be 0.2-0.5 nS (Anumonwo et al., 1992; Verheijck et al., 1998) and this is within the observed range above. For example, Fig. 3 from Cai et al. (1994) shows membrane potential throughout a 128×128 mesh of SA node cells with different intrinsic frequencies (randomly distributed) and different coupling conductances. With a coupling conductance of 0 nS there was no synchronisation (Fig. 3A), whereas there was rough synchronisation with 0.2 nS (Fig. 3B); with 50 nS the synchronisation was better and the membrane potential throughout the mesh was more uniform (Fig. 3D).

GAP JUNCTIONS IN THE SA NODE

Gap junctions have been seen in many ultrastrutural studies of the SA node (see Saffitz et al., 1997, for references). Here just two quantitative studies will be considered. Masson-Pévet et al. (1979) reported that the gap junctions of rabbit SA node are generally small and estimated that in leading pacemaker cells (presumably from the centre of the SA node) the gap junctions are about 10 times less numerous than in working myocardial cells.

Table 1. Analysis of gap junctions in the dog SA node

	LV	CT	SA node	LV:SA node ratio	CT:SA node ratio
ID length (µm) per 100 µm² cell area	3.5±0.7	4.4±1.3*	2.6±0.5	1.3	3.4
Number of GJ profiles per 100 µm ID length	15.5±3.8**	11.5±7.4*	5.6±2.4	2.8	2.1
Mean GJ profile length (µm)	0.82±0.36**	0.28±0.07**	0.17±0.07	4.8	1.6
Total GJ profile length (µm) per 100 µm ID length	12.7±2.8**	3.2±2.4*	1.0±0.7	12.7	3.2

ID, intercalated disk. GJ, gap junction. LV, left ventricle. CT, crista terminalis. *P<0.05 vs SA node; **P<0.01 vs SA node. From Saffitz et al. (1997).

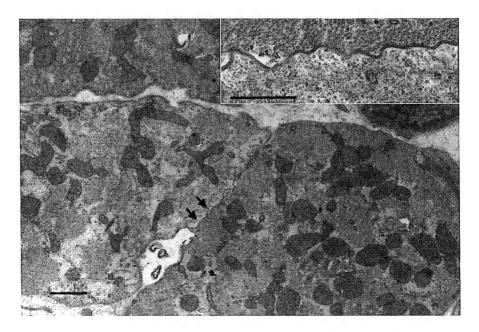

Figure 4. Electron micrographs of rabbit SA node tissue. Arrows and the inset show gap junctions. Scale bar in main panel, 1 μm. Scale bar in inset, 500 nm.

Typical gap junctions of the rabbit SA node are shown in Fig. 4. A more detailed study is that of Saffitz et al. (1997) who studied the gap junctions of dog heart. They reported that a typical SA node cell is connected to five neighbouring cells, whereas in the crista terminalis (atrial muscle) the cells are connected to six and in the left ventricle, 11. In the dog SA node, intercellular connections occur at small, simple intercalated disks located on cytoplasmic projections arising at various points along SA node cells. This arrangement provides opportunities for complex three-dimensional cell packing patterns. The aggregate gap junction profile length per unit cell area was five times greater in the crista terminalis and 27 times greater in the left ventricle than in the SA node. The individual gap junctions were statistically smaller in SA node cells than the other two cell types. Further statistics for the dog SA node are given in Table 1. The paucity and small size of gap junctions in the SA node are consistent with the weak electrical coupling in the SA node.

GAP JUNCTION SUBTYPES IN THE SA NODE

Each gap junction comprises clusters of serially linked hemichannels (connexons) contributed by the two apposing cell membranes, giving a way for small molecules (<1 kDa) to pass between the two cell interiors (Severs et al., 1990). Each connexon is composed of six transmembrane proteins called connexins, a multigene family of conserved proteins of which at least 13 members are known in mammals (Goodenough et al., 1996). Among the several connexins detected in the heart (Cx37, Cx40, Cx43, Cx45 and Cx46), Cx43 is ubiquitous and most abundant in the working myocardium (atrial and ventricular muscle), but this is not the case in the specialized conducting tissues (Gourdie et al., 1993; Coppen et al., 1998).

Many immunohistochemical studies have focused on connexin phenotypes in the SA node, but the results have been inconsistent and conflicting. Anumonwo et al. (1992) reported Cx43 in the rabbit SA node. Trabka-Janik et al. (1994) also reported Cx43 in the hamster SA node. Other studies on rabbit, mouse, rat, guinea-pig, dog, cow and human, however, have failed to detect Cx43 in the SA node (van Kempen et al., 1991; Oosthoek et al., 1993; Davis et al., 1994,1995; ten Velde et al., 1995; Kwong et al., 1998; Coppen et al., 1999; Verheule et al., 2001; Verheijck et al., 2001) (Fig. 5). Coppen et al. (1999) found that Cx45 and Cx40 are expressed in the Cx43-negative area of the rabbit SA node (Fig. 6). The dimensions and quantities of the Cx45 and Cx40 spots observed were much smaller than those of Cx43 spots in the atrial muscle, and this is consistent with the size and frequency of SA node cell gap junctions as revealed by electron microscopy (see above). Honjo et al. (2002) have shown in single SA node cells isolated from rabbit heart that small (putative central) cells express mainly Cx45 and a small amount of Cx40, but not Cx43; the labelled spots for Cx45 and Cx40 were small, punctate and dispersed over the cell surface (Fig. 7). Davis et al. (1994, 1995) also demonstrated the presence of Cx40.

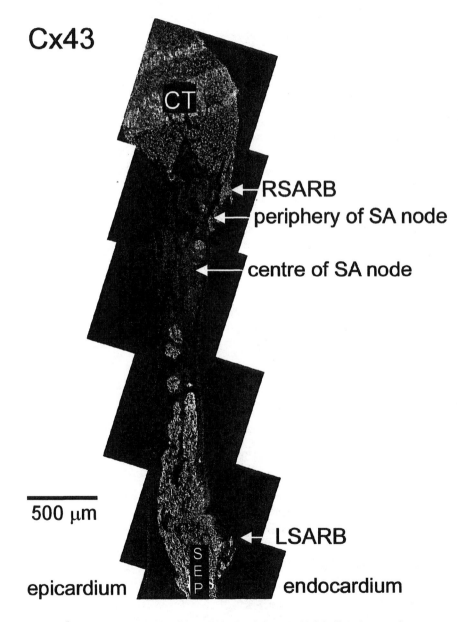

Figure 5. Connexin subtypes in the rabbit SA node - Cx43 labelling in a section
through the atrial muscle of the crista terminalis (CT) and the thinner intercaval
region where the centre of the SA node is located. RSARB, LSARB, right and left
branches of SA ring bundle. SEP, interatrial septum. From Coppen et al. (1999).

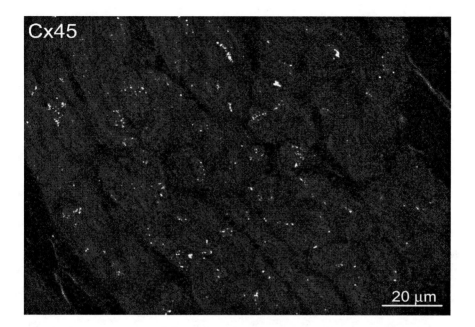

Figure 6. Connexin subtypes in the rabbit SA node - Cx45 expression in the centre of the SA node.

and Cx45 in the dog and human SA node region where Cx43 was undetectable. Verheule et al. (2001) reported the presence of Cx40 and Cx46 and the absence of Cx43 in the centre of rabbit SA node.

Discrepancies between different studies may be attributed in part to species differences in connexin expression in the SA node and in part to technical problems. Recognition of a specific immunohistochemical signal is more difficult in SA node cells than in atrial and ventricular cells, because the gap junctions are smaller and the cell-packing architecture is more complex. The mean number of channels in each SA node gap junction in rabbits is estimated to be ~90 channels (Masson-Pévet et al., 1979). This is close to the limit for detection by immunohistochemistry (ten Velde et al., 1995). Therefore, the absence of labelling does not necessarily mean the absence of the connexin. Unreliability of antibodies (cross reaction with other types of connexin) may also lead to false conclusions (Severs et al., 2001).

At the border between the SA node and atrial muscle in guinea-pig heart, ten Velde et al. (1995) demonstrated an intermingling (or inter-digitation) of strands of Cx43-positive atrial cells and Cx43-negative

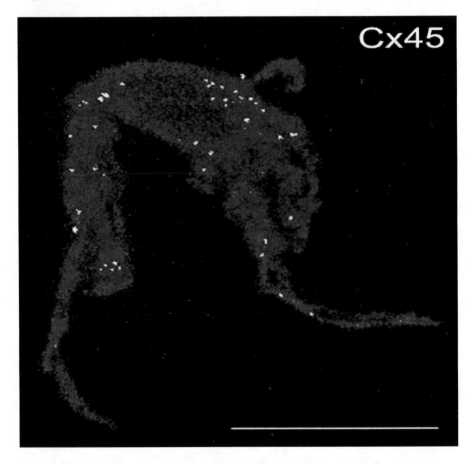

Figure 7. Connexin subtypes in the rabbit SA node - Cx45 expression in an isolated SA node cell. Scale bar, 20 μm. From Honjo et al. (2002).

node cells. A similar interdigitating arrangement at the periphery of the SA node was reported in a immunohistochemical study on rat, cow and human hearts (Oosthoek et al., 1993). In the rabbit SA node, Coppen et al. (1999) found that most boundaries between Cx43-positive cells and Cx43-negative (but Cx40-positive and Cx45-positive) SA node cells were sharply delineated, and no extensive interdigitation between the two cell types was apparent. Instead, in the periphery of the SA node both Cx43 and Cx45 were expressed. In the rabbit, whereas the centre of the SA node is in the thin intercaval region distant from the crista terminalis, the periphery of the SA node lies on the endocardial surface of the crista terminalis. The right branch of the SA ring bundle (seen in Fig. 5) can be a useful landmark to identify the periphery of the SA node, and it can be seen in Fig. 5 that Cx43, although absent from the centre of the SA node, is present in the periphery. An analogous transitional structure with both Cx43 and Cx45 has been reported in mouse SA node (Verheijck et al., 2001). In support of these observations, a population of large (putative peripheral) SA node cells from rabbits were shown to express both Cx43 and Cx45 (Honjo et al., 2002). Kwong et al. (1998) have shown in dogs that Cx43-positive SA node cells form bundles protruding into the Cx43-negative and Cx40-positive central SA node region.

Cx43 in the periphery of the SA node or that in bundles protruding into the centre of the SA node could serve an important role as the preferential conduction pathway for the propagation of the action potential from the SA node to the atrial muscle. This could represent the zone of intermediate coupling conductance proposed by Joyner and van Capelle (1986) that enables the SA node to drive the atrial muscle surrounding the SA node and yet not be suppressed by the atrial muscle.

In large (putative peripheral) SA node cells isolated from rabbit hearts, Honjo et al. (2002) showed that Cx43 and Cx45 often co-localised in the same gap junction plaque. This observation raises the possibility that heterotypic gap junction channels (in which one connexon is constructed from Cx43 and the partner connexon from Cx45) or heteromeric channels (comprising a mixture of Cx43 and Cx45) exist in the SA node. Whether such putative heterotypic or heteromeric channels, which are known to have different properties from homomeric channels in vitro (Valiunas et al., 2000; He et al., 1999), might contribute to modulation of electrical coupling at the periphery of the SA node to help maintain normal pacemaker function is at present unclear.

IMPORTANCE OF LIMITING THE CONTACT BETWEEN THE SA NODE AND ATRIAL MUSCLE

In various species, a connective tissue barrier has been described between the SA node and the adjoining atrial muscle of the crista terminalis: monkey (Alings et al., 1990), human and cow (Oosthoek et al., 1993), rabbit (Coppen et al., 1999) and mouse (Verheijck et al., 2001). Examples from mouse and rabbit are shown in Fig. 8 (highlighted by the arrows) and Fig. 9A (highlighted by the dashed line), respectively. In the case of the rabbit (Fig. 9A), there appears to be a connective tissue barrier between the two tissues where the periphery of the SA node overlaps the atrial muscle of the crista terminalis. The possible importance of this connective tissue barrier has been investigated by Zhang et al. (2001) using mathematical modeling. They developed a two-dimensional model (Fig. 9B) of the tissue section in Fig. 9A and varied the extent of connection between the SA node and atrial tissue in the region of overlap from no connection to full connection and the results are summarised in Fig. 10.

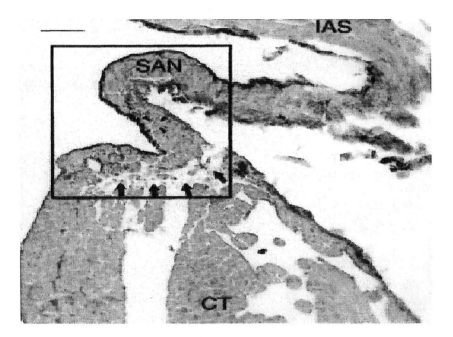

Figure 8. A connective tissue barrier (highlighted by arrows) between the atrial muscle of the crista terminalis (CT) and the SA node (SAN) in the mouse. IAS, interatrial septum. From Verheijck et al. (2001).

With no connection or too little connection, the SA node region showed pacemaker activity (5.6 Hz with no connection), but the SA node was unable to drive the atrial muscle of the crista terminalis. In this case, the leading pacemaker site was in the periphery of SA node. With a greater connection length, the SA node was able to show pacemaker activity and drive the atrial muscle. However, in this case, the pacemaker activity was slowed (e.g. the rate was 2.9 Hz with a connection length of 0.15 mm) and the leading pacemaker site was shifted from the periphery to the centre of the SA node. With an even greater connection length, the SA node was still able to show

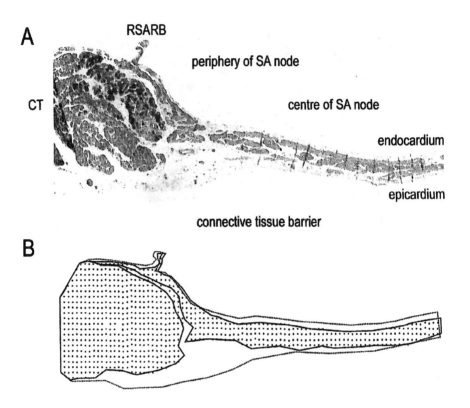

Figure 9. Modelling the connective tissue barrier between the atrial muscle and SA node in the rabbit. A, tissue section through atrial muscle of crista terminalis (CT) and SA node tissue of intercaval region. B, two dimensional model of the tissue section above. The tissue section was discretised and divided into "nodes" (the spots shown) and each node was assigned to be atrial muscle, connective tissue or SA node. RSARB, right branch of the SA ring bundle.

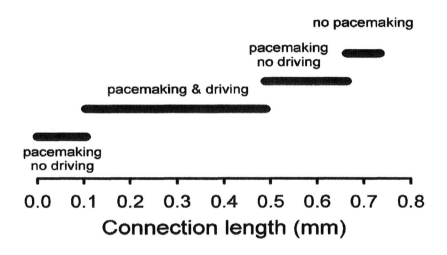

Figure 10. Effect of the extent of the connection between the atrial muscle and the SA node in the two dimensional model shown in Fig. 9B on the behaviour of the SA node.

pacemaker activity, but it was now unable to drive the atrial muscle. With full connection in the region of overlap, the greater suppressive effect of the atrial muscle on the SA node meant that the SA node did not even show pacemaker activity (Fig. 10).

CURVATURE OF THE EXCITING WAVEFRONT FROM THE SA NODE ARRIVING AT THE ATRIAL MUSCLE

Fig. 1 shows that, in the rabbit, from the leading pacemaker site the action potential preferentially propagates in an oblique cranial direction. This is perhaps the result of the orientation of the cells within the SA node: many of the cells, at least in the periphery, are orientated parallel to the crista terminalis. Such a preferential direction of propagation is also seen in other species (guinea-pig, cat, pig – Opthof et al., 1985, 1986, 1987). In the mouse and monkey the action potential propagates from the leading pacemaker site in an oblique caudal direction (Alings et al., 1990; Verheijck et al., 2001). However, regardless of the direction of propagation, in all species, the action potential arrives at the crista terminalis (the junction of the SA node and atrial muscle) as a broad wavefront (e.g. Fig. 1). The "curvature" of a wavefront governs the ability of a wavefront to depolarize the tissue ahead of it and the ability of a convex wavefront to propagate is weaker than the ability of a straight or concave one (Cabo et al., 1994; Fast and Kleber, 1997; Davidenko, 2001). If theaction potential was to radiate in a symmetrical fashion from the leading pacemaker site in the SA node, it would arrive at the crista terminalis as a convex wavefront and its ability to drive the atrial muscle would be expected to be weaker as a result. This problem is avoided, because the action potential arrives as an almost planar wavefront (e.g. Fig. 1).

RECONSTRUCTING THE SA NODE

A major factor affecting propagation from the SA node is the block zone: in the rabbit and other species (mouse, guinea-pig, cat, pig, monkey – Opthof et al., 1985, 1986, 1987; Alings et al., 1990; Verheijck et al., 2001), propagation of the action potential from the leading pacemaker site in the SA node towards the interatrial septum is blocked and the action potential must propagate around a block zone to reach the interatrial septum (e.g. Fig. 1). Theoretically, this block zone could be the result of an absence of coupling

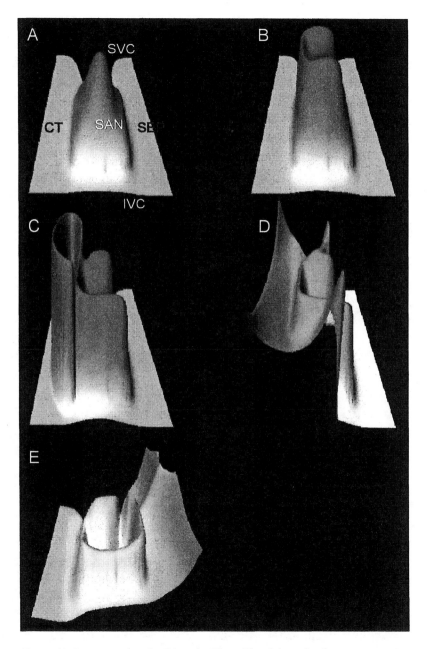

Figure 11. Reconstructing the SA node. Five stills of the activation sequence of a two dimensional mathematical model of the SA node and surrounding atrial muscle are shown. SAN, sinoatrial node. CT, crista terminalis. SVC, superior vena cava. SEP, interatrial septum. IVC, inferior vena cava.

between cells in this region. The activation sequence of the rabbit SA node has been modelled mathematically with the block zone modelled in this way (Michaels et al., 1987). However, in the rabbit the space constant in the block zone is the same as elsewhere in the SA node (Bleeker et al., 1982) and there is no absence of gap junctions in the block zone (Coppen et al., 1999).

Zhang et al. (1999) tentatively attributed the block zone to an absence of excitatory current (both Na^+ and Ca^{2+} currents). Fig. 11 shows membrane potential in a two-dimensional mathematical model of the SA node embedded in atrial muscle (five snapshots during the activation sequence of the SA node are shown). The model incorporates poor connectivity in the SA node and the block zone is modelled by an absence of excitatory current. The activation sequence is qualitatively similar to that in rabbit SA node (Fig. 1): the action potential is initiated in the centre of the SA node (Fig. 11A) and from here it propagates to the periphery of the SA node (Fig. 11B) and then into the atrial muscle of the crista terminalis (CT; Fig. 11C). From the leading pacemaker site, the action potential attempts to propagate towards the interatrial septum (SEP), but conduction is blocked (Fig. 11B, C). Propagation to the interatrial septum must wait for conduction around the block zone (Fig. 11D, E).

CLINICAL IMPLICATIONS

SA node dysfunction in humans, known as "sick sinus syndrome" is a common cause of symptomatic arrhythmias in elderly people (Ferrer, 1973). The syndrome is manifested by intermittent sinus bradycardia, sinus arrest, sinoatrial conduction block or alternating bradycardia and atrial tachy-arrhythmias. Sick sinus syndrome could be related to an age-related deterioration in the function of the SA node observed in humans and also other animal species (Alings et al., 1993): with age, the intrinsic heart rate (i.e. the heart rate in the absence of autonomic nerve activity) declines and SA node conduction time increases, perhaps culminating in SA node exit block. There are various possible explanations of the age-dependent deterioration. In the rabbit and cat SA node, Alings et al. (1993) showed that the total area of SA node does not change with age, but the region in which the upstroke velocity is low (a result of a low Na^+ channel density) increases; as a result the upstroke velocity of the action potential decreases in the periphery of the SA node (close to the crista terminalis) to a value similar to that in the centre of the SA node. This may account in part for the age-related increase of the SA node conduction time: Zhang et al. (1998) showed that, in a multicellular mathematical model of the SA node incorporating regional differences in ion channels, elimination of the Na^+ current from the periphery of the SA node slowed pacemaker activity and increased SA node conduction time; it could also result in SA node exit block. Jones and Boyett (2001) have shown that the Cx43-negative zone in the guinea-pig SA node increases with aging (from 1 to 38 months of age). Such a decrease in Cx43 expression could also help explain age-dependent SA node dysfunction. Further experimental studies will be required to shed light on this issue.

SUMMARY

This chapter has been concerned with how the SA node is connected and the implications of this on how the SA node fulfils its function of pacemaking and driving the surrounding atrial muscle. It is concluded that: (i) the SA node should be of sufficient size; (ii) coupling conductance should be low in the SA node; (iii) at the junction of the SA node with the atrial muscle, there should be a region of transitional conductance; (iv) at the junction of the SA node with the atrial muscle, the extent of the connection between the two tissues should be neither too large or too small; and (v) the wavefront from the SA node should arrive at the junction with the atrial muscle as a broad wavefront. Coupling in atrial muscle is good and is primarily provided by an abundance of large gap junctions made up of Cx43. However, coupling in the SA node is poor, because it is made up of a much lower abundance of small gap junctions made up of Cx45 and Cx40. The region of transitional conductance may correspond to the periphery of the SA node in which gap junctions are made up of both Cx43 and Cx45. The decline in conduction velocity within the SA node with ageing and the conduction problems in sick sinus syndrome might be the result of a loss of Cx43 from the SA node.

REFERENCE

Alings, A. M. W., Abbas, R. F., de Jonge, B., & Bouman, L. N. (1990). Structure and function of the simian sinoatrial node (Macaca fascicularis). J. Mol. Cell. Cardiol. **22**, 1453-1466.

Alings, A.M.W., & Bouman, L.N. (1993). Electrophysiology of the aging rabbit and cat sinoatrial node. Eur. Heart. J. **14**, 1278-1288.

Anumonwo, J. M. B., Wang, H.-Z., Trabka-Janik, E., Dunham, B., Veenstra, R. D., Dalmar, M., & Jalife, J. (1992). Gap junctional channels in adult mammalian sinus nodal cells. Immunolocalization and electrophysiology. Circ. Res. **71**, 229-239.

Bleeker, W. K., Mackaay, A. J. C., Masson-Pevet, M., Op't Hof, T., Jongsma, H. J., & Bouman, L. N. (1982). Asymmetry of the sino-atrial conduction in the rabbit heart. J. Mol. Cell. Cardiol. **14**, 633-643.

Bonke, F. I. M. (1973a). Passive electrical properties of atrial fibers of the rabbit heart. Pflügers Arch. **339**, 1-15.

Bonke, F. I. M. (1973b). Electrotonic spread in the sinoatrial node of the rabbit heart. Pflügers Arch. **339**, 17-23.

Bouman, L. N., Duivenvoorden, J. J., Bukauskas, F. F., & Jongsma, H. J. (1989). Anisotropy of electrotonus in the sinoatrial node of the rabbit heart. J. Mol. Cell. Cardiol. **21**, 407-418.

Boyett, M. R., Holden, A. V., Zhang, H., Kodama, I., & Suzuki, R. (1995). Atrial modulation of sinoatrial pacemaker rate. Chaos, Solitons & Fractals **5**, 425-438.

Boyett, M. R., Honjo, H., & Kodama, I. (2000). The sinoatrial node, a heterogeneous pacemaker structure. Cardiovasc. Res. **47**, 658-687.

Bukauskas, F. F., Gutman, A. M., Kisunas, K. J., & Veteikis, R. P. (1982). Electrical cell coupling in rabbit sinoatrial node and atrium. Experimental and theoretical evaluation. In Cardiac Rate and Rhythum, eds. Bouman, L. N. & Jongsma, H. J., pp. 195-214. Martinus Nijhoff Publishers, The Hague, Boston, London.

Cabo, C., Pertsov, A. M., Baxter, W. T., Davidenko, J. M., Gray, R. A., & Jalife, J. (1994). Wave-front curvature as a cause of slow conduction and block in isolated cardiac muscle. Circ. Res. **75**, 1014-1028.

Cai, D., Winslow, R. L., & Noble, D. (1994). Effects of gap junction conductance on dynamics of sinoatrial node cells: two cell and large scale networks. IEEE Trans. Biomed. Eng. **41**, 217-231.

Coppen, S.R., Dupont, E, Rothery, S., & Severs, J.N. (1998). Connexin45 expression is preferentially associated with the ventricular conduction system in mouse and rat heart. Circ. Res. **82**, 232-243.

Coppen, S. R., Kodama, I., Boyett, M. R., Dobrzynski, H., Takagishi, Y., Honjo, H., Yeh, H.-I., & Severs, N. J. (1999). Connexin45, a major connexin of the rabbit sinoatrial node, is co-expressed with connexin43 in a restricted zone at the nodal-crista terminalis border. J. Histochem. Cytochem. **47**, 907-918.

Davidenko, J. M. (2001). Spiral waves in the heart: experimental demonstration of a theory. In: Cardiac Electrophysiology: From Cell to Bedside. Edited by D. P. Zipes and J. Jalife. Philadelphia: W.B. Saunders Company, 478-488.

Davis, L.M., Kanter, F.H., Beyer E.C., & Saffitz, J.E. (1994). Distinct gap junction protein phenotypes in cardiac tissues with disparate conduction properties. J. Am. Coll. Cardiol. **24**, 1124-1132.

Davis, L.M., Rodefeld, M.E., Green, K., Beyer, E.C., & Saffitz, J.E. (1995). Gap junction phenotypes of the human heart and conduction system. J. Cardiovasc. Electrophysiol. **6**, 813-822.

Fast, V.G., & Kleber, A.G. (1997). Role of wavefront curvature in propagation of cardiac impulse. Cardiovasc. Res. **33**, 258-271.

Ferrer, M.I. (1973). The sick sinus syndrome. Circulation **47**, 635-641.

Goodenough, D.A., Goliger, J.A., & Paul, D.L. (1996). Connexins, connexons and intercellular communication. Ann. Rev. Biochem. **77**, 1156-1163.

Gourdie, R.G., Severs, N.J., Green, C.R., Rothery, S., Germroth, P., & Thompson, R.P. (1993). The spatial distribution and relative abundance of gap junctional connexin40 and connexin43 correlate to functional properties of the cardiac atrioventricular conduction system. J. Cell. Sci. **105**, 985-991.

He, D.S., Jiang, J.X., Taffet, S.M., & Burt, J.M. (1999). Formation of heteromeric gap junction channels by connexins 40 and 43 in vascular smooth muscle cells. Proc. Natl. Acad. Sci. USA **96**, 6495-6500.

Honjo, H., Boyett, M.R., Coppen, S.R., Takagishi, Y., Opthof, T., Severs, N.J., & Kodama, I. (2002). Heterogeneous expression of connexins in rabbit sinoatrial node cells: correlation between connexin isotype and cell size. Cardiovasc. Res. **53**, 89-96.

Jones, S.A., & Boyett, M.R. (2001). Ageing of the heart: a comparison of young and senescent guinea pigs. J. Physiol. **533P**.

Joyner, R. W., Kumar, R., Golod, D., Wilders, R., Jongsma, H. J., Verheijck, E. E., Bouman, L. N., Goolsby, W. N., & van Ginneken, A. (1998). Electrical interactions between a rabbit atrial cell and a nodal cell model. Am. J. Physiol. **274**, H2152-H2162.

Joyner, R. W. & van Capelle, F. J. L. (1986). Propagation through electrically coupled cells: how a small SA node drives a large atrium. Biophys. J. **50**, 1157-1164.

Kirchhof, C. J. H. J. & Allessie, M. A. (1992). Sinus node automaticity during atrial fibrillation in isolated rabbit hearts. Circulation **86**, 263-271.

Kirchhof, C. J. H. J., Bonke, F. I. M., Allessie, M. A., & Lammers, W. J. E. P. (1987). The influence of the atrial myocardium on impulse formation in the rabbit sinus node. Pflügers Arch. **410**, 198-203.

Kodama, I. & Boyett, M. R. (1985). Regional differences in the electrical activity of the rabbit sinus node. Pflügers Arch. **404**, 214-226.

Kodama, I., Boyett, M. R., Suzuki, R., Honjo, H., & Toyama, J. (1996). Regional differences in the response of the isolated sinoatrial node of the rabbit to vagal stimulation. J. Physiol. **495**, 785-801.

Kwong, K.F., Schuessler, R.B., Green, K.G., Laing, J.G., Beyer, E.C., Boineau, J.P., & Saffitz, J.E. (1998). Differential expression of gap junction proteins in the canine sinus node. Circ. Res. **82**, 604-612.

Masson-Pévet, M. A., Bleeker, W. K., & Gros, D. (1979). The plasma membrane of leading pacemaker cells in the rabbit sinus node: A quantitative ultrastructural analysis. Circ. Res. **45**, 621-629.

Michaels, D. C., Matyas, E. P., & Jalife, J. (1987). Mechanisms of sinoatrial pacemaker synchronization: a new hypothesis. Circ. Res. **61**, 704-714.

Oosthoek, P. W., Viragh, S., Mayen, A. E. M., van Kempen, M. J. A., Lamers, W. H., & Moorman, A. F. M. (1993). Immunohistochemical delineation of the conduction system. I: the sinoatrial node. Circ. Res. **73**, 473-481.

Opthof, T., de Jonge, B., Jongsma, H. J., & Bouman, L. N. (1987). Functional morphology of the pig sinoatrial node. J. Mol. Cell. Cardiol. **19**, 1221-1236.

Opthof, T., de Jonge, B., Mackaay, A. J. C., Bleeker, W. K., Masson-Pevet, M., Jongsma, H. J., & Bouman, L. N. (1985). Functional and morphological organization of the guinea-pig sinoatrial node compared with the rabbit sinoatrial node. J. Mol. Cell. Cardiol. **17**, 549-564.

Opthof, T., de Jonge, B., Masson-Pevet, M., Jongsma, H. J., & Bouman, L. N. (1986). Functional and morphological organization of the cat sinoatrial node. J. Mol. Cell. Cardiol. **18**, 1015-1031.

Saffitz, J. E., Green, K. G., & Schuessler, R. B. (1997). Structural determinants of slow conduction in the canine sinus node. J. Cardiovasc. Electrophysiol. **8**, 738-744.

Severs, N.J. (1990). The cardiac gap junctions and intercalated disc. Int. J. Cardiol. **26**, 137-173.

Severs, N.J., Rothery, S, Dupont, E., Coppen, S.R., Yeh, H.-I., Ko, Y.-S., Matsushita, T., Kaba, R., & Halliday, D. (2001). Immunocytochemical analysis of connexin expression in the healthy and diseased cardiovascular system. Micros. Res. Tech. **52**, 301-322.

Seyama, I. (1976). Characteristics of the rectifying properties of the sinoatrial node cell of the rabbit. J. Physiol. **255**, 379-397.

ten Velde, I., de Jonge, B., Verheijck, E.E., van Kempen, M.J.A., Analbers, L., Gros, D., & Jongsma, H.J. (1995). Spatial distribution of connexin43, the major cardiac gap junction protein, visualizes the cellular network for impulse propagation from sinoatrial node to atrium. Circ. Res. **76**, 802-811.

Toyama, J., Boyett, M. R., Watanabe, E.-I., Honjo, H., Anno, T., & Kodama, I. (1995). Computer simulation of the electrotonic modulation of pacemaker activity in the sinoatrial node by atrial muscle. J. Electrocardiol. **28** (supplement), 212-215.

Trabka-Janik, E., Coombs, W., Lemanski, L.F., Delmar, M., & Jalife, J. (1994). Immunohistochemical localization of gap junction protein channels in hamster sinoatrial node in correlation with electrophysiological mapping of the pacemaker region. Circ. Res. **71**, 229-239.

Valiunas, V., Weingart, R., & Brink, P.R. (2000). Formation of heterotypic gap junction channels by connexins 40 and 43. Circ. Res. **86**, e42-e49.

van Kempen, M.J.A., Fromaget, C., Gros, D., Moorman, A.F.M., & Lamers, W.H. (1991). Spatial distbution of connexin43, the major cardiac gap junction protein, in the developing and adult rat heart. Circ. Res. **68**, 1638-1651.

Verheijck, E. E., van Kempen, M. J., Veereschild, M., Lurvink, J., Jongsma, H. J., & Bouman, L. N. (2001). Electrophysiological features of the mouse sinoatrial node in relation to connexin distribution. Cardiovasc. Res. **52**, 40-50.

Verheijck, E. E., Wilders, R., Joyner, R. W., Golod, D., Kumar, R., Jongsma, H. J., Bouman, L. N., & van Ginneken, A. C. G. (1998). Pacemaker synchronization of electrically coupled rabbit sinoatrial node cells. J. Gen. Physiol. **111**, 95-112.

Verheule, S., van Kempen, M. J., Postma, S., Rook, M. B., & Jongsma, H. J. (2001). Gap junctions in the rabbit sinoatrial node. Am. J. Physiol. **280**, H2103-H2115.

Verheule, S., van Kempen, M. J., te Welscher, P. H., Kwak, B. R., & Jongsma, H. J. (1997). Characterization of gap junction channels in adult rabbit atrial and ventricular myocardium. Circ. Res. **80**, 673-681.

Watanabe, E.-I., Honjo, H., Anno, T., Boyett, M. R., Kodama, I., & Toyama, J. (1995a). Electrotonic modulation of pacemaking activity in the sinoatrial node by atrial muscle. Heart and Vessels Supplement **9**, 182-183.

Watanabe, E.-I., Honjo, H., Anno, T., Boyett, M. R., Kodama, I., & Toyama, J. (1995b). Modulation of pacemaker activity of sinoatrial node cells by electrical load imposed by an atrial cell model. Am. J. Physiol. **269**, H1735-H1742.

Yamamoto, M., Honjo, H., Niwa, R., & Kodama, I. (1998). Low frequency extracellular potentials recorded from the sinoatrial node. Cardiovasc. Res. **39**, 360-372.

Zhang, H., Boyett, M.R., Holden, A.V., Honjo, H., & Kodama, I. (1998). A hypothesis to explain the decline of sinoatrial node function with age. J. Physiol. **511**, 76P-77P.

Zhang, H., Dobrzynski, H., Kodama, I., Takagishi, Y., Holden, A. V., & Boyett, M. R. (2001). How does the sinoatrial node drive the atrium? J. Physiol. **536P**.

Zhang, H., Holden, A. V., Kodama, I., Honjo, H., Lei, M., Takagishi, Y., & Boyett, M. R. (1999). Hypothesis to explain the block zone protecting the sinoatrial node. Biophys. J. **76**, A368.

9

INWARD AND OUTWARD CURRENTS AND CARDIAC DISCONTINUOUS CONDUCTION

Mary B. Wagner and Ronald W. Joyner
Emory University, Atlanta, GA 30322

INTRODUCTION

In the normal heart, most of the individual cardiac cells are well coupled to adjacent cells through gap junctions. Because of this, the myocardium is referred to as an electrical syncytium such that excitation occurring at any location is able to spread throughout all parts of the heart which are not refractory to stimulation. The process of action potential propagation in the heart has generally been considered as a multi-dimensional analog of the continuous one-dimensional propagation observed in unmyelinated nerve fibers.

In the case of continuous conduction, the fast inward sodium current is responsible for both excitability and conduction. As charge is transferred to a cell which has not yet been activated, the depolarization which occurs, to bring the cell membrane potential to the voltage threshold for the fast sodium current, is largely determined by the input resistance of the cell and this input resistance is determined largely by the inward rectifier current, I_{K1}. Thus, for continuous conduction these two currents, the inward I_{Na} and the outward I_{K1}, along with the gap junctional conductance (G_c), are the predominant determinants of conduction. In contrast, in conditions where conduction is discontinuous due to either normal, regional differences or pathological conditions, the ionic determinants of conduction are altered.

It is difficult in syncytial tissue to clearly define the mechanisms by which action potentials are initiated and conducted. Several methodologies have been applied in an attempt to understand the roles that different ionic currents play in determining whether discontinuous conduction is successful. These include studies on the Purkinje-ventricular junction, patterned cultured cells, isolated cell pairs, and mathematical simulations. All of these studies have indicated that, while I_{Na} is indeed necessary for <u>activation</u> of a cell from a normal resting potential, this I_{Na} may not be a sufficient mechanism to produce <u>conduction</u> of the action potential to another cell. When conduction becomes discontinuous, with conduction delays of more than 3-4 msec, action potential conduction becomes dependent on another inward current (the L-type calcium current, I_{Ca}) and another outward current (the transient outward current, I_{to}).

INWARD CURRENTS AND DISCONTINUOUS CONDUCTION

In normal myocardium, the fast sodium current (I_{Na}) is responsible for excitability and conduction. Under conditions of discontinuous conduction, there can be delays between activation of connected cell groups of more than a few milliseconds. Because I_{Na} inactivates within a few milliseconds, other ionic currents become involved in the conduction process. To experimentally address this issue, we developed the "coupling clamp" technique (Tan, Joyner, 1990) which allowed us to connect two isolated cardiac cells, or a real cell and a real-time simulation of a cardiac cell, together with a controlled value of G_c. This allows the coupling conductance between the two cells to be controlled, the apparent size of the cells to be altered and also allows for pharmacologic modulation of one or both of the cells.

In our first study coupling together two isolated cardiac cells, we used the coupling clamp technique to investigate the role of I_{Ca} in discontinuous conduction (Sugiura, Joyner 1992). We simultaneously recorded Action potentials from two guinea pig ventricular cells and varied the coupling conductance between the cells. Figure 1 (top panel) shows an example of experimental recordings from isolated GP occurred, cell 2 had a rapid upstroke with a delay from the upstroke of cell 1 of about 16 msec. During conduction delay, there was a large partial repolarization of cell 1 due to the electrical load. After activation of cell 2, cell 1 has a recovery of potential up to the normal plateau level and subsequent waveforms of cells 1 and 2 are very similar. Figure 1 (lower panel) shows the potentials of cells 1 and 2 with cell 1 stimulated at BCL 130 msec with an 2:1

Cell 1 has a short action potential duration for each cycle in which cell 2 does not activate.

During conduction delay between the activation of the stimulated cell (leader cell) and delayed activation of the other cell

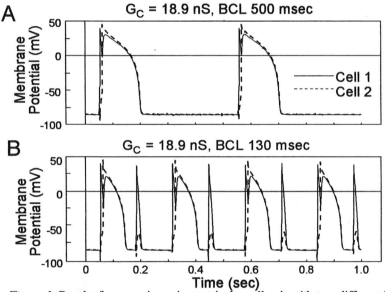

Figure 1. Results from a guinea pig ventricular cell pair with two different basic cycle lengths (BCLs) for stimulation of cell 1 with a coupling conductance (G_c) of 18.9 nS. Conduction fails intermittently with the shorter BCL. A: simultaneous recordings from cell 1 (solid line) and cell 2 (dashed line) at BCL 500 msec. B: simultaneous recordings from cell 1 (solid line) and cell 2 (dashed line) at BCL 130 msec.

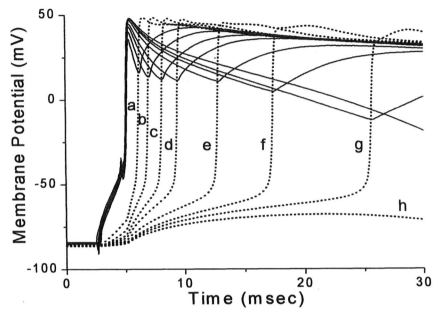

Figure 2. Recordings from a guinea pig ventricular cell (solid line) and a simultaneous real time computation of the LR ventricular cell model (dashed line)with a repetitive 1 Hz direct stimulation of the real cell. Values of G_c of 50, 30,20, 15, 10, 8, 7, and 6 nS are indicated by the letters a, b, c, d, e, f, g, and h, respectively on the dashed traces.

(follower cell) there was a substantial partial repolarization of the leader cell which then reversed quickly when the follower cell activated. Action potential peak amplitude and excitability of the leader cell were not affected by the electrical load that determined conduction failure or success. This suggested that I_{Ca} was much more important in the conduction process than previously considered, at least for cells with discontinuous conduction. We coupled pairs of isolated guinea pit ventricular cells over a wide range of G_c and compared the conduction delay and the extent of the partial repolarization of the leader cell in normal Tyrode's solution versus that observed for the same cell pairs with submaximal concentrations of nifedipine, a blocker of I_{Ca}. The critical G_c below which conduction blocked was increased significantly by nifedipine and, at a given G_c, the conduction delay and extent of the early repolarization was increased by nifedipine.

In a collaboration with Dr. Ronald Wilders (Wilders et al 1996), we modified the coupling clamp technique so that one of the real cells was replaced by a real time simulation of a ventricular cell, and were able to study the effects of G_c, asymmetry in the size of coupled cells, and modulation of I_{Ca} over a wide range of G_c. The use of the model cell as the follower cell in a cell pair made the electrical load that each real cell saw exactly the same, decreasing the variability in the experiments. Additionally, pharmacologic modulation of the real cell did not change the properties of the follower cell, which removes that complication from the analysis. In this study, the follower cell was the Luo-Rudy ventricular action potential model (Luo, Rudy 1994) (LR model). Figure 2 shows results for stimulating a guinea pig ventricular cell coupled to the LR model while varying G_c but maintaining equal size between the real cell and the model (Joyner et al 1996). Data for

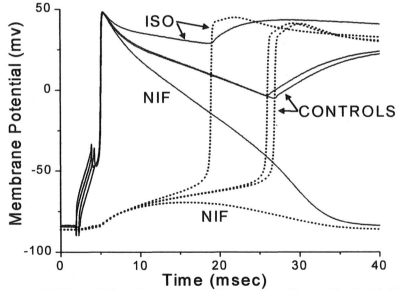

Figure 3. Effects of 20 nM isoproterenol (ISO) and the effects of 1 µM nifedipine (NIF) on conduction between a guinea pig ventricular cell (solid line) and the LR model cell (dashed line). For this cell, in control solution, conduction block occurred for G_c less than 6.6 nS. Results are illustrated for a G_c of 6.6 nS for the initial control, the washout after ISO and the washout after NIF (CONTROLS), as well as the response to ISO and to NIF. Note that the conduction delay is decreased with ISO and that conduction fails with NIF.

the real cell is plotted as solid lines while data for the LR model cell is plotted as dotted lines. Conduction delay progressively increases as G_c is decreased from 50 nS (trace 'a') to 6 nS (trace 'h'), with the delay at 50 nS being only 1.0 msec. Note that the early repolarization of the real cell becomes progressively less steep as G_c is lowered. This is due to the decrease in the electrical load on the leader cell with the smaller values of G_c. For values of G_c below 7 nS (trace 'g') for this cell there was conduction failure from the real cell to the LR model cell.

To investigate how I_{Ca} is involved in discontinuous conduction, we used pharmacological modulation (Joyner et al 1996)of I_{Ca} of a guinea pig ventricular cell that was the leader cell of a hybrid cell pair in which the follower cell was the LR model cell. Figure 3 illustrates the effects of nifedipine and isoproterenol applied separately to the real ventricular cell. For this cell pair, after normalizing the size of the real cell, the critical G_c was 6.6 nS, which is the value of G_c used in Figure 3. The three traces for the real cell (solid lines) and the model cell (dotted lines) labeled as 'CONTROLS' were recorded during the initial control period, after the washout of the isoproterenol solution, and after the washout of the nifedipine solution, respectively. Each of these pairs of recordings show a conduction delay of 21-22 msec. When we applied 20 nM isoproterenol the critical value of G_c was reduced to 4.5 nS. For a G_c of 6.6 nS, as shown by the set of traces labeled 'ISO', the conduction delay was decreased from the control conditions (22 msec) to 14 msec. This effect was completely reversible. Note that the early repolarization of the leader cell is less in the isoproterenol solution than in the control solution. Thus, during the early plateau of the action potential, when I_{Ca} is turned on, with isoproterenol, more I_{Ca} is available. Therefore during this time there is more inward current than control which results in a slower early repolarization and larger driving force for the coupling current. More current is supplied for the same value of G_c and the follower cell is brought to threshold earlier, resulting in a shorter delay between activation of the two cells. In contrast, when we applied 1 μM nifedipine to the same cell to block I_{Ca} (after the recovery from the isoproterenol effects) critical G_c increased to 8.5 nS, with the pair of curves labeled 'NIF' showing conduction failure with a G_c of 6.6 nS. Conduction failure produced by nifedipine at this value of G_c was completely reversible, as shown by the nearly identical three sets of recordings made in the control solution. Note that because there is less I_{Ca} available due to the nifedipine, the early repolarization of the action potential in the leader cell occurs at a more rapid rate. Thus, the driving force for the coupling current is decreased and is insufficient to bring the follower cell to threshold, resulting in conduction failure. Control values of critical G_c (n=17) were 6.8 ± 0.1 nS. Critical G_c was significantly decreased by 20 nM isoproterenol (5.3 ± 0.2 nS, n=8, p < 0.001) and increased by 1 μM nifedipine (8.8 ± 0.2 nS, n=9, p < 0.0001) (mean $\pm$ SEM). The extent of the early repolarization in the leader cell also suggested that the actual magnitude of I_{Ca} which flowed during the action potential might be asymmetrical, with more I_{Ca} for the leader than for the follower cell due to differences in the early part of the action potential waveform and we confirmed this prediction experimentally (17) by using action potentials recorded from coupled cells as time-varying command potentials for other cells in voltage clamp mode

The relative contributions of I_{Na} and I_{Ca} to conduction were examined by Shaw and Rudy (1997) in a simulation study using a multicellular fiber model consisting of 70-100 model cells serially coupled by a resistive gap junctions. They defined the safety factor for conduction as the ratio of the charge generated by the fiber excitation to the smallest amount of charge needed for fiber excitation and investigated how the safety factor varied with the coupling conductance. As they decreased the coupling conductance they found that the safety factor first increased and then decreased. With lower values of coupling conductance less current is shunted downstream, so more current is available for local depolarization, thereby increasing the safety factor. Further decreases in the coupling conductance and thus the coupling current, cause a long subthreshold excitation phase which inactivates I_{Na} before it reaches threshold, thus decreasing the safety factor. They then repeated their simulations but set I_{Ca} to zero to investigate how I_{Ca} alters the safety factor for conduction. They found that the safety factor curve was depressed and shifted to higher conductance values, so that the critical value of conductance that allowed propagation was more than three times larger for the fiber without I_{Ca} than the fiber with I_{Ca} (19.7 uS vs. 5.6 uS, respectively), consistent with our experimental results from the coupled cell pairs. They were also able to calculate the theoretical relative contributions of I_{Na} and I_{Ca} at different values of coupling conductance by calculating the charge contributed by each current (by integrating the current over time). They found that as the coupling conductance decreased from 20 to 10, 6, and 5.7 nS the ratio of charge contributed by the I_{Na} to the charge contributed by I_{Ca} decreased from 1.47 to 0.81, 0.26 and 0.16 respectively. Thus, I_{Ca} becomes increasingly important in the conduction process at low coupling conductances. Indeed, at very low coupling conductances, I_{Na} is required to bring the membrane potential into the activation range of I_{Ca} but I_{Ca} is the dominant current that sustains propagation. In fact, in their simulations, I_{Ca} influenced the safety factor at values of coupling conductance as high as 500 nS (20% of control) where the conduction delay was only 0.3 msec.

The contribution to conduction by I_{Ca} has also been studied in multicellular preparations. Rohr and Kucera (1997) used patterned growth cultures of rat ventricular myocytes to investigate how pharmacologic modulation of I_{Ca} altered propagation from a narrow strand into a large rectangular tissue area. Although they did not alter the coupling conductance between the cells, they created conduction delay at the area of size (and therefore current-to-load) mismatch and hypothesized that I_{Ca} is necessary for successful propagation. A microsuperfusion system was used to supply nifedipine (a I_{Ca} blocker) or Bay K 8644 (a I_{Ca} enhancer) to the narrow strand just before the expansion. They found cultures that displayed successful but delayed propagation from the strand to the expansion, decreasing I_{Ca} by nifedipine created unidirectional conduction block. The ability of nifedipine to induce conduction block depended on the conduction delay in control conditions. If the delay was greater than 1 msec than conduction block was more likely to occur with nifedipine. This delay is even smaller than the required delays we had reported for cell pairs (Sugiura., Joyner 1992). The authors attributed this to the fact that there is greater loading in the tissue culture because the conductance is higher, thus the nifedipine effect is seen with shorter conduction delays. Additionally, cultures that displayed unidirectional conduction block under control conditions, were converted to successful bidirectional propagation if Bay K 8644 was applied to the superfusate.

One region of normal ventricular tissue that has been characterized both with anatomical and electrophysiological studies as showing discontinuous conduction is the junctional region between the Purkinje cells and the underlying endocardial ventricular muscle cells. While most of the Purkinje cells on the endocardial surface are electrically insulated from the underlying ventricular muscle cells, the Purkinje-ventricular junctions are sites where sufficient electrical coupling allows action potential conduction from the Purkinje cells to the ventricular muscle cells. The Purkinje-ventricular junction was first characterized as a "funnel" of increasing electrical load based on measuring 5 to 25

msec delays in asymmetrical conduction from the Purkinje to the
ventricular muscle cells (Alaniz, Benitez 1967; Alaniz, Benitez
1970; Mendez et al 1969; Mendez et al 1970; Myerburg et al
1985; Myerburg et al 1972). We used two-dimensional activation
studies of the Purkinje and ventricular muscle cell layers with
surface electrodes combined with microelectrode recordings to
more precisely locate junctional sites and to show that action
potential conduction could be characterized as a "resistive barrier"
in which transitional cells coupled Purkinje cells to underlying
ventricular muscle cells (Overholt et al 1984; Rawling, Joyner
1997; Veenstra et al 1984). Recent histological studies(Martinez-
Palomo et al 1970; Tranum-Jensen et al 1991), have confirmed
these findings and described the Purkinje-ventricular junction of
the rabbit papillary muscle as a region in which an "intermediate
sheet of transitional cells" couples the Purkinje cells to the
ventricular muscle cells as specific junctional sites (Tranum-
Jensen et al 1991).

We have extended our work on the determinants of discontinuous
conduction done with the coupling clamp to a study of the
Purkinje-ventricular junction. We hypothesized that conduction at
the Purkinje-ventricular junction would be more sensitive to
modulations of I_{Ca} than conduction in either the Purkinje or
ventricular muscle layer of the canine papillary muscle
(Weidmann et al 1996), because the Purkinje-ventricular junction
is an area that normally displays long conduction delays. We
recorded surface electrograms every 2 mm over the muscle
surface using bipolar electrodes and created separate activation
maps of the Purkinje layer and the ventricular muscle layer. We
applied cadmium at several concentrations to block I_{Ca} and
measured the changes in the conduction delay at the Purkinje-
ventricular junction and the conduction velocity in the Purkinje
and/or ventricular muscle layer. We found 400 µM cadmium
caused 6 of 16 sites that were junctional to become reversible
nonjunctional. The conduction delay at the sites that remained
junctional increased by 117.4% while the conduction delay at the
sites that became nonjunctional increased by 263.9%. In contrast,
the conduction velocity decreased by only 27.1% in the Purkinje
cell layer and by 18.39% in the ventricular muscle layer in
response to 400 µM cadmium. Application of 2 µM isoproterenol,
which increases I_{Ca}, decreased the conduction delay by 18.51%,
while the conduction velocity in the Purkinje layer increased only
6.15%. The increase in the conduction delay at the Purkinje-
ventricular junction caused by cadmium was partially reversed by
the addition of isoproterenol. These results show that modulation

of I_{Ca} can alter the conduction delay that normally exists at the Purkinje-ventricular junction, demonstrating that in intact tissue displaying discontinuous conduction, I_{Ca} is an important ionic current in propagation.

There is also indirect evidence for I_{Ca} as an important player in discontinous propagation from whole heart studies of infarction. Zuanetti *et al.* (Zuanetti et al 1990) showed that slow conduction by a premature stimulus in the epicardial tissue of a healed infarct was modulated by β-stimulation with isoproterenol. Although isoproterenol did not change the activation pattern and velocity for stimulations at the basic drive frequency, for premature stimulations it reduced the slowing of conduction, changed the conduction pattern and prevented the occurrence of functional block in tissues. A recent study by Cabo *et al.* (2000) investigated whether increasing I_{Ca} could prevent reentrant activity in the epicardial border zone of healing canine infarcts. They found that Bay Y 5959, a cardiac specific calcium channel enhancer, prevented reentrant activity in 7 of 14 experiments. They found that conduction slowed and block occurred in regions of slow nonuniform conduction in response to Bay Y 5959. They attributed this to further cellular uncoupling caused by the increase in intracellular calcium due to the increase in I_{Ca}. Additionally, they found that premature impulses conducted faster in response to Bay Y 5959, so that lines of unidirectional block were unable to form and reentry could not be initiated. This effect occurred in regions where conduction was not as depressed. They attributed the increase in conduction of premature impulses to the contribution that the increased I_{Ca} makes to the plateau of the action potential, therefore enhancing conduction.

OUTWARD CURRENTS AND DISCONTINUOUS CONDUCTION

Our work using the coupling clamp circuit to investigate the role of I_{Ca} in discontinuous conductions emphasized the importance of the early plateau of the action potential, following the fast upstroke, in maintaining the driving force for conduction. These studies were done in guinea pig ventricular cells where the early plateau is maintained primarily by I_{Ca}. In some species and cell types, the early plateau of the action potential is determined by the interaction between I_{Ca} and the transient outward current, I_{to}. Numerous studies have demonstrated the variable magnitude of I_{to} (Escande et al 1987) in different species and in different regions of the heart. I_{to} has been recorded in a wide range of cardiac tissues, including: ventricular cells from rat (Wahler, Dollinger 1994), ferret (Campbell et al 1993), dog (Litovsky, Antzelevith 1988), and rabbit (Hiraoka, Kawano 1989); atrial cells from rabbit (Clark er al 1988) and dog (Wang et al 1993); atrial and ventricular cells of human (Shibata er al 1989; Wettner et al 1993) and rabbits (Giles, Imaizumi 1988), with a variable density and kinetics.

In a recent study, we investigated the role of I_{to} in discontinuous conduction by coupling two isolated rabbit atrial cells together using our coupling clamp technique (Wang et al 2000). The shape of the action potential in atrial cells is fundamentally different

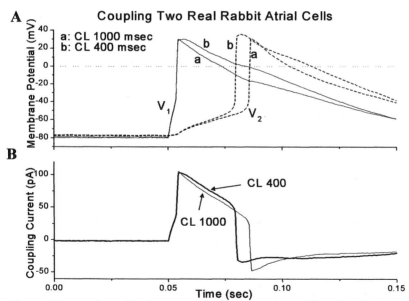

Figure 4. Comparison of action potentials from a coupled rabbit atrial cell pair paced at two different cycle lengths (CL). A. The action potentials of the leader cell (solid line, V_2) and the follower cell (dashed line, V_2) are superimposed. Results from CL 1000 msec are labeled 'a' and CL 400 are labeled 'b'. Horizontal dashed line is the zero reference line. B. The coupling current ($Ic=GcX(V1-V2)$ where $Gc=1.0$ nS) that was applied during the experiment as a current added to the follower cell and subtracted from the leader cell through the pipettes attached to the real cells.

than ventricular cells. Atrial cells have a very rapid early repolarization phase produced by the activation of I_{to} (Escande et al 1987). Since the I_{to} of atrial cells has been shown to be frequency dependent, with less I_{to} at higher frequencies of pacing (Fermini et al 1992), we hypothesized that at increased pacing frequencies a pair of atrial cells would have successful propagation at values of coupling conductance which did not allow successful propagation at lower pacing frequencies.

For these experiments we coupled two isolated atrial cells together at a fixed value of coupling conductance and increased the pacing frequency, from a cycle length (CL) of 1000 msec to a CL of 400 msec. Figure 4A (upper panel) shows the results for an experiment where the coupling conductance was set to 1.0 nS. The membrane potential of the leader cell (V_1, solid lines) and the follower cell (V_2, dashed lines) are plotted for the last stimulation at CL 1000 msec (labeled 'a') and for the 13th stimulation at CL 400 msec (labeled 'b'). For the leader cell, the action potential amplitude is nearly the same for the two values of CL, but the early repolarization occurs much more quickly at CL 1000 msec than at CL 400 msec. The slowed early repolarization at CL 400 msec produces a greater voltage difference between the leader cell and the follower cell during the propagation process. Figure 4B shows the coupling current (positive in the direction from the leader cell to the follower cell). The peak value of coupling current is the same at the two values of CL, but the decline in coupling current is much slower for CL 400 msec. Thus the charge transferred from the leader cell to the follower cell (the time integral of the coupling current), which produces the depolarization of the follower cell, occurs more quickly at CL 400 msec than at CL 1000 msec and the conduction delay between the leader cell and the follower cell is decreased.

Figure 5 shows recordings from the same two cells with the coupling conductance lowered to 0.9 nS. The top panel is the recording from the leader (stimulated) cell and the bottom panel is the recording from the follower cell. At this lower value of conductance, propagation fails at CL 1000 msec (the first 3 stimulations) but succeeds as soon as CL was decreased to 400 msec. The first two stimulations (marked with asterisks) after the return to CL 1000 msec also propagate, but the rest at CL 1000 msec fail. When we analyzed the action potential duration at 30% repolarization (APD_{30}) for isolated atrial cells (no coupling) at CL 1000 and 400 msec, we found an increase in APD_{30} from 19.4 ± 2.5 to 40.7 ± 2.6 msec ($p<0.01$). This increase in APD_{30} is the result of decreased I_{to} due to incomplete recovery from inactivation and this slower early repolarization provides additional current that is able to bring the follower cell to threshold at the faster pacing rates. In 8 cell pairs, the mean value of critical coupling conductance for successful propagation decreased from 1.21 ± 0.11 nS at CL 1000 msec to 0.77 ± 0.10 nS at CL 400 msec ($p<0.001$). Compared to the critical coupling conductance at CL 400 msec, the increase in CL to 1000 msec required a 57% increase in the critical value of coupling

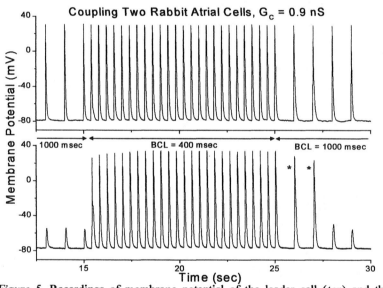

Figure 5. Recordings of membrane potential of the leader cell (*top*) and the follower cell (*bottom*) of the same atrial cell pair as for Figure 4 but now coupled with G_c=0.9 nS as the CL for stimulation is changed from 1000 to 400 msec and then back to 1000 msec. The data shown are the last three stimulations at a CL of 1000 msec, 25 stimulations at a CL of 400 msec and the first four stimulations after the return to a CL of 1000 msec. Note that propagation fails at CL 1000 msec but succeeds at CL 400 msec. *Successful propagation of the first 2 action potentials after the switch back to CL 1000 msec.

conductance required for propagation, demonstrating that conduction was <u>facilitated</u> at CL 400 msec compared to CL 1000 msec.

To determine if the facilitation of propagation by increases in the frequency of stimulation is due to I_{to} we repeated these experiments but blocked I_{to} with 2 mM 4-AP. We found that in an isolated cell (with no coupling) at a CL of 1000 msec, the APD_{30} is increased from 20.1 ± 2.5 msec in control to 35.4 ± 8.4 msec in 2 mM 4-AP (n=5, p< 0.03). When the CL was changed to 400 msec, the APD_{30} was 41.4 ± 2.5 msec in control solution (an increase of 106% over the APD_{30} at CL 1000 msec, n=14, p<0.001) and was 36.7 ± 9.3 msec in 2 mM 4-AP (n=5, CL 400 msec, not significantly different from the APD_{30} values at CL 1000 msec in 4-AP or to APD_{30} values at CL 400 msec in control solution). When we exposed cell pairs to the 4-AP solution we found that the critical coupling conductance required to sustain conduction at CL 1000 msec was 0.52 ± 0.05 nS, significantly decreased from control solution (p<0.05 compared to control solution, CL 1000 msec). Additionally, unlike the control solution, the critical coupling conductance in the 4-AP solution was unchanged by decreasing CL to 400 msec. These results with 4-AP showed that blocking I_{to} resulted in action potentials with less steep early repolarization and thus the driving force for conduction is greater resulting in a lower value of conductance that will still sustain propagation. Additionally, blocking I_{to} inhibits the facilitation of propagation by increases in the frequency of stimulation.

In ventricular cells from human, canine and rabbit, I_{to} is responsible for the rapid phase one repolarization that gives rise to the 'spike and dome' shape of the action potential (Binah 1970; Campbell etal 1995). Huelsing *et al.* (2001) recently investigated the role of I_{to} in ventricular action potential conduction. They coupled two isolated rabbit ventricular cells using the coupling clamp circuit and investigated the effect of 2 mM 4-AP on the conduction delay and critical value of resistance required for pair, in control and 4-AP solution, with the leader cell plotted as the solid line and the follower cell as the dashed line. In control solution, the critical value of resistance required for conduction to propagation between the cells. Figure 6 shows the results of a cell occur was 126 MΩ (Figure 6A). At this value of resistance, the conduction delay was 14.4 msec and the early partial repolarization of the leader cell was 48.7 mV. By keeping the resistance fixed and applying 2 mM 4-AP to the bath solution, the conduction delay decreased to 12.0 msec and the early partial repolarization decreased to 17.3 mV (Figure 6B). Figure 6C shows that the critical resistance for conduction increased to 168 MΩ when I_{to} was blocked with 4-AP. Additionally, by blocking

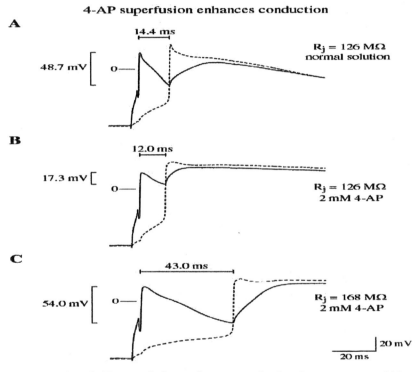

Figure 6.   4-AP superfusion enhances conduction between two rabbit ventricular cells. Initial phase of the action potentials are plotted. A. Action potentials during conduction at the critical value of coupling resistance, R_j, during control conditions, B. at the same value of R_j with superfusion of 4-AP and C. at the critical value of R_j measured during 4-AP superfusion. Conduction delay is indicated above and early repolarization is indicated to the left of each set of action potentials. Adapted from Huelsing et al., *Cardiovasc Res,* 49 (2001) 779-789, with permission.

I_{to}, a much larger conduction delay could be supported (43 msec). For 6 cell pairs studied, they found that the critical value of resistance required for conduction was increased from 132 ± 13

MΩ in control solution to 180 ± 19 MΩ in 2 mM 4-AP solution (p<0.05).

Because I_{to} in rabbit ventricular cells has slow recovery kinetics, increased frequency of pacing results in an action potential with an increased early plateau. Huelsing et al. (13) examined how increased pacing frequency altered propagation when the resistance between a pair of rabbit ventricular cells was relatively high so that conduction was discontinuous. Their results are shown in Figure 7. In part A of Figure 7 they paced the leader cell of a cell pair with a basic cycle length (BCL) of 2 seconds and the coupling resistance is set to the critical value of 116 MΩ. The conduction delay is 14.6 msec and the early repolarization is 44.7 mV. When the BCL is decreased to 0.5 seconds and the coupling resistance is kept constant, the action potential propagates with a shorter delay (10.3 msec) and less early repolarization (10.6 mV) as seen in part B. At this faster rate the critical value of resistance that supported conduction was increased to 168 MΩ (see part C). A conduction delay of 33.0 msec could also be supported at this pacing frequency. For 6 cell pairs studied, they found that the critical value of resistance required for conduction was increased from 106 ± 8 MΩ at BCL 2.0 seconds to 138 ± 12 MΩ at BCL 0.5 seconds (p<0.05). These results are consistent with a decrease in I_{to} at higher pacing frequencies because I_{to} is unavailable due to incomplete recovery from inactivation at these pacing rates. They found similar facilitation of propagation when they applied a premature stimulus. The conduction delay was decreased and early repolarization was decreased for a premature beat. They then inhibited I_{to} with a 4-AP and this facilitation was blocked, confirming that I_{to} was responsible for the facilitation of propagation of premature beat.

In cells that have both I_{to} and I_{Ca}, the interplay between the two currents can be very important in determining conduction success or failure. Additionally both currents can be altered in physiological and pathophysiological conditions. For example, it has been shown that I_{to} has differences in both density and kinetics in human subendocardial versus subepicardial ventricular cells (Wettner et al 1994). There are also age-related changes (Wang, Duff 1997) and alterations in pathological conditions such as myocardial infarction or ischemia (Jeck et a; 1995),cardiac hypertrophy (Tomita et al 1994), terminal heart failure and atrial dilatation (Beuckelmann et al 1993; Le Grand et al 1994)

Rate-acceleration enhances conduction

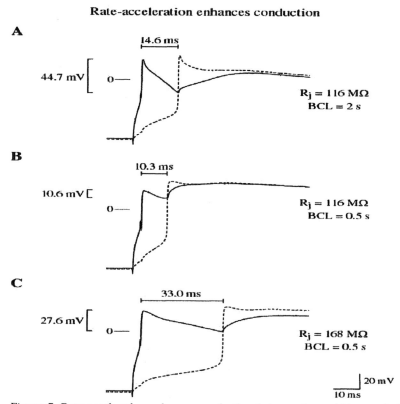

Figure 7. Rate-acceleration enhances conduction between two rabbit ventricular cells. Initial phase of the action potentials are plotted. A. Action potentials during conduction at the critical value of coupling resistance, Rj, measured during pacing at BCL=2.0 s, B. at the same value of Rj during pacing at BCL=0.5 s and C. at the critical value of Rj measured during pacing at BCL=0.5 s. Adapted from Huelsing et al., *Cardiovasc Res,* 49 (2001) 779-789, with permission.

Interactions between coupled myocytes during the early plateau phase were studied by Huelsing *et al.* (14), showing that the greater I_{to} magnitude of rabbit Purkinje cells compared to rabbit ventricular cells produced an intrinsically more rapid repolarization of the Purkinje cell and thus caused complex interactions during the early repolarization period, but in these experiments the cells were simultaneously stimulated such that propagation of the action potential was not studied. Although many of these studies have focused on either the magnitude of the current or the duration of the action potentials, few previous studies have focused on the effects of I_{to} on action potential propagation. Since action potential propagation between two adjacent cardiac cells with high levels of coupling conductance occurs with very short delays, the activation of I_{to} does not play a role in propagation under these conditions, since conduction occurs before activation of I_{to}. However, the long delays associated with discontinuous conduction (with lower levels of coupling conductance) make early plateau currents, such as I_{Ca} and I_{to}, important components of the propagation process.

SUMMARY

Action potential conduction in cardiac tissue is always "discontinuous" to some degree, due to the discrete nature of the cells. As the gap junctional conductance decreases, at some regions, with respect to the input conductance of the cells, there is a spectrum of changes in the conduction properties. Experimental studies on cell pairs, cultured monolayers, and the Purkinje-ventricular junction, as well as theoretical computations, have shown that discontinuous conduction for which delays between individual cells or well coupled cell groups get as long as a few milliseconds produces conduction phenomena dependent on the magnitudes of the inward I_{Ca} and the outward I_{to} currents. The dependence of discontinuous conduction on I_{Ca} may help to explain the changes in conduction produced by β-adrenergic stimulation and may be important in determining differences in epicardial versus endocardial conduction. The alterations in conduction seen with changes in I_{to} can help to explain the apparently paradoxical phenomena of increased ability to conduct action potentials as the frequency of stimulation or the degree of prematurity is increased in some tissues. These findings may have implications for clinical arrhythmias under pathophysiological conditions. In regions of the atrium with low coupling conductance, some premature beats may be conducted with decreased delay and require less conductance. This could facilitate the initiation of atrial arrhythmias because the premature beat may be able to propagate along a pathway that was blocked for the regular excitations, thus changing the spatial pattern of the activation wavefront. I_{to} was found to be substantially decreased in atrial cells from patients with atrial fibrillation (van Wagoner et al 1997) and in ventricular cells from patients with heart failure (Beuckelmann et al 1993). The decreased I_{to} in the atrial cells following atrial tachycardia or fibrillation may actually facilitate action potential conduction at regions of low coupling conductance and may encourage the re-initiation of atrial tachycardia or fibrillation.

REFERENCE

Alanis, J. and D. Benitez. 1967 Transitional potentials and the propagation of impulses through different cardiac cells. In Sano, T., V. Misuhira, and K. Matsuda, eds. Electrophysiology and Ultrastructure of the Heart. Tokyo,Japan, Bunkoko Co.,Ltd.

Alanis, J. and D. Benitez. 1970 Purkinje and transitional cells action potential and the propagation across the purkinje-ventricular junction. *Jpn.J Physiol* 20: 217-232

Beuckelmann, D. J., M. Nabauer, and E. Erdmann. 1993 Alterations of K+ currents in isolated human ventricular myocytes from patients with terminal heart failure. *Circulation Research* 73: 379-385.

Binah, O. 1990 The transient outward current in the mammalian heart. In Rosen, M. R., M. J. Janse, and A. L. Wit, eds. Cardiac electrophysiology: a textbook. Mount Kisco, NY, Futura Press, 93-106.

Cabo, C., H. Schmitt, and A. L. Wit. 2000 New mechanism of antiarrhythmic drug action: increasing L-type calcium current prevents reentrant ventricular tachycardia in the infarcted canine heart. *Circulation* 102: 2417-2425.

Campbell, D. L., R. L. Rasmusson, M. B. Comer, and H. C. Strauss. 1995 The cardiac calcium-independent transient outward potassium current: Kinetics, molecular properties and role in ventricular repolarization. In Zipes, D. P. and J. Jalife, eds. Cardiac electrophysiology: from cell to bedside. Philadelphia, W.B. Saunders, 83-96.

Campbell, D. L., R. L. Rasmusson, Y. Qu, and H. C. Strauss. 1993 The calcium-independent transient outward potassium current in isolated ferret right ventricular myocytes. I. Basic Characterization and kinetic analysis. *J.Gen.Physiol.* 101: 571-601.

Clark, R. B., W. R. Giles, and Y. Imaizumi. 1988 Properties of the transient outward current in rabbit atrial cells. *J.Physiol.(London)* 405: 147-168.

Escande, D., A. Coulombe, J. Faivre, E. Deroubaix, and E. Coraboeuf.(1987) Two types of transient outward currents in adult human atrial cells. *Am.J Physiol.* 252: H142-H148.

Fermini, B., Z. Wang, D. Duan, and S. Nattel. 1992 Differences in rate dependence of transient outward current in rabbit and human atrium. *Am.J Physiol.* 263: H1747-54.

Giles, W. R. and Y. Imaizumi. 1988 Comparison of potassium currents in rabbit atrial and ventricular cells. *J.Physiol.(London)* 405: 123-145.

Hiraoka, M. and S. Kawano. 1989 Calcium-sensitive and insensitive transient outward current in rabbit ventricular myocytes. *J.Physiol.(Lond)* 410: 187-212.

Huelsing, D. J., A. E. Pollard, and K. W. Spitzer. 2001 Transient outward current modulates discontinuous conduction in rabbit ventricular cell pairs. *Cardiovasc.Res* 49: 779-789.

Huelsing, D. J., K. W. Spitzer, J. M. Cordeiro, and A. E. Pollard. 1999 Modulation of repolarization in rabbit Purkinje and ventricular myocytes coupled by a variable resistance. *Am.J Physiol.* 276: H572-H581.

Jeck, C. D., J. M. Pinto, and P. A. Boyden. 1995 Transient outward currents in subendocardial purkinje myocytes surviving in the infarcted heart. *Circulation* 92: 465-473.

Joyner, R. W., R. Kumar, R. Wilders, H. J. Jongsma, E. E. Verheijck, D. A. Golod, A. C. van Ginneken, M. B. Wagner, and W. N. Goolsby. 1996 Modulating L-type calcium current affects discontinuous cardiac action potential conduction. *Biophys.J.* 71: 237-245.

Kumar, R. and R. W. Joyner. 1995 Calcium currents of ventricular cell pairs during action potential conduction. *Am.J.Physiol.* 268: H2476-H2486.

Le Grand, B., S. Hatem, E. Deroubaix, J. P. Couetil, and E. Coraboeuf. 1994 Depressed transient outward and calcium currents in dilated human atria. *Cardiovasc.Res.* 28: 548-556.

Litovsky, S. H. and C. Antzelevitch. 1988 Transient outward current prominent in canine ventricular epicardium but not endocardium. *Circ.Res.* 62: 116-126.

Luo, C. H. and Y. Rudy. 1994 A dynamic model of the cardiac ventricular action potential. I. Simulations of ionic currents and concentration changes. *Circ.Res.* 74: 1071-1096.

Martinez-Palomo, A., J. Alanis, and D. Benitez. 1970 Transitional cells of the conduction system of the dog heart. *J.Cell.Biol.* 47: 1-17.

Mendez, C., W. J. Mueller, J. Meredith, and G. K. Moe. 1969 Interaction of transmembrane potentials in canine purkinje fibers and at purkinje fiber-muscle junctions. *Circ.Res.* 24: 361-373.

Mendez, C., W. J. Mueller, and X. Urguiaga. 1970 Propagation of impulses acreoss the purkinje fiber-muscle junctions in the dog heart. *Circ.Res.* 26: 135-150.

Myerburg, R. J., J. S. Cameron, N. J. Lodge, S. Kimura, N. Saoudi, P. L. Kozlovskis, and A. L. Bassett. 1985 The papillary musle preparation in a study of cardiac electrophysiology, electropharmacology, and disease models. In Zipes, D. P. and J. Jalife, eds. Cardiac electrophysiology and arrhythmias. Orlando, FL, Grune & Stratton, 225-231.

Myerburg, R. J., K. Nilsson, and H. Gelband. 1972 Physiology of canine interventricular conduction and endocardial excitation. *Circ.Res.* 30: 217-243.

Overholt, E. D., R. W. Joyner, R. D. Veenstra, D. Rawling, and R. Weidmann. 1984 Unidirectional block between purkinje and ventricular layers of papillary muscle. *Am.J.Physiol.* 247: H584-H595.

Rawling, D. A. and R. W. Joyner. 1987 Characteristics of the junctional regions between Purkinje and ventricular muscle cells of the canine ventricular subendocardium. *Circ.Res.* 60: 580-585.

Rohr, S. and J. P. Kucera. 1997 Involvement of the calcium inward current in cardiac impulse propagation: induction of unidirectional conduction block by nifedipine and reversal by Bay K 8644. *Biophys.J.* 72: 754-766.

Shaw, R. M. and Y. Rudy. 1997 Ionic mechanisms of propagation in cardiac tissue. Roles of the sodium and L-type calcium currents during reduced excitability and decreased gap junction coupling. *Circ.Res.* 81: 727-741.

Shibata, E. F., T. Drury, H. Refsum, V. Aldrete, and W. Giles. 1989 Contributions of a transient outward current to repolarization in human atrium. *Am.J.Physiol.* 257: H1773-H1781.

Sugiura, H. and R. W. Joyner. 1992 Action potential conduction between guinea pig ventricular cells can be modulated by calcium current. *Am.J.Physiol.* 263: H1591-604.

Tan, R. C. and R. W. Joyner. 1990 Electrotonic influences on action potentials from isolated ventricular cells. *Circ.Res.* 67: 1071-1081.

Tomita, F., A. L. Bassett, R. J. Myerburg, and S. Kimura. 1994 Diminished transient outward currents in rat hypertrophied ventricular myocytes. *Circ.Res.* 75: 296-303.

Tranum-Jensen, J., A. A. Wilde, J. T. Vermeulen, and M. J. Janse. 1991 Morphology of electrophysiologically identified junctions between Purkinje fibers and ventricular muscle in rabbit and pig hearts. *Circ.Res.* 69: 429-437.

Van Wagoner, D. R., A. L. Pond, P. M. McCarthy, J. S. Trimmer, and J. M. Nerbonne. 1997 Outward K+ current densities and Kv1.5 expression are reduced in chronic human atrial fibrillation. *Circ.Res.* 80: 772-781.

Veenstra, R. D., R. W. Joyner, and D. A. Rawling. 1984 Purkinje and ventricular activation sequences of canine papillary muscle. Effects of quinidine and calcium on the purkinje-ventricular conduction delay. *Circ.Res.* 54: 500-515.

Wahler, G. M. and S. J. Dollinger. 1994 Time course of postnatal changes in rat heart action potential and in transient outward current is different. *Am.J.Physiol.* 267: H1157-H1166.

Wang, L. and H. J. Duff. 1997 Developmental changes in transient outward current in mouse ventricle. *Circ.Res.* 81: 120-127.

Wang, Y. G., M. B. Wagner, R. Kumar, W. N. Goolsby, and R. W. Joyner. 2000 Fast pacing facilitates discontinuous action potential propagation between rabbit atrial cells. *Am.J Physiol.* In Press.

Wang, Z., B. Fermini, and S. Nattel. 1993 Mechanism of flecainide's rate-dependent actions on action potential duration in canine atrial tissue. *J.Pharmacol.Exp.Ther.* 267: 575-581.

Wettwer, E., G. J. Amos, H. Posival, and U. Ravens. 1994 Transient outward current in human ventricular myocytes of subepicardial and subendocardial origin. *Circ.Res.* 75: 473-482.

Wiedmann, R. T., R. C. Tan, and R. W. Joyner. 1996 Discontinuous conduction at Purkinje-ventricular muscle junction. *Am.J.Physiol.* 271: H1507-16.

Wilders, R., R. Kumar, R. W. Joyner, H. J. Jongsma, E. E. Verheijck, D. Golod, A. C. van Ginneken, and W. N. Goolsby. 1996 Action potential conduction between a ventricular cell model and an isolated ventricular cell. *Biophys.J.* 70: 281-295.

Zuanetti, G., R. H. Hoyt, and P. B. Corr. 1990 Beta-adrenergic-mediated influences on microscopic conduction in epicardial regions overlying infarcted myocardium. *Circ.Res.* 67: 284-302.

10

CELLULAR ELECTRICAL UNCOUPLING DURING ISCHEMIA

Michiel J. Janse, Hanno L. Tan,
Lukas R.C. Dekker and André G. Kléber
Department of Clinical and Experimental Cardiology, Academic Medical
Center, University of Amsterdam, and the Interuniversity Cardiology Institute,
The Netherlands * Department of Physiology University of Bern, Switzerland

INTRODUCTION

In 1875 T.W. Engelmann wrote: "Solche Zellen, die whrend des Lebens mit Verlust ihrer eigenen physiologischen Individualitt mit anderen zu einem Individuum hoherer Ordnung verschmolzen sind, erhalten beim Absterben ihre Individualitt zuruck ... Die Zellen leben zusammen, aber sterben einzeln". (Engelmann, 1875) In our translation: "Such cells, which during life, at the expense of their own identity, are Joined with other cells to form an entity of higher order, regain their individuality when dying ... The cells live together, but die alone." Thus, Engelmann formulated on the one hand the concept that the normal heart functions as a syncytium, on the other hand that lethally injured cells become isolated from the rest of the heart, a phenomenon that later became known as *"healing-over"*.

Important studies showing that healing-over is due to an increase in the resistance of gap junctions that normally provide low resistance pathways between cardiac cells are those of De Mello and associates (De Mello et al, 1969, De Mello, 1975) and of Déleze (1970). These studies also emphasized the important role of calcium ions in causing cellular uncoupling. Later studies showed that both hypoxia and ischemia eventually result in an increase in coupling resistance (Wojtczak, 1979; Ikeda, Hiraoka, 1988; Kleber et al 1987; Rieggen et al, 1989). Apart from a rise in intracellular calcium concentration, other factors have been identified that may play a role in ischemia-induced uncoupling: an increase in intracellular protons (Reber, Weingart, 1982; Spray et al 1981; De Mello, 1983; Pressler 1987; Noma, Tsuboi, 1987) accumulation of long-chain acylcarnitines (Wu et al, 1993) and lysophosphatidylcholile (Dalean, 1996), and a fall in ATP concentration (Sugiura et al, 1990).

In the present chapter we will 1) describe the time course of electrical uncoupling during ischemia; 2) describe various interventions that can delay the moment of uncoupling, such as ischemic preconditioning, activation of the ATP sensitive K-channel, and reduction of cellular calcium overload; 3) discuss the central role of cellular calcium in uncoupling.

METHODS

In essence, the methods originally developed by Kléber and co-workers were used (Kléber et al, 1987; Kleber, Riegger, 1987). Briefly, rabbits were anesthetized and heparinized, and the hearts were rapidly removed and submerged in cooled Tyrode's solution (4° C). The atria, free left ventricular wall and basal part of the ventricular septum were removed and the septal artery was cannulated and perfused. The delay between respiratory arrest and cannulation averaged 4 mm. After removal of the free wall of

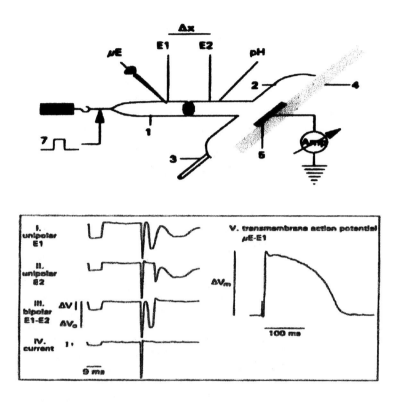

Figure 1. Upper panel shows schematic drawing of preparation and recording method Papillary muscle (1) and interventricular septum (2) are perfused via a cannula (3) inserted in the septal artery and mounted on a silicone covered perspex plate (4) containing a large electrically grounded Ag/AgCl electrode *(5)*. The papillary muscle is horizontally hooked to a force transducer (6). Subthreshold and excitatory current pulses are injected at the muscle apex (7). El and E2 = extracellular electrodes; μE = extracellular microelectrode; pH = extracellular pH electrode; Amp = current meter, Ax = distance between electrograms from El and E2, respectively; channel III = bipolar electrogram (El minus E2); IV = current signal from current meter; V = transmembrane action potential (E1 minus E2); AV = drop of extracellular voltage between El and E2; ΔV_0 = amplitude of bipolar electrogram; I current strength of subthreshold pulse; ΔV_m = amplitude of transmembrane action potential Records are plotted with a 2 kHz resolution. Note that the time scale of channel V different from channels I to IV. (Reproduced with permission from Tan, 1993.)

the right ventricle, the preparation was positioned in a recording chamber and a right ventricular papillary muscle (length 4-6 mm, diameter 0.8-1.4 mm) with a single insertion of the tendon was horizontally hooked to a force transducer. The muscle was enclosed by a water-saturated gas mixture of 95% $O_\sim$ +5% CO_2 at 37° C. Extracellular and intracellular electrodes for recording and stimulation were placed as indicated in Figure 1. Ischemia was induced by stopping perfusion and by changing the gas mixture inside the chamber to 95% N_2 + 5 Co_2.

Calculation of electrical resistance

The determination of tissue resistance is based on cable theory first applied to cardiac muscle by Weidmann (1970). To determine total tissue resistance and its two components, intra- and extracellular resistance, two sequential measurements must be made (Kléber et at1987; Kléber, Riegger, 1987). First, a subthreshold constant current pulse was applied between apex and septum (7 and 5 in Figure 1), and the voltage drop between extracellular electrodes E_1 and E_2 was measured. The subthreshold current will divide itself between intra and extracellular compartments while spreading electrotonically along the long axis of the muscle. The transmembrane current approaches zero at three space constants of the membrane (i.e. approximately 1.5 mm) from' the point of current injection. Beyond this point, extra- and intracellular voltages will decrease linearly. Therefore, longitudinal tissue resistance r_t, composed of intracellular (r_1) and extracellular (r_0)

resistance in parallel can be calculated as follows:

$$r_t = \frac{r_i \cdot r_o}{r_i + r_o} = \frac{\Delta V}{\Delta x \cdot I}$$

where AV is the voltage drop between the two extracellular electrode(r_1) and extracellular (r_0) the distance between these two electrodes, and I the strength of subthreshold current pulse.

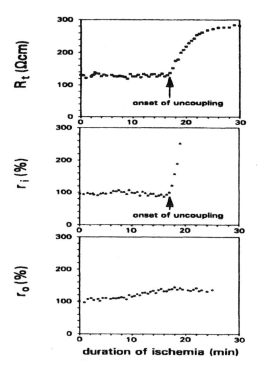

Figure 2. Graphs show method for determining onset of cellular electrical uncoupling one representative experiment. Upper panel shows total specific resistance R~ d sustained ischemia, central and lower panels show relative values of intracellular resistance.

For the second set of measurements, an excitatory current pulse was applied (30 msec after the subthreshold pulse), resulting in an action potential propagating from apex to septum. During propagation, the extracellular bipolar electrogram between B_1 and $E._2$ was measured and the transmembrane potential between an intracellular floating microelectrode and extracellular electrode F_1 (Figure 1). The ratio of extra- to intracellular resistance was obtained from the amplitudes of the bipolar electrograms (AV_0) and the transmembrane action potential (AVm):

$$\frac{r_o}{r_i} = \frac{\Delta V_o}{\Delta V_m - \Delta V_o}$$

From these two equations, r_i and r_0 can be calculated.

Measurement of intracellular Ca^{2+}

The method to determine intracellular Ca^{2+} transients by means of indo 1 fluorescence has been described in detail elsewhere (Dekker et al; Dekker 1996). Briefly, muscles were loaded with indo 1 during a 30 min period of perfusion. A circular area on the surface of the papillary muscle of 1.3 n-mi was Illuminated by 340 nm excitation light and emitted light was simultaneously measured by two photomultipliers at 405 nm and 495 nm. The ratio R of the 405 nm and *495* nm signals, after subtraction of the autofluorescence at both wavelengths, was used as an indicator of $[Ca^{2+}]i$.

RESULTS

Time course of electrical uncoupling during ischemia

Figure 2 shows the changes in total tissue resistance (R_t), and of intra- and extracellular resistances, in a representatwe experiment (Tan;1993). Following the arrest of coronary flow, and changing the gaseous atmosphere to 95% N_2 and 5% CO_2, extracellular resistance rises by about 30% in the course of 15 to 20 min while intracellular resistance remains constant, in this experiment until 18 min. The rise m extracellular resistance is most likely due to osmotic cell swelling and the consequence reduction of the extracellular space (Tranum, Jense et al, 1981). The abrupt increase in both and intracellular resistance marks the beginning of cellular uncoupling which in this preparation occurs on average after 15 mm of ischemia (Kléber, Riegger, 1987; Tan, 1993;Tan et al 1993). This moment correlates well with the moments at which first morphological changes at the intercalated disk are observed, such a dissociation of the gap junctional membranes (McCallister et al, 1993) and with the second phase of the increase in extracellular potassium concentration (Hill Getter, 1980; three phenomena can be regarded as markers for the onset of irreversible injury.

Delaying the onset of cellular uncoupling

Brief episodes of ischemia protect the heart from damage caused by a subsequent longer period of ischemia. Most often the effects of this so-called ischemic preconditioning is assessed by a reduction of infarct size following a certain period of ischemia, preceded by a brief episode of ischemia followed by reperfusion. The protection is not absolute, but consists of a delay in the onset of irreversible injury, as is apparent from the title of the first paper demonstrating ischemic preconditioning (Murry et al, 1986). The effects of ischemic preconditioning can therefore also be assessed by determining the delay in onset of electrical uncoupling (Kléber, Riegger, 1987; Dekker 1996; Tan, 1993). Figure 3 shows the results of five experimental protocols: 1) sustained ischemia; 2) sustained ischemia preceded by 10 min of ischemia and 10 min of reperfusion (preconditioning); 3) the same protocol as in 2), except for the addition of 20 µM glibenclamide (a blocker of the ATP-sensitive K^+ channel) at the start of reperfusion; 4) sustained uncoupling after preconditioning ischemia induced 15 min after addition of 20 µM cromakalim (an activator of the ATP-sensitive $K\sim$ channel) to the perfusate; 5) sustained ischemia induced 10 nun after the addition of 20 µM glibenclamide to the perfusate. In all protocols the first intervention was made after an equilibration period of at least 60 min

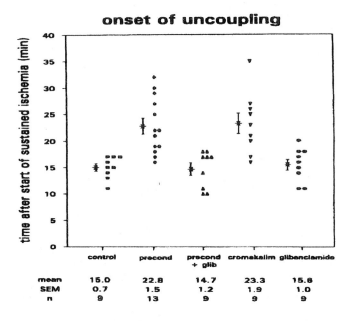

Figure 3. Onset of electrical uncoupling in all individual experiments is plotted alo Y-axis (in minutes after the start of sustained ischemia). Experiments are horizontally grouped according to the protocol. Every symbol represents one experiment. Asterisk each group represent mean values. Bars are standard error bars. Mean values and (minutes) are also shown below the graph. From left to right: control, sc preconditioning, diamonds; preconditioning + 20 μM glibenclamide, triangles; 20 cromakalirn, inverted triangles; circles, 20 μM glibenclamide. The graph shows a sign delay of onset of electrical (p<0.001 vs. control). The is completely abolished when glibenclamide is added after the reconditioning occlusion Cromakalim delays onset of uncoupling significantly in the absence of preconditioning (p <0.002 vs. control). Glibenclamide has no effect on the onset of uncoupling in the absence of preconditioning. (Reproduced with permission from Tan et al, 1993).

As can be seen, both preconditioning and the addition of cromakalim to the perfusate result in a significant delay in the onset of electrical uncoupling by 7 to 8 min. Glibenclamide, added to the perfusate during reperfusion after the first episode of ischemia, completely abolished the effect of preconditioning, but was without effect when added 10 min before sustained ischemia. From these data it was concluded that preconditioning delays the onset in electrical uncoupling and that this effect may be caused by activation of ATP-sensitive K^+ channels. This last conclusion should be viewed with caution because the use of so-called specific blockers and activators of the ATP-sensitive K^+ channels is fraught with pitfalls. Thus, glibendamide has many other effects besides blocking the K_{ATP} channel: it blocks chloride channels, it blocks other K-channels, it affects calcium release from the sarcoplasmatic reticulum, it stimulates lactate production in normoxic conditions, it inhibits lactate production during hypoxia and ischemia, and finally, the efficacy of the drug to block the K_{ATP} channel may be lost during ischemia (for discussion and references see Wilde and Aksnes (1995).

Cromakalim in the concentration used causes extreme shortenin; of the action potential duration during ischemia and leads to inexcitability after about 5 min (Tan et al, 1993). Later, it was shown that both mechanical am electrical arrest significantly delay the onset of uncoupling (Tan, Jense, 1994).

The finding that the compound R 56865, which reduces cellular calcium overload secondary to reducing sodium overload (Ver Donck et al, 1993), significantly delays cellular uncoupling (Tan et al, 1993), pointed to an important role of ai increase in intracellular calcium in causing ischemia-induced uncoupling. (Kléber, Riegger, 1987).

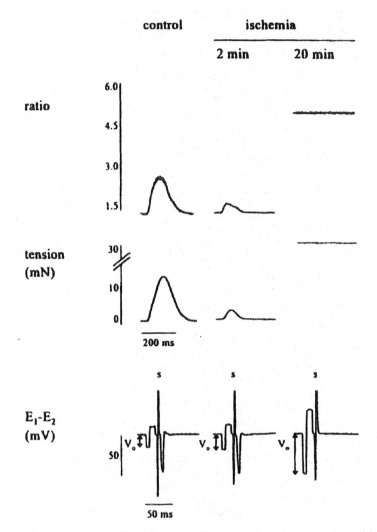

Figure 4. Simultaneous recordings from a papillary muscle during control conditions (left panels) and after 2 and 20 minutes of ischemia (middle and right panels). After 2 minutes ischemia the Ca^{2+} transient and the developed tension have declined and subthreshold voltage drop has increased by 20%. After 20 minutes of ischemia Ca^{2+} transients and contractions have disappeared and diastolic Ca^{2-} and resting tension are high. Cellular uncoupling is indicated by the large increase of the subthreshold voltage drop. Note that the time scale for the electrograms is different from Indo-ratio and tension. (Reproduced with permission from Dekker et al, 1996).

Calcium and ischemia-induced electrical uncoupling

Figure 4 shows simultaneous recordings of the indo 1 ratio, the developed tension and the bipolar electrogram during control perfusion and after 2 and 20 min of ischemia. After 2 min of

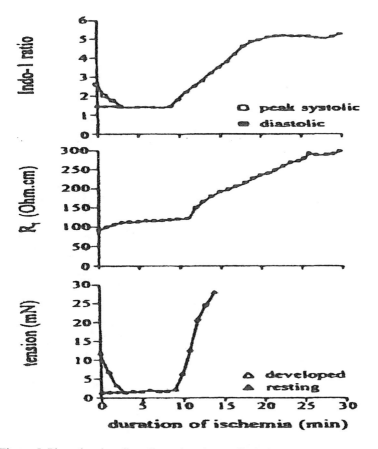

Figure 5. Plots showing diastolic and peak systolic indo 1 ratio (top panel), tissue resistance, R, (middle panel), and resting and developed tension (bottom panel) during ischemia in one experiment. Values at t=0 are preischemic control values. Systolic Ca^{2+} levels and developed tension rapidly decline after the induction of ischemia. Small initial increase of R_t is caused by a rise in the extracellular longitudinal resistance. Diastolic Ca^{2+} and resting tension start to increase at 10 minutes of ischemia followed by an abrupt increase of R_t at 12 minutes of ischemia indicating the onset of uncoupling. (Reproduced with permission from Dekker et al, 1993).

ischemia the systolic ratio and the developed tension have substantially decreased, whereas the diastolic ratio and resting tension are unchanged. The subthreshold voltage drop between the two extracellular electrodes (V_0) has increased by 20%, corresponding to a rise in r_o. After 20 minutes R_t has increased to 230% of control and local electrical activation following the suprathreshold stimulus is absent. Diastolic ratio and resting tension are high. These changes indicate that after 20 min of ischemia the muscle has become inexcitable, myocytes have become uncoupled at a high intracellular Ca^{2+} concentration, and contracture has developed. The time course of the changes in indo 1 ratio, tissue resistance and tension are shown in Figure 5.

The relationship between the diastolic indo 1 ratio and tissue resistance is depicted in Figure 6. On average (n = 6) the diastolic indo ratio started to increase after 12.6 ± 1.3 min, the onset of uncoupling occurred at 14.5± 1.2 min. and contracture at 12.6 ± 1.5 min. The effects of ischemic preconditioning are shown in Figure 7. On average (n = 6), in preconditioned muscles the rise in intracellular calcium started at 21.5 ± 4.0 min, uncoupling at 24.0 ± 4.1 mm contracture at 23.0 ± 5.3 min of ischemia. Since both occurred at 14.5 ± 1.2 min, and contracture at 12.6 ± 1.5 min. a rise in intracellular calcium and a decrease in intracellular pH have been implicated factors that could cause uncoupling during ischemia, a set of experiments was performed in which ischemia was preceded by metabolic inhibition caused by pretreatment with 1 mmol/L iodoacetic acid. This substance blocks glycolysis, causes

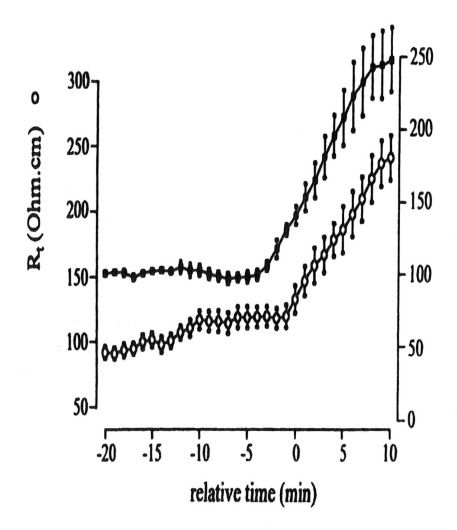

Figure 6. Average R~ and diastolic ratio of control preparations (n=6) during ischemia plotted on a relative time scale. Moment at which uncoupling started was assigned **t=0** for each experiment. See text for further details. (Reproduced with permission from Dekker et al, 1996)

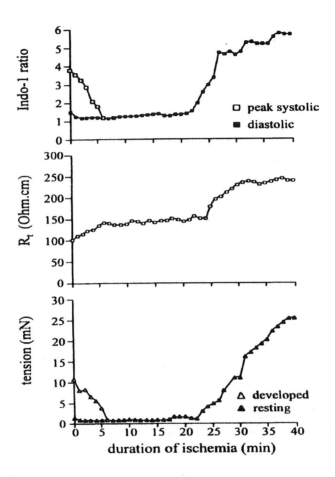

Figure 7. Effect of ischemic preconditioning on peak systolic and diastolic indo 1 ratio (top panel), tissue resistance R, (middle panel), and resting and developed tension (bottom panel) during ischemia in a papillary muscle. Values at t=O indicate values after preconditioning just before sustained ischemia. Systolic Ca^{2+} and developed tension rapidly decrease after induction of ischemia. Diastolic Ca^{2+} and resting tension start to increase after 23 minutes of ischemia. The rise in R, after 25 minutes of ischemia marks the onset of uncoupling. (Reproduced with permission from Dekker et al, 1996).

a rapid depletion of ATP, and impairs anaerobic metabolism and acidification during ischemia (Jennings et al,1989). This was indirect shown in our experiments by measuring extracellular pH. After 20 min ischemia in untreated preparations, pH_o was on

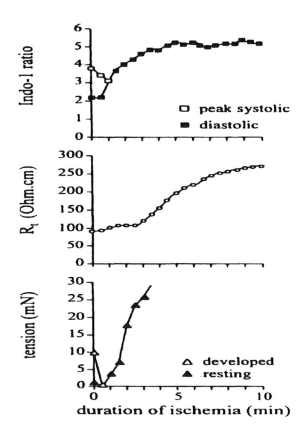

Figure 8. Effect of pretreatment with 1 mmol/L iodoacetate on peak systolic and diastolic fluorescence ratio (top panel), tissue resistance (middle panel) and resting and develop tension (bottom panel) during ischemia in a papillary muscle. Values at t = 0 indicate preischemic values after pretreatment with iodoacetate. Decreasing systolic Ca^{2+} and developed tension merge into the terminal increase of diastolic Ca^{2+} and resting tension 1.0 minute of ischemia. The increase of R, at 3.0 minutes of ischemia indicates the onset uncoupling. (Reproduced with permission from Dekker et al, 1996).

1.4 ± 0.05 pH units lower than during control perfusion. In metabolically inhibited muscles, pH_o maximally decreased by 0.15 pH units. As shown in Fig.8, the effect of pretreatment with iodoacetic acid leads to a very early rise in $Ca^{2\sim}$ and a very early onset of uncoupling and con tracture.

In all three experimental groups (control ischemia, preconditioning and metabolic inhibition) the rise in intracellular calcium occurred significantly earlier than cellular uncoupling (paired t-test, p< 0.01), whereas the start of contracture was not significantly different from the moment of Ca^{2+} rise. This is shown in Figure 9, where the onset of rise in Ca^{2+} is plotted against the onset of uncoupling: all points are above the line of identity, indicating that uncoupling always followed the rise in Ca^{2+}. The average delay was 2.1 ± 0.2 mm.

DISCUSSION

Calcium and ischemic injury

The first minutes of myocardial ischemia are characterized by increasing extracellular K^+ accumulation, acidification, depolarization of the cell membrane, development of inexcitability and contractile failure (1989). The cardiac arrhythmias that occur during this early, reversible phase of ischemia, the so-called 1-A arrhythmias, are related to the changes in excitability, notably the decrease in conduction velocity and the inhomogeneities in refractory period (Janse, Wit, 1989; Coronel et al. 1995; Kléber et al 1986).

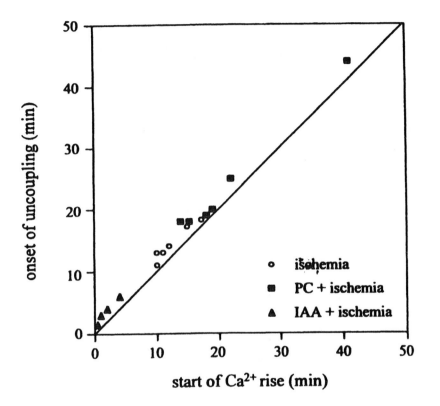

Figure 9. The relation between the moment of diastolic Ca^{2-} rise (on the abscissa) and the moment of the onset of uncoupling (on the ordinate) after the induction of isohemia for all experiments. Isohemia: sustained ischemia in control preparations; *PC* + ischeinia: sustained ischemia in ischemically preconditioned preparations; IAA + ischemia sustained ischemia in preparations pretreated with 1 mmoVL indoacetate. The oblique line is the line of identity. Uncoupling always follows the increase of $(Ca^{2+})_i$. The average interval is 2.1±0.2 minutes. (Reproduced with permission from Dekker et al, 1996).

After about 15 minutes of complete ischemia changes become irreversible. The transition to irreversible damage coincides with the secondary decline of the cytosolic phosphorylation potential (Fiolet et al, 1984), contracture and enzyme release (Steenbergen et al 1990), the secondary increase in extracellular K^+ accumulation and electrical cellular uncoupling (Kléber et al,1987 Cascio et al 1990). The second type of ischemia-induced arrhythmias, the 1-B arrhythmias, are associated with the onset of electrical uncoupling (Smith et al, 1995). Most hypotheses on the pathogenesis of irreversible ischemic injury center on intracellular calcium overload (Steenbergen et al, 1990; Poole-Wilson et al, 1984; Katz, Reuter, 1979). Our findings also show that the increase of intracellular calcium is closely coupled to the onset of irreversible ischemic damage even in the absence of acidification (Dekker et al, 1996;Dekker, 1996).

Calcium overload in ischemia could in principle be caused by an enhanced influx of calcium from the extracellular space via the voltage sensitive $Ca^{2\sim}$ channels or the Na^+/Ca^{2+} exchanger, or by release of calcium from the sarcoplasmatic reticulum.

A possible way leading to increased intracellular Ca^{2+} is via the Na^+/Ca^{2+} exchanger which is stimulated by an increase of intracellular Na^+, which in its turn is caused by an increase of Na^+/H^+ exchange secondary to acidosis. It is, however, unlikely that this is the main source of calcium influx. The rate of Na^+ dependent Ca^{2+} exchange is inhibited during ischemia (Dixon et al, 1987), and in our experiments cytosolic calcium accumulation still occurred in the absence of acidification (Dekker et al, 1996).

The calcium entry blocker verapamil postpones the onset of uncoupling, the secondary rise in extracellular $K\sim$ accumulation and the rise in resting tension (Cascio et al. 1996). However, this could be due to a variety of factors, such as a decrease in energy requirement with preservation of energy-rich phosphate compounds, and a decreased calcium concentration in the sarcoplasmatic reticulum. This would reduce the energy required to maintain a given level of cytosolic Ca^{2+} and, consequently, the cells would tolerate a lower ATP potential.

The most likely cause for the increase in cytosolic calcium during ischemia is a net release of calcium from the sarcoplasmatic reticulum (Klébber, Oetliker, 1992). Normally, the Ca^{2+} pump of the sarcoplasmatic reticulum has to maintain a difference in calcium concentration of about a factor 100,000 over the sarcoplasmatic reticulum membrane. This is close to the thermo-dynamic limit imposed on a very efficient Ca^{2+} pump by the cytosolic phosphorylation potential (free energy change of ATP hydrolysis) (Hasselbach, Oetliker, 1992; Marban et al, 1989). As the cytosolic phosphorylation potential decreases during ischemia (Fiolet et al ,1984), it will set the thermodynamic threshold value to a smaller maximal calcium gradient. This will result in a depletion of Ca^{2+} from tiw. satcoplasm~atic reticulum and an increase in the cytosol, initiating the development of irreversible ischemic injury.

Cardioprotection by reduction of sarcoplasmatic reticulum calcium loading

Cardioprotection, by ischemic preconditioning or by pharmacological preconditioning by cromakalim, is related to postponement of the rise in cytosolic calcium and this may be due to a delay in release of calcium from the sarcoplasmatic reticulum (Dekker , 1996). This is shown in a diagrammatic form in Figure 10.

There are three reasons why in preconditioned myocardium the release of calcium by the sarcoplasmatic reticulum may be delayed:

1) In preconditioned myocardium, creatine phosphate levels, and thus the cytosolic phosphorylation potential ΔG_{ATP}, are higher at the start of sus tained ischemia than in control hearts *(Fiolet et al, 1984, Steenbergen et al, 1993; Kida et al1991).*
2) Both ischemic preconditioning and postponement of uncoupling by croma kalim are associated with a reduction in calcium loading of the sarcoplas matic reticulum (Dekker 1996). Moreover, reducing the sarcoplasmatic reticulum content with cydopiazonic acid protects the heart during subsequent

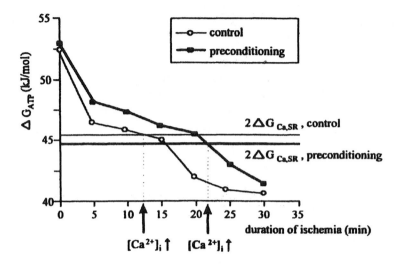

Figure 10. Theoretical diagram of relative decline of ΔG_{ATP} during ischemia in control (open circles and thin lines) and preconditioned (filled squares and thick lines) hearts. Horizontal lines represent proposed threshold ΔG_{ATP} (equivalent to 2 times ΔG_{caSR}) for control (thin line) and preconditioned (thick line) hearts. See text for further details. Dotted vertical lines represent moment of $[Ca^{2+}]_i$ rise during isohemia in control (thin) and preconditioned hearts (thick). (Reproduced with permission from Dekker, 1996)

ischemia (Dekker 1996). Because of lowering of the calcium gradient across the sarco plasmatic reticulum membrane, energy consumption in preconditioned hearts is reduced, and the decline in ATP is decreased (Fiolet et al, 1984; Steenbergen et al, 1993; Kida et al, 1991; Murry et al 1990).

3) The lower calcium gradient across the sarcoplasmatic reticulum membrane can be maintained at a lower ΔG_{ATP} and the threshold beyond which the sarcoplasmatic reticulum will release calcium is lower. The threshold ΔG_{ATP} at which a net calcium efflux into the cytosol will occur equals 2 ΔG_{ATP} (the electrochemical gradient for calcium across the sarcoplasmatic reticulum membrane) *(Fiolet et al, 1984).*

In summary, the hypothesis based on the thermodynamic consider-ations described above, states that the reduction of calcium loading of the sarcoplasmatic reticulum attenuates the decline of ΔG_{ATP} and decreases the thermodynamic limit, which determines the sarcoplasmatic calcium gradient during ischemia. As a result, during ischemia in hearts with prior reduced calcium content of the sarcoplasmatic reticulum, ΔG_{ATP} reaches the threshold for Ca^{2+} depletion at a later moment compared to hearts with a normal calcium content of the sarcoplasmatic reticulum (Dekker. 1996).

A great many hypotheses have been put forward to explain the protective effects of preconditioning: activation of adenosine 1 receptors (A_1), alpha 1 adrenoreceptors (i). muscarinic receptors (M_2), stimulation and translocation of protein kinase C (PKC), opening of ATP sensitive K channels and activation of heat shock proteins. Activation of A_1, 1 and M_2 receptors may lead to a G-protein-dependent activation of PKC, which reduces the field to two main candidates: activation of PKC and activation of ATP sensitive K channels. The ultimate mechanism underlying preconditioning is still unclear (Lawson, Downey, 1993), but it is worthwhile to consider a low sarcoplasmatic reticulum calcium content as the final common pathway. PKC inhibits calcium accumulation in the sarcoplasmatic reticulum (Rogers et al, 1990) and extracts calcium from the cytosol by stimulating the Na^+/Ca^{2+} exchanger and inhibiting sarcolemmal Ca^{2+} channels (Brecheler et al, 1990; Lacerda et al, 1988). It is more difficult to link activation of ATP-sensitive K^+ channels to sarcoplasmatic Ca^{2+} content. As already mentioned, glibenclamide and cromakalim have other effects besides blocking and activating Al sensitive K^+ channels. Moreover, there is evidence that pharmacologic preconditioning with openers of ATP-sensitive K^+ channels occurs independently from activation of sarcolemmal K_{ATP} channels. Pronounce alterations of calcium transients during exposure to cromakalim have been observed, indicative of calcium release from the sarcoplasmatic reticulum without concomitant shortening of action potential duration (Dekker,1996). Also the K_{ATP} channel opener bimakalim offered cardioprotection in if absence of action potential shortening (Yao, Grant, 1994).

Since only a tiny fraction of sarcolemmal K_{ATP} channels need to be activated to produce a substantial shortening of the action potential (Weiss, 1996) these data indicate that these K channel openers have other action besides activating sarcolemmal K_{ATP} channels. K channel openers direct decrease sarcoplasmatic reticulum calcium loading in smooth muscle cells (Chopra et al, 1992;Bray et al, 1991) and probably do so as well in cardiac cells (Dekker, 1996). Clearly, future research on the cardioprotective effect of reduced calcium loading of the sarcoplasmatic reticulum is needed to unravel the relationship between calcium transients, protein kinase C activity, activation of adenosine alpha adrenergic and muscarinic receptors, the actions of K_{ATP} channel blockers and openers, the subcellular pathways involved and sarcoplasmatic calcium content.

REFERENCE

Bray KM. Weston All, Duty 5, Nargreen DT, Longmore J, Edwards G, Brown TJ. (1991) Differences between the effects of cromakalim and nifedipine on agonist-induced responses in rabbit aorta. Br J Pharmacol 102:337

Brechler V, Pavoine C. Lotersztajn S, Garbare E, Pecker F. (1990) Activation Na/Ca exchanger by adenosine in the ewe heart sarcolemma is mediated pertussis toxin sensitive G protein. J Biol Chem; 265:16851-16855.

Cascio WE, Yan G, Kléber AG. (1990) Passive electrical properties, mechanical activity, and extracellular potassium in arterially perfused and ischemic rabbit ventricular muscle. Effects of calcium entry blockade or hypocalcemia. Circ Res 66:1461-1473.

Chopra LC, Twort CHC, Ward JPT. (1992) Direct action of BRL 38227 and glibenclanide on intracellular calcium stores in cultured airway smooth muscle cells of rabbit. Br J Pharmacol 105:259-260.

Coronel R, Wilms-Schopman FJG, Dekker LRC, Janse MJ. (1995) Heterogeneitis in [K+]o and TQ potential and the inducibility of ventricular fibrillation during acute regional ischemia in the isolated porcine heart. Circulation; 92:120-19.

Daleau P. (1996) Effects of lysophosphatidyleholine on intercellular resistance of guinea pig ventricular cell pairs (abstract). Circulation 94:1-9.

De Mello WC, Motta GE, Chapeau M. (1969) A study on the healing-over of myocardial cells of toads. Cire Res; *24:475487.*

De Mello WC. (1975) Effect of intracellular injection of calcium and strontium on cell communication in heart. J Physiol 250:231-245.

De Mello WC. (1983) The influence of pH on the healing-over of mammalian cardiac muscle. I Physiol 339:299-307.

Dekker LRC, Fiolet JWT, Van Bavel E, Coronel R, Opthof T, Spaan JAE, Janse MJ. (1996) Intra cellular $Ca^{2~}$, intercellular coupling resistance, and mechanical activity in ischemic rabbit papillary muscle. Effects of preconditioning and metabolic blockade. Circ Res; 79:237-246.

Dekker LRC. (1996) Role of intracellular calcium in ischemic damage and preconditioning in cardiac muscle. Thesis, University of Amsterdam (ISBN 90-9009992-1),

Déleze J. (1970) The recovery of resting potential and input resistance in sheep heart injured by knife or laser. 3 Physiol; 208:547-562.

Dixon IM, Eyolfson DA, Dhalla NS. (1987) Sarcolemmal Na^{+}/Ca^{2+} exchanger activity in hearts subjected to hypoxia reoxygenation. Am J Physiol;253: 111026-111034.

Engelmaun TW. (1875) Ueber die Leitung der Erregung im Herzniuskel. Pfluegen Arch; 11: *465-480.*

Fiolet JWT, Baartscheer A, Schumacher CA, Coronel R, Ter Welle HF. (1984) The change of the free energy of ATP hydrolysis during global ischemia and anoxia in the rat heart. J Mol Cell Cardiol 16:1023-1036.

Hasselbach W, Qetliker H. (1983) Energetics and electrogenicity of the sarcoplasmatic reticulum calcium pump. Annu Rev Physiol; 45:325-339.

Hill JL, Gettes LS. (1980) Effects of acute coronary artery occlusion on local myocardial extracellular K^{+} activity in swine. Circulation 61:768-778.

Ikeda K, Hiraoka M. (1982) Effects of hypoxia on passive electrical proper ties of canine ventricular muscle. Pfluegers Arch; 393:45-50.

Janse MJ, Wit AL. (1989) Electrophysiological mechanisms of ventricular arrhythmias resulting from myocardial ischemia and infarction. Physiol Rev 69:1049-1169.

Jennings RB, Reimer KA, Steenbergen Jr C, Schaper J. (1989) Total ischemia I effect of inhibition of anaerobic metabolism. J Mol Cell Cardiol 21 (Suppl 1): 37-54.

Katz AM, Reuter H. (1979) Cellular calcium and cardiac cell death. Am J Cardiol 44:188-190.

Kida M, Fujiwara H, Ishida M, Kawai C, Ohura M, Miura I, Yabuuchi Y. (1991) Ischemic preconditioning preserves creatine phosphate and intracellular pH. Circulation 84:2495-2503.

KIéber AG, Riegger CB. (1987) Electrical constants of arterially perfused rabbit papillary muscle. J Physiol 385:307-324.

Kléber AG, Janse MJ, Wilms-Schopman FJG, Wilde AAM, Coronel R. (1986) Changes in conduction velocity during acute ischemia in ventricular myocardium in the isolated porcine heart. Circulation 73:189-198.

Kléber AG, Oetliker H. (1992) Cellular aspects of early contractile failure in ischemia, in Fozzard HA, Haber E, Jennings RB, Katz AM, Morgan HE (eds): The heart and cardiovascular system, 2nd edition, New York, Raven Press, pp 1975-1996.

Kléber AG, Riegger CB, Janse MJ. (1987) Electrical uncoupling and increase of extracellular resistance after induction of ischemia in isolated, arterially perfused rabbit rapillary muscle. Circ Res 61:271-279.

Lacerda AE, Romyze D, Brown AM. (1988) Effects of protein kinase C activators on cardiac Ca^{2+} channels. Nature 333:249-251.

Lawson CS, Downey IM. (1993) Preconditioning: state of the art of myocardial protection. Cardiovasc Res 27:542-550.

Marban B, Koretsune Y, Corretti M, Chacko VP, Kusuoka H. (1989) Calcium and its role in myocardial cell injury during ischemia and reperfusion. Circulation 80 (Suppl IV): 17-22.

McCallister LP, Trapudki 5, Neely JR. (1979) Morphometric observation on the effects of ischemia in the isolated perfused rat heart. J Mol Cell Cardiol 11:619-630.

Murry CE, Jennings RB, Reimer KA. (1986) Preconditioning with ischemia: a delay of lethal cell injury in ischemic myocardium. Circulation 74:1124-11

Murry CE, Richard VJ, Reimer KA, Jennings RB. (1990) Ischemic preconditioning slows energy metabolism and delays ultrastructural damage during a sustained ischemic episode. Circ Res 913-931.

Noma A, Tsuboi N. (1987) Dependence of junctional conductance on proton, calcium and magnesium ions in cardiac paired cells of guinea-pig. J Physiol 382:193-211.

Poole-Wilson PA, Harding DP, Bourdillon PDV, Tones MA. (1984) Calcium out of control. J Mol Cell Cardiol 16:175-187.

Pressler ML (1987) Effects of pCa_1 and pH, on cell-to-cell coupling. Experientia 43:1084-1092.

Reber WR, Weingart R. (1982) Ungulate cardiac Purkinje fibres: the influence of intracellular pH on electrical cell-to-cell coupling. J Physiol 328:87-104.

Riegger CR, Alperovich G, Kléber AG. (1989) Effect of oxygen withdrawal on active and passive electrical properties of arterially perfused rabbit ventricular muscle. Circ Res 64:532-541.

Rogers RB, Gaa ST. Massey C, D6semeci A. (1990) Protein kinase C inhibits Ca^{2+} accumulation in cardiac sarcoplasmatic reticulum. J Biol Chem 265:4302-4308.

Smith WT, Fleet WF, Johnson TA, Engle CL, Cascio WE. (1995) The lb phase of ventricular arrhythmias in ischemic in situ porcine heart is related to changes in cell-to-cell coupling. Circulation 92:3051-3060.

Spray DC, Stern HJ, Harris AL, Bennett MVL. (1981) Gap junctional conductance: comparison of sensitivities to H and Ca ions. Proc Nat. Acad Sci USA 79:441445

Steenbergen C, Murphy E, Waths JA, London RE. (1990) Correlation between cytosolic free calcium, contracture, ATP, and irreversible ischemic injury in perfused rat heart. Circ Res *66:135-146.*

Steenbergen C, Perlman ME, London RE, Murphy B. (1993) Mechanism of preconditioning: ionic alteration. Circ Res 72:112-125.

Sugiura H, Toyama J, Tsuboi N, Kamiya K, Kodama I. (1990) ATP directly affects junctional conductance between paired ventricular myocytes isolated from guinea pig heart. Circ Res 66:1095-1102.

Tan HL, Janse MJ. (1994) Contribution of mechanical activity and electrical ad to cellular uncoupling in ischemic rabbit papillary muscle. J Mol Cell Cardio 26:733-742.

Tan HL, Maz6n P, Verbeme HJ, Sleeswijk ME, Coronel R, Opthof T, Ja MJ. (1993) Ischemic preconditioning delays ischemia-induced cellular electrical uncoupling in rabbit myocardium by activation of ATP-sensitive K^+ channels Cardiovasc. Res 27:644-651.

Tan HL, Netea AC, Sleeswijk ME, Maz6n P. Coronel R, Opthof T, Janse (1993) *R56865* delays cellular electrical uncoupling in ischemic rabbit papillary muscle. J Mol Cell Cardiol 25:1059-1066.

Tan HL. (1993) Cellular electrical uncoupling and protection of isehemic myocardium. Thesis, University of Amsterdam (ISBN 90-9006433-8),

Tranum-Jensen J, Janse MJ, Fiolet J'WT, Krieger WJG, Naumann d'Alnc court C, Durrer D. (1981) Tissue osmolality, cell swelling, and reperfusion in acu regional myocardial isehemia in the isolated porcine heart. Circ Res 49:364-381.

Ver Donck L, Borgers M, Verdonek F. (1993) Inhibition of Na^+ and Ca^{2+} overload in the myocardium: a new cytoprotective principle. Cardiovasc Res 37:349-357.

Weidmann S. (1970) Electrical constants of trabecular muscle from mammalian heart. I Physiol 210:1041-1054.

Weiss JN. (1996) ATP-sensitive K channels in myocardial ischemia, in Vereecke Van Bogaert PP (eds): Potassium channels in normal and pathological conditions, Leuven, Leuven University Press, pp 119-132.

Wilde AAM, Aksnes G. (1995) Myocardial potassium loss and cell depolarization ischemia and hypoxia. Cardiovasc Res 29:1-15.

Wojtczak J. (1979) Contractures and increase in internal longitudinal resistance of cow ventricular muscle induced by hypoxia. Circ Res 44:88-95.

Wu J, McHowat J, Saftitz JE, Yamada KA, Con- PB. (1993) Inhibition of gap
    junctional conduction by long-chain acetylcarnitines and their
    preferential accumulation in junctional sarcolemma during hypoxia. Circ
    Res 72:879-889.
Yao Z, Garrett JG. (1994) Effects of the KATP channel opener bimakalim in
    coronary blood flow, monophasic action potential duration, and infarct
    in dogs. Circulation *89:1769-1775.*

11

CELL COUPLING AND IMPULSE PROPAGATION IN THE FAILING HEART:THE ROLE OF THE RENIN ANGIOTENSIN SYSTEM.

Walmor C. De Mello

Department of Pharmacology, Medical Sciences Campus, UPR

It is known that myocytes from the failing heart present several abnormalities of ion pumps, calcium re-uptake by the sarcoplasmic reticulum, hormone receptors, etc (Morgan,Baker,1991).

In cardiomyopathic hamsters a calcium overload of the heart cells has been considered a possible etiologic factor. The mechanism of this overload is not completely clear but there is evidence that the calcium uptake by the cell is enhanced (Lossnitzer et al,1975; Wrogeman,Nylen,1978) leading to a calcium-determined necrotic process with myocytolysis and typical fibrillar disarray (Jasmin,Proschek,1984). As emphasized by Weismand and Weinfeldt (1987), the cardiomyopathic hamster represents an important model for cardiomyopathy and hypertrophy in humans. Indeed, ventricular hypertrophy followed by progressive cardiac dilation and death by congestive heart failure is seen in cardiomyopathic hamsters at late stage of the disease (Bajusz,1969; Gertz 1992).

Our present knowledge of the electrophysiological properties of the failing heart is meager, particularly of the alterations in cell

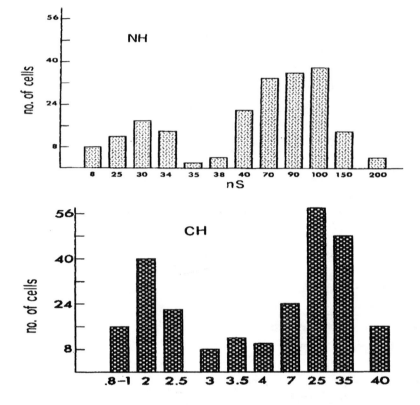

Figure 1. Distribution of gj values found in several ventricular cell pairs of normal hamsters (NH, top) and CM hamsters (CH, bottom). From De Mello,1996, with permission.

coupling. In the present chapter I will discuss some relevant aspects of this problem and recent findings.

Measurements of gj performed in cell pairs isolated from normal hamsters (11 months old) indicated predominant values in the rage from 40 to 100 nS (Fig. 1). In the ventricle of cardiomyopathic hamsters, at an advanced stage of the disease, the values of gj are very low. Two major populations of cells in terms of values of gj were found: one in which the value of gj is very low (0.8-2.5 nS) and the other in which the values are higher (7-35 nS) but still smaller than the controls (see Fig. 1) (De Mello,1996).The values of membrane resistance are in the range of 1.4 -1.8 GΩ.

The very low values of gj and the high membrane resistance found in CM hamsters cell pairs, particularly at an advanced stage of the disease, provide a reliable condition for the determination of gj. These two major populations of CM myocytes were classified not only by their different values of gj but also by some morphological characteristics. The group of cells presenting very low values of gj showed clear alterations in cross striations as previously described by Sen et al (1990) while the other group with higher values of gj showed an internal normal structure but the cell length was increased. In normal hamsters of same age (11 months old) no such morphological abnormalities were found among the ventricular myocytes. Histological studies performed in normal and CM hamsters indicated extensive areas of interstitial fibrosis and calcification in the myopathic ventricle but not in the normal animal (see Figs. 2) (De Mello et al,1997) and severe destruction of intercellular contacts can be seen in the right and left ventricle of cardiomyopathic hamsters (11 months old) using confocal microscopy (Cherry, De Mello,1996). This alteration of ventricular morphology, which is more pronounced near calcified zones or in areas in which intense interstitial fibrosis can be detected, represents an important detrimental factor for electrical synchronization and ventricular contractility. Electronmicroscopic studies performed on the myocardium of another strain of cardiomyopathic hamsters (UM-X7.1) indicated smaller intercalated discs with an abnormal orientation and distribution (Luque et al,1994).

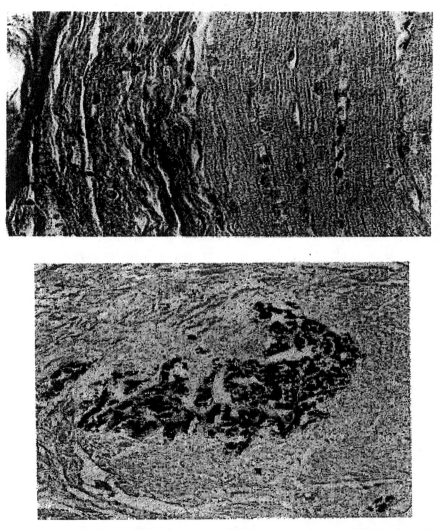

Figure 2. Top-Histopathology of the right ventricle of cardiomyopathic hamster (11 months old) showing extensive interstitial fibrosis with Masson trichrome. Magnification 50x. Bottom-Von Kossa's stain of the left ventricle of cardiomyopathic hamster (11 months old) showing central lesion with Ca depots. From reference De Mello et al,1997, with permission.

The mechanism of the impairment of cell coupling in the failing myocardium is not known. Electrophysiological observations performed on transfected cell pairs showed that different connexins form gap junctions with different channel gating properties (Kanter et al,1993). In the hypertensive rat heart, for instance, the expression of connexin 43 is reduced but the expression of connexin 40 is enhanced (Bastide et al,1993). The possibility exists that the impairment of cell coupling seen in the failing heart be, in part, related to an alteration in the expression of different connexins. A decline in the expression of connexin43 has been considered by Severs (1994) as responsible for some electrophysiological abnormalities of the diseased heart. An alternative explanation of the decline in gj is the calcium overload which is one of the characteristics of this cardiomyopathy. The intracellular calcium concentration measured in isolated myocytes from the BIO-T02 cardiomyopathic hamsters at late stage of the disease (11 months), for instance, indicated an average value of 480 (SEM ± 28) nM compared with 143 (SEM ± 24) nM in the control hamster (F1B) of the same age (De Mello, unpublished). This result is in accord that those found in other strain of myopathic hamster (BIO 14.6) (8 months old) (Sen et al,1990).

The mechanism of the calcium overload is not known. An increase in the permeability of the surface cell membrane to calcium has been described (Sen et al,1990) but the possibility that excess catecholamine damage the surface cell membrane with consequent increase in intracellular calcium has been proposed by Fleckenstein (1971). A deficiency of ATP caused by excessive activation of calcium-dependent ATPases and mitochondrial damage by excessive calcium accumulation inside might not be related to a primary defect of the sarcolemma but due to a exhausted hypokinetic state that favor Ca accumulation with progressive deterioration of structural proteins (Jasmin,Proschek,1984). Measurements of the membrane resistance made in isolated myocytes from CM hamsters indicated values in the range of 1.4 – 1.8 G Ω which is not different from controls(P>0.05).

It has been found that during depolarization a large slowly inactivating inward current is activated in ventricular myocytes of cardiomyopathic hamsters and that this current seems to be generated by the Na-Ca exchanger (Hatem et al,1994) suggesting that the Na/Ca exchanger plays a major role in the regulation of heart contractility and calcium sequestration in the cardiomyopathic hamsters .

An alternative explanation for the decline in cell coupling is a decrease in size of the gap junctions.

Connexin distribution in the heart of cardiomyopathic hamster

In 2 month-old cardiomyopathic hamsters specimens swatches of anomalous tissue could be seen in the wall of the left ventricle. These anomalous sectors were evident even without magnification. Under magnification the sectors appeared as scallop-shapes sectors of dying myocardium located at evenly spaced intervals. The sectors started 10-200 μm from the epicardium and seemed to penetrate all the way through the subendocardium in serial sections (Gourdie and De Mello, unpublished).

The connexin distribution in the heart of CM hamsters at 2 month of age,indicated that the surviving myocardial tissue within and bordering of the anomalous zone displayed disorganized patters of connexin 43 distribution (Fig 3).

Also associated with the fibrotic zones, aberrant-looking vascular structures, showing Cx40 immunolabelled endothelial tissues can be seen(Fig 3). Cx43 appears disorganized and not particularly disk-localized in myocytes surviving within and adjacent to the fibrotic zones(Fig 3). Low levels of Cx45 were apparent in normal-looking sectors of the myocardium in 10 month-old cardiomyopathic hamsters, but was reduced and disorganized in myocytes in surviving the fibrotic zones (Fig 3).In the left ventricle of control hamsters Cx45 was localized at low levels between the working myocardium (Fig 3).

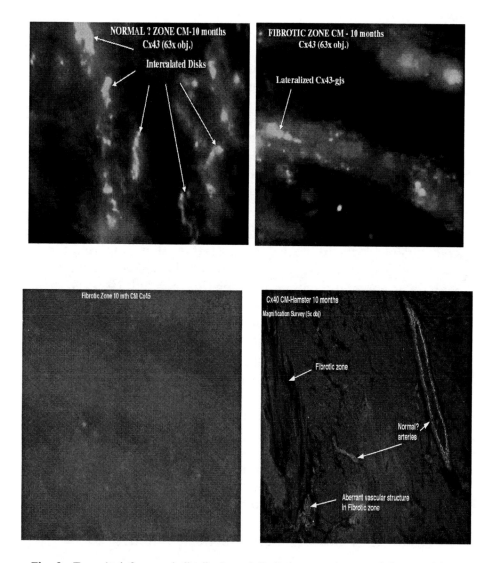

Fig. 3 Top- At left normal distribution of Cx43 in normal zone of the ventricle of cardiomyoapathic hamster (CM-TO2)10 month- old. At right- abnormal distribution (lateral)of Cx43 near damaged zone from the same preparation shown at left.Bottom-distribution of Cx45 in the ventricle of CM hamsters(10 month-old). At right aberrant vascular structure in the ventricle of CM hamster (10 month-old). From Gourdie and De Mello, unpublished.

Interestingly, studies performed on the LV of 30 day-old CM hamsters indicated no zones of fibrosis or necrosis and the distribution of Cx43 is limited to the intercalated discs as found in normal controls (Gourdie and De Mello, unpublished).Moreover, no signs of interstitial fibrosis or calcification are seen at this age. This finding indicates that the changes in cell communication found in the failing heart of cardiomyopathic hamsters are not manifested before the first month of age.

Studies of Severs (1994) showed a disturbance in spatial distribution of gap junctions at the border of healed infarcts and a decreased quantity of immunodetectable Cx43 in regions of normal gap junction distribution distant from the infact scars. At the epicardial borders of healed canine infarcts, the distribution of Cx43 has been reported to be altered and this change is correlated with the location of reentrant rhythms (Peters et al . 1997).

In human congestive heart failure, a significant reduction in levels of Cx43 was found but the Cx40 expression was enhanced (Dupont et al 2001). More recently, it was found that in Cx43 deficient mice there is an increased incidence, frequency and duration of ventricular tachyarrhythmias after coronary ligation (Lerner et al, 2000),an expected result considering the decline in intercellular junctions.

These findings as well as those reported above in the failing heart of CM hamsters, indicate that an abnormal Cx43 distribution is probably involved in the generation of malignant reentrant rhythms seen in this model of heart failure as well as in patients with congestive heart failure (see also De Mello, 2001).

Since it is known that an increment in Cai lead to a decline in gj (De Mello,1975) ,it is justified to think that the fall in gj seen in the myopathic ventricle be related to calcium overload. Although there is an increment in the intracellular calcium concentration in myopathic myocytes, it has been found that these cells present a remarkable capacity to buffer changes in Cai induced by variations of external Ca (Sen et al,1990), a phenomenon probably related to an increased sarcoplasmic reticulum described in these cells(Francis,Cohn,1986).Experiments performed in our laboratory indicated that when cell pairs from cardiomyopathic animals are dialyzed with high Ca solution, the junctional conductance is less affected when compared with normal hamsters of same age. As shown in Fig. 4 (De Mello, unpublished) the dialysis of Ca (0.5 μM) into the cells of normal hamster caused a suppression of cell coupling within 12 min while in cardiomyopathic hamster the administration of the same concentration of Ca to the cytosol and using pipettes with the same tip diameter, caused a decline of gj of only 65% in about 18 min. (p<0.05). It is not known if that the gap junction proteins in myopathic hamsters are less sensitive to calcium or whether the buffer capacity of the cytosol for Ca, particularly near the junctions is enhanced in this model of heart failure.

The control of junctional conductance by beta-adrenergic receptor activation is impaired in the failing heart.

It is well known that the adrenergic receptors-G protein-adenyl cyclase complex is involved in an important signaling system entailed in the control of heart contractility (Covell et al, 1966; Bristow et al, 1982; Fowler et al, 1986).

Evidence is available that cardiac failure is accompanied by changes in autonomic regulation including a decreased parasympathetic tonus and an enhanced sympathetic control (Feldman et al 1990; Bohm et al, 1990). It is also known that with the progress of the disease, the cardiac muscle becomes quite insensitive to sympathetic stimulation (Feldman et al,1988; De Mello,1996; Fowler et al,1986) -a finding that has been attributed to the down regulation of beta-adrenoreceptor activation in the failing heart and also to a defective coupling of G-proteins to adenyl cyclase (Feldman et al,1990). An increase in the alpha -

subunit of the inhibitory G protein was confirmed by pertussis toxin-catalyzed ADP ribosylation (Bohm et al,1990; Feldman et al,1988). Moreover, myocardial Gi mRNA levels are elevated in terminal cardiac failure (Bohm et al,1990).

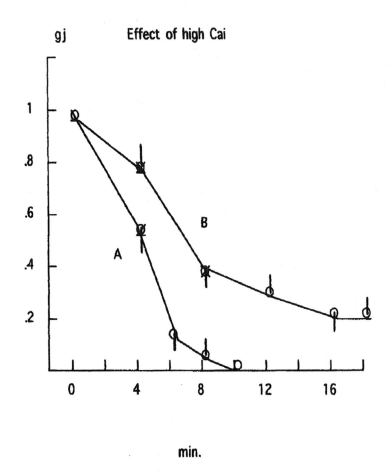

Figure 4. Effect of intracellular dialysis of 0.5 µM Ca on gj of normal hamsters (A) and cardiomyopathic hamster (B) 11 months old. Values of gj were normalized. Vertical line at each point - SEM.

Studies made on the influence of beta-adrenergic receptor activation in cell pairs isolated from the ventricle of cardiomyopathic hamsters at late stage of the disease (11 months), indicated that isoproterenol $(10^{-6}\,M)$ or forskolin $(10^{-7}\,M)$ had no influence on gj (De Mello, 1996). These findings

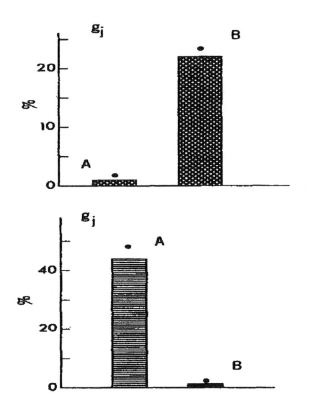

Figure 5. Bottom-Negligible effect of isoproterenol (10-6 M) on gj of CM cell pairs from hamsters 11 months old (B). At A-effect of the drug on gj of control of same age. Each bar is the average of 15 experiments. Black dot indicate SEM. Top - Small effect of forskolin (10-' M) on gj of myopathic cell pairs (A) and controls (B) (n=14). From De Mello,1996 , with permission.

contrast with those obtained in cell pairs of normal hamsters of same age in which isoproterenol and forskolin, at the same drug concentration, increased gj by $45 \pm 3\%$ (n=13) and $23 \pm 2.8\%$ (n=16), respectively. The inhibition of phosphodiesterase with isobutylmethylxanthine (10^{-6} M) which increased gj in the controls by $38 \pm 1.5\%$ (n=12), was unable to increment gj in the myopathic cell pairs (De Mello,1996). However, dibutyryl-cAMP (10^{-6}M) incremented gj by $58 \pm 2.1\%$ (n=14) in the cardiomyopathic hamster - an effect similar to that found in the normal hamster (Fig. 5). These findings indicate that the activation of cAMP dependent protein kinase by cAMP is able to increment gj as found in the normal heart (De Mello,1996) supporting the notion that the lack of control of gj by the cAMP cascade is related to down regulation of beta adrenergic receptors and to a defect of the adenyl cyclase. Measurements of the time constant of cell membrane performed in isolated myocytes before (21 ± 3 ms) and after (20.7 ± 2.1 ms) dibutyryl cAMP (10^{-6} M) indicated that the drug is not altering the surface cell membrane resistance ($p>0.05$). The effect of the compound on gj, however, is inhibited by intracellular administration of an inhibitor of cAMP-dependent protein kinase (see also De Mello,1988).

These observations indicate that sympathetic stimuli are unable to increase gj in cardiomyopathic myocytes at a late stage of the disease. Consequently, the enhanced conduction velocity and electrical synchronization usually seen under beta-adrenergic activation in the normal heart, is not present in the failing myocardium what creates a serious impairment of autonomic

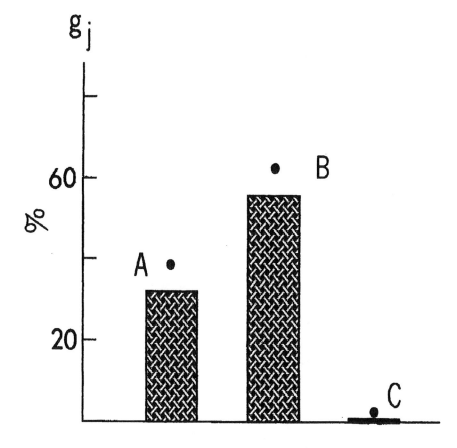

Figure 6. Effect of dibutyryl-cAMP (10-' M) on gj of CM cell pairs from 11 months old hamsters (A) and controls of same age (B). At C suppression of the effect of dB-CAMP caused by intracellular dialysis of an inhibitor of PKA (20 ug/ml). Each bar is the average from 14 experiments. Black dot - SEM. From De Mello,1996 with permission.

regulation preventing cardiovascular adjustments that are essential for cardiovascular homeostasis.

The role of the renin-angiotensin system on the regulation of gj and impulse propagation

Evidence is available that a local renin-angiotensin system(RAS) exists in the heart (Dzau, 1988; see for review De Mello,Danser,2000; Bader et al ,2001). Moreover, angiotensin II and renin activity have been demonstrated in aphrenic patients (Campbell,1985).

There are several lines of evidence supporting the notion that there is a local renin-angiotensin system in the heart: 1) angiotensin II receptors have been localized in cultured heart cells (Rogers et al,1986); 2) angiotensin I is converted to angiotensin II in the isolated and perfused rat heart (Linz et al,1986); 3) genes of renin and angiotensinogen are coexpressed in cardiac muscle (Dzau et al,1986). An additional and important finding is that the beneficial effect of angiotensin converting enzyme inhibitors in patients with essential hypertension and congestive heart failure, is not only dependent on the blockade of the plasma RAS but is also due to an effect on the cardiac RAS (Linz et al, 1986).

Although it is known that angiotensin II increases heart contractility (Koch-Weser,1965), the influence of the peptide and of the renin angiotensin system, as a whole, on intercellular communication was not known at the moment we started these studies.

Influence of extracellular angiotensin II on heart cell coupling

In cell pairs isolated from normal adult rats, angiotensin II (Ang II) (10^{-8} M) added to the bath, caused a decline in gj of 60% within 45 sec. The effect of the peptide was blocked by losartan what indicates that the activation of AT1 receptors is essential for the effect of Ang II (De Mello,Altieri,1992). The effect of the peptide on gj requires the activation of protein kinase C because staurosporine abolished the effect of angiotensin II. The activation of the kinase was probably related to the hydrolysis of phosphatidyl-inositol-4-5-biphosphate with consequent formation of diacylglycerol. Since the synthesis of inositol triphosphate leads to the release of calcium from intracellular stores, the possibility that the increment in Cai be involved in the effect of the peptide cannot be discarded. However, in our experiments the use of high concentration of EGTA (10 mM) and HEPES (l0mM) in the internal solution seems to indicate that the participation of changes in (Ca)i or pHi on the decline of gj is unlikely.

Conceivably, the decline in cell-to-cell coupling caused by Ang II can increase the intracellular resistance in muscle trabeculae with consequent impairment of impulse propagation. We have carried on studies on the influence of the peptide on the electrical properties of intact normal rat heart muscle and the results showed that the peptide causes a decrease in conduction velocity from 59.5 ± 2.5 cm/s to 35 ± 3.5 cms (De Mello et al,1993) while enalapril -an angiotensin converting enzyme inhibitor, reduced the intracellular resistance and increased the conduction velocity appreciably (De Mello et al,1993).

In cardiomyopathic hamsters (11 month- old) Ang II (10^{-8} M) added to the extracellular fluid , caused a maked decline of gj or even a total suppresion of cell coupling as shown in Fig 6 . The effect of Ang II on cell communication is not related to a fall in surface cell membrane resistance which (1.4 – 1.8 G Ω) remained unchanged during the experiments.

Angiotensin converting enzyme inhibitors, cardiac failure and cell communication

Several clinical studies indicate that angiotensin converting enzyme (ACE) inhibitors reduce the mortality of patients with congestive heart failure (CONSENSUS,1987). The mechanism of

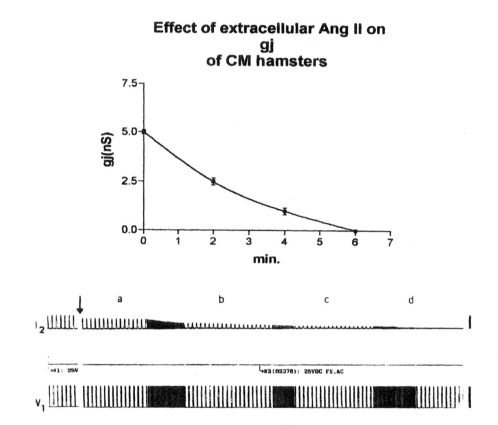

Figure 7. Top - Effect of angiotensin 11 (Ang II) (10-8 M) on CM cell pairs with very low gj (n=18) at an advanced stage of the disease. Vertical line at each point SEM..Bottom- effect of Ang II on single cell pair from the failing heart of the CM hamster .Fom De Mello1996, with permission.

action of these compounds is not limited to the decline in afterload and preload. There is evidence that these drugs prevent or reduce the ventricular hypertrophy elicited by aortic banding using low doses of the compounds which do not cause a decline of the arterial blood pressure (Linz et al,1986). These findings support the view that a decrease in the synthesis of Ang II in the heart is involved in the effect of the ACE inhibitors. In rats with left ventricular infarction, for instance, the content of angiotensin converting enzyme as well as the mRNA levels of angiotensinogen and ACE are enhanced in the hypertrophied myocardium (Dzau et al,1986; Hirsch et al, 1991). In cardiomyopathic hamsters (TO-2) similar increment of ACE activity was found during the late stages of the disease (De Mello and Crespo,1999). Furthermore, it is known that Ang II is a growth factor even in cultured heart cells,an effect mediated by the enhanced expression of proto-oncogenes such as c-myc and c-fos-and mediated by the activation of protein kinase C (Izumo et al,1988).

It has been shown that enalapril-an angiotensin converting enzyme inhibitor, increases the junctional conductance in rat isolated heart cell pairs (De Mello,Altieri,1992). The effect of enalapril was seen within 4 in after its addition to the bath solution -a period of time probably needed to its conversion in enalaprilat. The effect of the ACE inhibitor is not related to cAMP formation or to an effect on bradykinin metabolism. It is then conceivable that in presence of elevated levels of Ang II in plasma, enalapril can change gj by suppressing the synthesis of Ang II.

The increment in gj with enalapril (10^{-8} M) was also seen in normal and cardiomyopathic hamsters. In cardiomyopathic ventricle, the effect of enalapril was appreciable ($219 \pm 20.3\%$) in cell pairs with very low values of gj (0.8-2.5 nS) compared with controls ($33 \pm 5.4\%$) (De Mello,1996). Although the mechanism of action of enalapril is not known, the possibility exists that the compound increases gj by inhibiting the synthesis of Ang II in the heart.

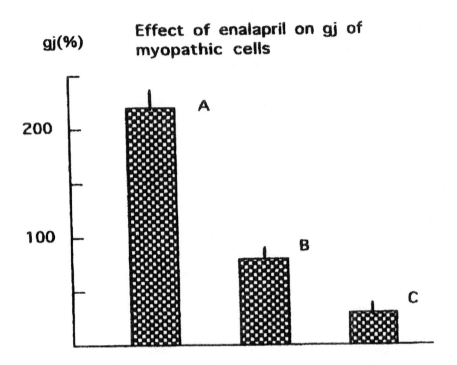

Figure 8. Effect of enalapril -an angiotensin converting enzyme inhibitor, (10-8 M) on gj of CM cell pairs with very low gj (0.8 - 2.5 nS) (A), in CM pairs with higher gj (7-35 nS) (B) and in control hamsters (C). Each bar is the average of 18 experiments.

The increment of gj elicted by the ACE inhibitor ,in part, responsable, for the increase in conduction velocity seen with the drug in muscle trabeculae isolated from the ventricle of CM hamsters (De Mello et al,1997) (see Table 1   ). This finding and the increment of cardiac refractoriness elicited by enalapril in the ventricle of cardiomyopathic hamsters, indicate that the drug has antiarrhythmic properties (De Mello,2001)

TABLE 1.

Conduction Velocity (cm/s) of Normal and Cardiomyophatic Isolated Right Ventricular Muscle

Control Hamsters* (n=5)	Cardiomyopathic Hamsters* (n=5)
42.7	36.9
(±1)	(±3)
P <.05	
Control* Hamsters* (n=5)	Cardiomyopathic Hamsters* (n=5)
22.5	77.1
(±0.75)	(±2.1)
P <.05	

* Difference between the influence of enalapril on conduction velocity in control and cardiomyopathic ventricular muscle

+ Numbers indicate increase in conduction velocity elicited by enalapril. An average of 4 measurements were made in each animal. From De Mello et al,1997, with permission.

Furthermore, enalapril caused a hyperpolarization (6.8 mV) (p < 0.05) of myopathic ventricular fibers with consequent increase of the action potential amplitude and facilitation of impulse propagation. The hyperpolarizing action of enalapril, which is seen in normal or hypoxic ventricular cells (De Mello et al,1997) as well as in normal pig ventricular muscle, is related to the activation of the sodium potassium pump because ouabain and K-free solution suppressed the effect of the drug. (De Mello ,unpublished) Moreover, evidence has been provided that enalapril reduces the slope of diastolic depolarization in pig's Purkinje fibers beating spontaneously (De Mello,unpublished).

The following diagram illustrates the influence of the activation of the renin angiotensin system on the process of cell coupling and consequent generation of reentrant rhythms.

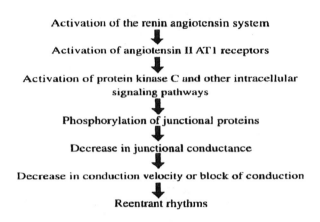

Fig. 9   Diagram showing the possible consequences of activation of the rennin-angiotensin system on cell coupling and impulse propagation in the failing heart.From De Mello,2001,with permission.

2.3 An intracellular renin-angiotensin system is involved in the control of gap junction conductance

The major difficulty of characterizing local renin-angiotensin systems was the possibility of contamination with the plasma RAS and the lack of appropriate biochemical methods. The use of recombinant DNA technology has provided definitive information on the cardiac RAS. Renin and angiotensinogen transcripts have been localized in atria and ventricles of neonatal rat heart and angiotensin I (Ang I), angiotensin II (Ang II) as well as the angiotensin converting enzyme (ACE) have been found inside cultured cardiac myocytes using immunofluorescent technique (see for review De Mello,Danser,2000). The fact that these peptides have been found using in situ hybridization indicates that the elements needed for the synthesis of the compounds are inside the heart cell.

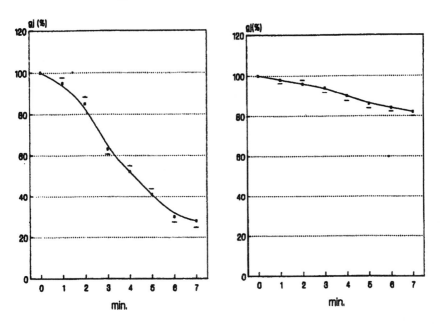

Figure 10. Effect of intracellular dialysis of Ang 1 (10-8 M) on gj of normal adult rat heart cell pairs (Left). At right the peptide was administered after enalapril (10-8 M). Each point average from 10 experiments. Vertical line - SME. From De Mello,Altieri,1992, with permission.

However, some there are controversies concerning the synthesis of some elements of the renin angiotensin system inside the heart cell. Because the cardiac renin RNA levels are extremely small or even undetectable in nephrectomized animals (Danser et al,1994) and because there is a close relationship between the plasma and the cardiac levels of renin , there is the possibility that cardiac renin results from plasma renin uptake.

Under pathological conditions, however, it is not unlikely that renin and angiotensinogen genes are switched on. Recently, an additional renin transcript was found to be expressed in different tissues in which the coding sequence for the prefragment is absent what means that it must remain intracellular (Clausmeyer et al,1999;Lee-Kirch et al,1999).The alternative transcript is expressed only within the heart. It is important to add that >75% of cardiac Ang II levels and >90% of cardiac Ang I is synthesized at tissue sites (see De Mello Danser ,2000). Local synthesis of the angiotensin converting enzyme (ACE) which is responsible for the convertion of Ang I to Ang II, is present in normal heart cell, but its activity is appreciably increased in the rat model of heart failure (Hirsh et al,1991)as well as in cardiomyopathic hamsters (De Mello, Crespo 1999). The findings of ACE RNA levels found in diseased heart are in full agreement with the changes in protein levels under these conditions (De Mello Danser 2000).

The concept of an intracrine RAS implies that the hormone as well as the chemical machinery including its specific receptor are available inside the cell.It is the intracellular action of the hormone that fulfills the difinition of intracrine.

To investigate the possible role of the intracrine renin angiotensin system on the process of cell communication, Ang I (10^{-8} M) was dialyzed into the cytosol of cardiac cells. The results indicated that gj was reduced by 76% within seven minutes (De Mello,1994).). During these experiments the membrane resistance remained high ($1.4 - 1.7$ GΩ). The possibility that this effect of Ang I on gj was related to its conversion to Ang II was investigated by adding enalaprilat to the pipettes solution prior to the addition of Ang I to the internal solution. In these experiments an electrode similar to that described by Irisawa and Kokubun (1983) was used. Since the effect of Ang I was greatly reduced (but not abolished) by enalaprilat (Fig 9) it is reasonable to think that the effect of Ang I on gj was mainly related to its conversion to Ang II. The finding that the effect of Ang I was not completely suppressed by enalaprilat probably means that other enzyme (probably a chymase) is also involved in the conversion of Ang I to Ang II (Urata et al,1990).

The question remains whether Ang II, by itself, is able to reduced gj. The dialysis of Ang II into the cell also reduced gj by 60% within 45 sec (De Mello,1996) - an effect abolished by losartan given intracellularly. This result was quite appealing because not only indicates that the synthesis of Ang II inside the cardiac myocyte can control intercellular communication but also suggests that the activation of an intracellular receptor similar to AT1 is required for the effect of Ang II on gj. Moreover, the activation of protein kinase C is also involved in the effect of Ang II because the dialysis of the pseudo-substrate of protein kinase C (20 ug/ml) - an inhibitor of the kinase, into the cell abolished the effect of the peptide on gj (De Mello,1994). The fall in gj elicited by the activation of this kinase is probably related to the phosphorylation of gap junction proteins (De Mello,1987). It is known that PKC is a potent inhibitor of gap junctional communication(Kwak,Jongsma,1996) and that phosphorylation of connexin43 on serine 368 by PKC regulates the junctional communication (Lampe et al,2000).

Tyrosine protein kinases represent a quite large family of molecules which play an important role on signal transduction and are involved on regulatory mechanisms such as growth and differentiation (Hunter,1996).Its has been shown that viral scr tyrosine protein kinase suppresses gap junction communication in fibroblasts (Atkinson et al,1981;Azarnia,Loewenstein,1984). Ulterior studies indicated that connexin43 is a MAP kinase substrate in vivo and that phosphorylation of Ser255,Ser 279 and Ser 282 initiates the down regulation of gap junctional communication(Zhou et al,1999).Immunoprecipitation and immunoblot analyses revealed that levels of tyrosine phosphorylated Cx43 were increased in the heart of cardiomyopathic hamsters,at an advanced stage of the disease(Toyofuku et al,1999).These and other findings open the possibility that intracellular Ang II reduces gj in the failing heart, in part, through tysonine phosphorylation (De Mello,1999),an idea supported by the evidence that tyrosine phosphorylation is involved in Ang II-mediated signal transduction in different systems (Haendeler,Berk,2000).

Further support to the hypothesis that there is an intracrine RAS in the heart was provided by studies of the intracellular dialysis of renin (De Mello,1995). When renin (0.2 pmol/L) was added to the pipette solution and the compound was dialyzed in to the cell a fall in gj of 29 ± 3.8% (p<0.05) was found in seven minutes (see Fig. 10). Enalaprilat dialyzed previously into the cell reduced appreciably the effect of renin on gj what indicates that the effect of renin on gj was related to the synthesis of Ang II. Moreover,the simultaneous dialysis of angiotensinogen (0.4 pmol/L) and renin (0.2 pmol/L) caused an much greater decline of gj (see Fig. 10. It is then possible to conclude that when the genes of renin and angiotensinogen are concomitantly expressed in heart cells, an appreciable decline in gj is produced, particularly when the ACE activity is enhanced like in the case of heart failure.(see De Mello, Crespo 1999).

The question whether the activation of the cardiac RAS is in part responsible for the abnormalities of cell communication and impulse propagation seen in the failing heart is of capital importance.

Intracellular dialysis of Ang I (10^{-8} M) on cell pairs of CM hamsters characterized by very gj (0.8-2.5 nS) caused cell uncoupling within 2 min (see Fig. 11) .

The effect of intracellular administration of Ang I was reduced by previous administration of enalaprilat (10^{-9} M) into the cell and the intracellular dialysis of Ang II (10^{-9} M), by itself, reduced gj by 48 ± 4.2% (n=8) within 2.5 min. This effect of Ang II was similar to that seen in the control animals (40 ± 5.6%; n=9)(De Mello,1996).

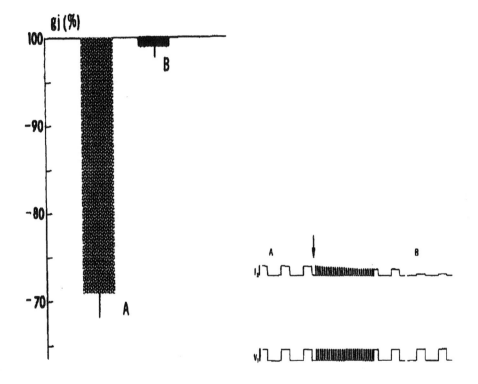

Figure 11. Left - (A) Effect of intracellular dialysis of renin (02 pmol/L) on gj of normal adult rat heart cell pairs. B - reduction of the effect of intracellular renin on gj elicited by enalaprilat. Each bar is the average from 11 experiments. Vertical line at each bar SEM. From reference 55, with permission. Right - effect of intracellular dialysis of renin (0.2 pmol/L) plus angiotensinogen (0.4 pmol/L) on gj of single ventricular cell pair of the rat. IZ - junctional current; VI - transjunctional voltage. The polarity of 12 was changed at the recorder. Calibration at IZ - and V, - 2 nA and 20 mV, respectively. From De Mello,1995 with permission.

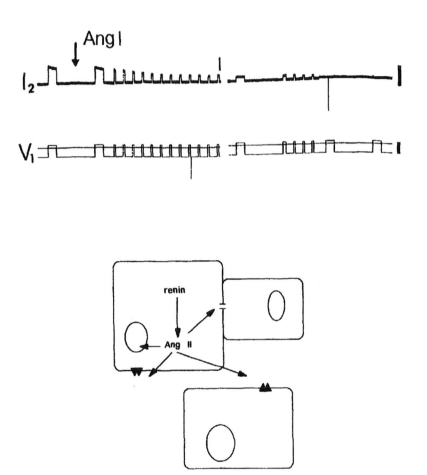

Figure 12. Top - Cell uncoupling elicited by intracellular dialysis of Ang I (10-8 M) in single cell pair of CM ventricle (11 months old). Calibration at 1, - 0.05 nA; at VI - 40 mV. Polarity of 1, chahged at the recorder. From reference 8 with permission. Bottom - diagram illustrating the intracrine and paracrine action of Ang 11. Small triangles at cell membrane represent Ang 11 receptors. From De Mello,1996 with permission.

Here as in the case of normal controls, the effect of Ang I or Ang II seems to be unrelated to changes in Cai or pHi because high concentrations of EGTA and HEPES were used in the internal solution.

The interesting aspect of these experiments is that the effect of intracellular administration of Ang II was suppressed by the addition of losartan (10^{-8} M) to the cytosol (see De Mello,1996). Since losartan is an specific AT1 Ang II receptor antagonist, it is possible to conclude that, in the failing heart, as well as in the controls there is an intracellular Ang II receptor similar to AT1 whose activation is essential for the effect of the peptide on cell communication. Evidence is available that there is an intracellular Ang II receptor in other systems. Indeed, cytoplasmic Ang II receptors and a soluble angiotensin– binding protein with a molecular weight of 75 KD has been described in liver cells (Sugiura et al, 1992; Tang et al, 1992). Further studies will be necessary to clarify the physiological and pathological role of this "receptor" on the alteration of cell coupling seen in the failing heart.

Concerning the physiological meaning of the intracrine RAS in the heart, recent observations indicate that intracellular administration of Ang II in single rat cardiac myocytes, in which the peptide has a negative inotropic action, reduces the inward calcium current while in hamsters myocytes the I_{Ca} was incremented by the same concentration of the petide (De Mello,1998). These observations indicated that a possible role of the intracrine renin angiotensin system in the heart is the regulation of cell contractility.

Atrial natriuretic peptide reduces gj in cardiomyopathic hamster heart

Atrial natriuretic factor reduces cell coupling in the failing heart, an effect mediated by cyclic GMP. Atrial natriuretic factor is a 28-aminoacid peptide that was originally found to be secreted from atrial myocytes after a preliminary storage in granules(Jamilson and Palade,1964; de Bold et al,1981).More recently, evidence has been provided that the ANF is also expressed in ventricular myocytes. The intraventricular conduction system of the rat seems to be rich in ANF (Cantin et al ,1989).Moreover, transcription of ANF has been found in the ventricle of cardiomyopathic hamsters (Lattion et al,1986) .An enhanced gene expression of ventricular ANF has been described in patients with hypertrophic cardiomyopathy without clinical signs of congestive heart failure. It is known that ANF has a powerful natriuretic activity, regulates extracellular fluid volume, causes relaxation of vascular smooth muscle and inhibits the activity of the renin angiotensin system (Brenner et al,1990).

In cardiomyopathic hamsters with congestive heart failure,ANF-specific granules were found in about of 20% of ventricular myocytes (Nardo et al,1993).The meaning of this observation is not known.

It is then of interest to investigate the possible effect of ANF on the junctional conductance in ventricular muscle of cardiomyopathic hamsters. For this male TO-2 cardiomyopathic hamsters at an advanced stage of the disease (11 months old) and healthy male F1B control hamsters were used. As shown in Fig 12 the gj was reduced by ANF (10^{-8} M) administered to extracellular fluid. Average results from 15 cell pairs indicated a decline of gj from 10 ± 2.1 nS to 5.2 ± 1.98 nS(P<0.05),which represents a decrease of gj of 48% within 90 seconds.De Mello 1998).The effect of ANF on gj was dose-dependent and was completely reversible. The series resistance was compensated electronically and did not change during the experiments and the membrane resistance (Rm) remained high (1.4 - 1.8 G Ω) and stable throughout these experiments.

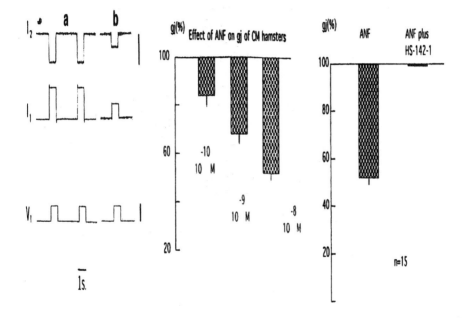

Fig 13. Left: Effect of ANF (10-8 M) on gj recorded from single cell pair of CM hamster 11 months old.;Middle: dose-dependent effect of ANF on gj(n=15).Vertical line at each bar SEM.Right: suppression of the effect of ANF on gj elicited by HS-142-1 (25 ug/ml),an antagonist of ANF receptor.From De Mello,1998,with permission.

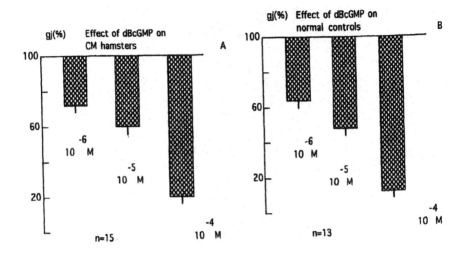

Fig 14. A-Effect of different doses of dibutyryl-cyclicguanosine monophosphate (cGMP) on gj of 11 months old CM hamsters.Each bar(n=15) ,vertical line SEM.B-effect of different doses of dB-cGMP on gj of normal controls.From De Mello,1998, with permission.

A major question is how ANF reduces gj. To investigate the participation of a specific ANF receptor on the effect of the peptide, cell pairs were exposed to HS-142-1 (25 ug/ml) for 5-7 min prior to the administration of ANF to bath solution. As shown in Fig 12 the effect of ANF (10-8 M) on gj was completely suppressed by the receptor antagonist(De Mello,1998).

Because it is known that cGMP is produced by ANF in several systems(Smith and Lincoln,1987), it is conceivable that the decline in gj seen with the peptide is related to the synthesis of cGMP. On the other hand, cGMP reduces gj in the failing heart of cardiomyopathic hamsters (see Fig 13). To investigate the possible role of cGMP on the effect of ANF on gj, cell pairs were incubated with zaprinast (100 μM), a selective inhibitor of cGMP phosphodiesterase for 7 min and then ANF was added to the bath containing zaprinast. Under these conditions the effect of ANF was enhanced by $20 \pm 1.9\%$ while zaprinast by itself had no effect on gj (De Mello,1998).

The present results lead to the conclusion that ANF has a direct effect on cardiac muscle. Because ANF is released from the LV of patients with hypertrophic cardiomyopathy, from cultured heart cells under hypoxia (Ichi et al 1997;Ruskoaho,1992) and during ischemia- reperfusion (Lochsner et al,1992), the question remains whether cardiac arrhythmias seen during myocardial ischemia or in the failing heart are related to the effect of ANF on gj. Further studies will be needed to clarify this point.

3. Conclusion

The development of heart failure is a complex process involving different aspects. The present review provides evidence that the process of cell communication is greatly impaired, especially at late stages of the disease, when a decrease in gap junction conductance and abnormalities of Cx43 distribution associated with severe destruction of the ventricular parenquima, represent important factors in the generation of slow conduction, cardiac arrhythmias and the decline in heart contractility. The sequestration of large masses of ventricular myocytes from the normal process of excitation induced by the decrease in gj, reduces the number of active cells involved in the process of ventricular contraction and contributes to the impairment of ventricular function. Moreover, the down regulation of beta-adrenergic receptors and the impairment in function of adenyl cyclase prevent the extrinsic regulatory mechanism of cardiac adjustment so necessary for the cardiovascular homeostasis.

The plasma as well as the cardiac renin angiotensin system play an important role on the regulation of gj in the failing heart and are probably involved in the generation of slow conduction and malignant ventricular arrhythmias ,a cause of sudden death in patients with congestive heart failure. Here I presented evidence that there is an intracrine renin angiotensin system in the failing heart and that its activation has a regulatory role on cell coupling, on impulse conduction and on inward calcium current. More recently, I found that intracellular Ang II reduces the rate of repolarization of the action potential and increases refractoriness in the failing heart (De Mello, in preparation). These observations demonstrate, by the first time, that an intracrine renin angiotensin system modulates intercellular communication and other important cellular processes. Moreover, the effect of ANF on gj of CM hamsters demonstrates that this hormone has a direct effect on heart muscle. Its possible contribution to the generation of cardiac arrhythmias must be carefully evaluated.

REFERENCE

Atkinson MM, Menko AS, Jonhson RG, Sheridan JD(1981) Rapid and reversible reduction of junctional permeability in cells infected with a temperature-mutant of avian sarcoma virus. J Cell Biol 91: 573-578

Azarnia R, Lowenstein WR (1984) Intercellular communication and control of growth.X Alteration of junctional permeability by scr gene.A study with temperature sensitive mutant sarcoma virus. J Membrane Biol. 82: 191-205

Bader M, Peters J, Baltatu O, Muller DN, Luft FC, Ganten D (2001) Tissue renin-angiotensin systems : new insights from experimental animal models in hypertension research.J.Mol Med. 79: 76-102

Bajusz E (1969). Dystrophic calcification of myocardium as conditioning factor in genesis of congestive heart failure: an experimental study. Am Heart J; 78:202-209.

Bastide B, Neyses L, Ganten D and Traub O (1993). Gap junction protein connexin 40 is preferentelly expressed in vascular endothelium and conductive bandles of rat myocardium and is increased under hypertensive condictions. Circ Res, 73:1138-1149

Bohm M, Gierschik P, Jakobs KH, Pieske B, Schnabel P, Ungerer M, Erdmann E (1990). Increase in Giv in human heart with dilated but not ichemic cardiomyopathy. Circulation, 82:1249-1265.

Brenner BM, Ballerman BJ,Gunning ME,Ziedel ML (1990)Diverse biological action of atrial natriuretic peptide.Physiol.Rev 70:665-699

Bristow MR, Ginsburg R, Minobe WA, Cubicciotti RS, Sageman WS, Luric K, Billingham ME, Harrison DC and Stinson EB (1982). Decreased catecholamine sensitivity and beta-adrenergic receptor density in failing human hearts. N Engl J Med; 307:205-211.

Campbell DJ (1985). The site of angiotensin production. J Hypertens, 3:199-207.

Cherry JR and De Mello WC (1996). Confocal microscopy and intercellular communication in failing cardiomyopathic heart. FASEB J, April 14th, Abstract 2275.

Clausmeyer S,Sadoshima J,Brosius FC, Izumo S (2000) Tissue-specific expression of rat renin transcript lacking the coding sequence,the prefragment and its stimulation by myocardial infarction. Endocrinology 141: 2963- 2970

CONSENSUS Trial Study Group (1987) Effects of enalapril on mortality in severe congestive heart failure: Results of the Cooperative North Scandinavian Enalapril Survival Study. N Engl J Med 1987, 316:1429-1435.

Covell JW, Chidsey CA and Braunwald E. Reduction in the cardiac response to postganglionic sympathetic nerve stimulation in experimental heart failure. Circ Res 1966; 19:51-66.

Danser AHJ,van Katz JP,Admiraal PJJ,Dekx FHM,Lamers JMJ,Vendouw PD,Saxena PR,Schalekamp MADH (1994) Cardiac renin and angiotensins: uptake from plasma versus in situ synthesis. Hypertension 24:37-48

de Bold AJ,Boresntein HB,Veress AT,Sonnenburg H (1981) 32: 976-982 A rapid and potent natriuretic response to intraveneous injection of atrial myocardial extracts in rats. Life Sci 28: 89-94

De Mello WC (1975). Effect of intracellular injection of calcium and strontium on cell communication in heart. J Physiol (London) 250:231245.

De Mello WC (1984). Effect of intracellular injection of cAMP on the electrical coupling of mammalian cardiac cells. Biochem Biophys Res Commun, 119:1001-1007.

De Mello WC (1987). Modulation of junctional permeability. Fed Proc, 43:2692-2696.

De Mello WC (1988). Increase in junctional conductance caused by isoproterenol in heart cell pairs is suppressed by cAMP-dependent protein kinase inhibitor. Biochem Biophys Res Comm, 154:509-514.

De Mello WC (1996). Impaired regulation of cell communication by beta adrenergic receptor activation in the failing heart. Hypertension 27: 265-268

De Mello WC (1995). Influence of intracellular renin on heart cell communication. Hypertension, 25:1172-1177.

De Mello WC (1996). Renin-angiotensin system and cell communication in the failing heart. Hypertension, 27:1267-1272.

De Mello WC (1998) Intracellular angiotensin II regulates the inward calcium current in cardiac myocytes. Hypertension 32: 976-982

De Mello WC (2001) Cardiac arrhythmias; the possible role of the renin angiotensin system. J. Mol Med 79: 103-108

De Mello WC and Altieri P (1992). The role of the renin-angiotensin system in the control of cell communication in the heart; effects of angiotensin II and enalapril. J Cardiovasc Pharmacol 20:643-651.

De Mello WC and Crespo M (1993). Effect of angiotensin II and enalapril on cardiac refractoriness and conduction velocity. American Heart Association, 66th Scientific Session, November.

De Mello WC, 1994. Is an intracellular renin-angiotensin system involved in the control of cell communication in heart? J Cardiovasc Pharmacol 23:640-646.

De Mello WC, Cherry R and Manivannan S (1997). Electrophysiologic and morphologic abnormalities in the failing heart; effect of enalapril on the electrical properties. Cardiac Failure 3:53-62.

De Mello WC, Crespo MJ and Altieri P (1993). Effect of enalapril on intracellular resistance and conduction velocity in rat ventricular muscle. J Cardiovasc Pharmacol 22:259-263.

De Mello WC,Crespo M (1995) Cardiac refractoriness in rats is reduced by angiotensin II. J. Cardiovasc.Pharmacol 25: 1-6

De Mello WC (1999) Gap junctional conductance in cardiomyopathic hamsters.The role of c-scr. Circ. Res 85: 661- 662

De Mello WC,Danser AHJ (2000) Angiotensin and the heart. On the intracrine renin angiotensin system. Hypertension 35:1183-1188

Dupont E,Matsushita T,Kaba RA,Vozzi C, Coppen SR,Khan N,Yacoub MH, Severs NJ 2001 Altered connexin expression in human congestive heart failure J Mol Cell Cardiol. 33:359-371

Dzau VJ (1988). Cardiac renin-angiotensin system. Am J Med, 84:22-27.

Dzau VJ, Ingelfinger J, Pratt RE and Ellison KE (1986). Identification of renin and angiotensinogen RNA sequences in mouse and rat brains. Hypertension, 8:544.

Feldman AM, Cates AE, Veazey WB, Hershberger RE, Bristow M, Baughman KI, Baungartner WA and van Dop C (1988). Increase in the 40.000-mol-wt pertussis toxing substrate (G-protein) in the failing human heart. J Clin Invest, 82:189-197.

Feldman AM, Rowena GT, Kessler PD, Weisman HF, Schulman SP, Blumenthal RS, Jackson KDG and Van Dop C (1990). Diminished beta-drenergic receptor responsiveness and cardiac dilation in heart of myopathic Syryan hamsters are associated with functional abnormality of the G stimulatory protein. Circulation, 81:1341-1352.

Fleckenstein A (1971). Specific inhibitors and promoters of calcium action in the excitation-contraction coupling of heart muscle and their role in the prevention or production of myocardial lesions. In: Calcium and the Heart, P Harris and LH Opie, Eds pp 135-188, Londong Academic Press.

Fowler MB, Laser JA, Hopkins GL, Minobe W and Bristow MR (1986). Assessment of the beta-adrenergic receptor pathway in the intact failing hfiman heart: Progressive receptor down-regulation and subsensitivity to agonist response. Circulation, 74:1290-1302.

Francis GS and Cohn JN (1986). The autonomic nervous system in congestive heart failure. Ann Rev Med; 37:235-247.

Gertz EW (1992). Cardiomyopathic Syrian hamster; a possible model of human disease. Prog Exp Tumor Res 16; 242-247.

Haendeler J, Berk B (2000) Tyrosine phosphorylation is involved in Ang II-mediated signal transduction. Reg Pept 95: 1-7

Hatem SN, Sham JSK and Morad M (1994). Enhanced Na+-Ca 2+ exchange exchange activity in cardiomyopathic Syrian hamster. Circ Res, 74:253-261.

Hirsh AT, Talsness CE, Schunkert H, Paul H and Dzau V (1991). Tissue-specific activation of cardiac angiotensin converting enzyme in experimental heart failure. Circ Res, 69:475-482.

Hunter T (1996) Tyrosine phosphorylation; Past,present and future. Biochem Soc Trans Hopkins Medical Letter 24: 307- 327

Ichii Y, Kawashima E, Kawabe J,Kikuchi K (1997) Secretion of atrial natriuretic factor from the left ventricle and heart in patients with hypertrophic cardiomyopathy: relationship with hemodynamic and echocardiographic prolfiles J Cardiol 30:19-28

Irisawa H and Kokubun S (1983). Modulation by intracellular ATP and cyclic AMP of the slow inward current in isolated single ventricular cells of the guinea-pig. J Physiol (London) 338:321-337

Izumo S, Nadal-Ginard B and Mahdavi V (1988). Proto-oncogene induction and reprogramming of cardiac gene expression produced by pressure overload. Proc Nat Acad Sci, USA, 85:339-343.

Janielson JD,Palade GE (1964) Specific granules in atrium muscle cells J.Cell Biol 23:151-156

Jasmin G and Proschek L (1984). Calcium and myocardial cell injury. An appraisal in the cardiomyopathic hamster. Can J Physiol Pharmacol; 62:891-900.

Kanter HL, Laing JG, Beyer EC, Greeen KG and Saffitz JE (1993). Multiple connexins colocalize in canine ventricular myocyte gap junctions. Circ Res 73:344-350.

Koch-Weser J (1965). Nature of the inotropic action of angiotensin on ventricular myocardium. Circ Res, 16:230-237.

Kwak BR, Jongsma HJ (1996) Regulation of cardiac gap junction channel permeability and conductance by several phosphorylating condictions. Mol Cell Biochem 157: 93-99

Lampe PD,TenBroek, Burt JM, Kurata WE,Jonhson RG, Lau AF (2000) Phosphorylation of connexin43 on serine 368 by protein kinase C regulates gap junctional communication J Cell Biol 149: 1503- 1512

Lattion AL,Michel JB, Aauld E,Corvol P, Soubrier F (1986) Myocardial recruitment during ANF mRNA increase with volume overload in the rat. Am J Physiol 25:H890-H896

Lee-Kirch M,Gaudet F, Cardoso M, Lindpaintner K (1999) Distinct renin isoforms generated by tissue-specific transcription initiation and alternative splicing.Circ.Res. 84: 240-246

Lerner DL,Yamada KA, Schuessler RB, Saffitz JE (2000) Accelerated onset and increased incidence of ventricular arrhythmias induced by ischemia in Cx43 deficient mice. Circulation 101: 547-552

Linz W, Scholkens BA, Han JF (1986). Beneficial effects of the converting enzyme inhibitor ramipril in ischemic rat hearts. J Cardiovasc Pharmacol 8: (Suppl 10) S91-S99.

Lochner A,Genade S, Mouton R,(1992) Massive atrial natriuretic peptide (ANP) release in ischemia reperfusion.Cardiovasc Drugs Ther 6:447-458

Lossnitzer K, Janke J, Hein B, Stauch M and Fleckenstein A (1975). Disturbed myocardial calcium metabolism: a possible pathogenic factor in the hereditary cardiomyopathy of the Syrian hamster. In Fleckenstein A, Rona G, eds., Recent Advances in Studies on Cardiac Metabolism. Baltimore; Vol. VI, 207-215, University Park Press.

Luque EA, Veenstra R, Beyer E and Lemanski LF (1994). Localization and distribution of gap junctions in normal and cardiomyopathic hamster heart. J Morphol 222:203-213.

Morgan ME and Baker MM (1991). Cardiac hypertrophy: mechanical, neural and endocrine dependence. Circulation 1991; 83:23-25

Nardo PD,Minieri M,Carbone A et al.(1993) Myocardial expression of atrial natriuretic factor gene in early stages of hamster cardiomyopathy. Mol Cell Biochem 125:179-192

Peters NS, Coromilas J, Severs NJ,Wit AL (1997) Disturbed connexin 43 gap junction correlates with the location of reentrant circuits in the epicardial border zone of healing canine infarcts that cause ventricular tachycardia. Circulation 95: 988-996

Rogers TB, Gaa AH and Allen IS (1986). Identification and characterization of functional angiotensin II receptors on cultured heart myocytes. J Pharmacol Exp Ther, 36:438-444.

Ruskoaho H (1992) Atrial natriuretic peptide: synthesis, release and metabolism .Pharmacol Rev 44:479-487

Sen L, ONeill M, Marsh JD and Smith TW (1990). Myocyte structure, function and calcium kinetics in the cardiomyopathic hamster heart. Am J Physiol; 259:H1533-H1543.

Severs NJ (1994). Pathophysiology of gap junctions in heart disease. J Cardiac Electrophysiol, 5:462-475.Smith JB,Lincoln TM (1987) Angiotensin decreases cyclic GMP accumulation produced by atrial natriuretic factor.Am J Physiol 253(Cell Physiol 22) C147-150

Sugiura N,Hagiwara H, Hirose S (1992) Molecular cloning of porcine soluble angiotensin binding protein.J Biol Chem 267: 18067- 18072

Tang SS,Rogg H, Schumaker R,Dzau VJ (1992) Characterization of nuclear angiotensin II-binding sites in rat liver and comparison with plasma membrane receptors.Endocrinology 131: 347- 375

Toyofuku T, Yabuki M, Otsu K, Kuzuya T, Tada M, Hori M (1999) Functional role of c-scr in gap junctions of the cardiomyopathic heart. Circ. Res 85: 672- 681

Urata H, Kinoshita A, Hisono KS, Bumpus FM and Husain A (1990). Identification of a highly specific chymase as the major angiotensin II -forming enzyme in the human heart. J Biol Chem, 265:22348-22357.

Weismand HF and Weinfeldt ML (1987). Toward an understanding of the molecular basis of cardiomyopathies. J Am Cell Cardiol; 10:1135-1138.

Wrogemann K and Nylen EG (1978). Mitochondrial calcium overloading in cardiomyopathic hamsters. J Mol Cell Cardiol; 10:185-195.

Zhou L, Kasparek EM, Nicholson BJ(1999) Dissection of the molecular basis of pp-60(v-scr) induced gating of connexin 43 gap junction channel J Cell Biol. 144: 1033-1045

12

GAP JUNCTIONS AND CONNEXIN EXPRESSION IN HUMAN HEART DISEASE

Nicholas J. Severs
National Heart and Lung Institute, Faculty of Medicine,
Imperial College, Royal Brompton
Hospital Sydney Street, London SW3 6NP, UK

INTRODUCTION

Sequential contraction of the cardiac chambers depends on orderly spread of the wave of electrical excitation from one cardiomyocyte to the next, throughout the heart. As discussed in earlier chapters of this volume, the pathways enabling this cell-to-cell current flow are formed by the gap junctions that link individual cardiomyocytes into a functional syncytium. Gap junctions are essentially clusters of transmembrane channels that span the paired plasma membranes of neighboring cells, linking their cytoplasmic compartments together to form pathways for direct cell-to-cell communication. The component proteins of the gap-junctional channel, connexins, are assembled into hexamers which form hemi-channels termed connexons, the complete channel being formed by the docking of a pair of connexons across the adjacent plasma membranes. Twenty different connexin genes have now been identified in the human (Willecke et al., 2001), and most tissues, including those of the cardiovascular system, express two or more connexin isoforms. Three principal isoforms – connexin43, connexin40 and connexin45 – are expressed in cardiomyocytes (reviews, Beyer et al., 1997; Severs, 1999; Severs et al., 2001), and further isoforms such as connexin46 (Paul et al., 1991) and connexin57 (Manthey et al., 1999) may also be present in trace amounts. Gap-junctional channels composed of different connexins exhibit distinctive biophysical properties *in vitro* (review, Bruzzone et al., 1996), and studies on transgenic mice demonstrate that the precise functional properties of gap junctions *in vivo* may depend in part on the specific connexins from which they are constructed, though there is also considerable capacity for functional compensation of one connexin isoform by another (Kirchhoff et al., 2000; Krüger et al., 2000; Plum et al., 2000; Tamaddon et al., 2000; van Rijen et al., 2001). Different subsets of cardiomyocyte express different combinations and relative quantities of connexins 43, 40 and 45, potentially providing for regional differentiation of electrophysiological properties. The concept has thus developed that gap junction organization and spatially defined patterns of connexin expression may preside over the precisely orchestrated patterns of current flow that govern the normal heart rhythm.

Mutations in genes that encode connexins are now known to underlie a number of human diseases (e.g., Cohn and Kelley, 1999; Mackay et al., 1999; Scherer et al., 1999), and in the heart are associated with some forms of congenital abnormality (Dasgupta et al., 1999). Distinct from these primary defects are alterations in gap junction organization and expression that accompany the pathogenesis of acquired, adult heart disease. Such changes, referred to as gap junction remodelling, have attracted attention and debate as potential contributory factors in the development of arrhythmia, a major cause of death and disability in heart disease (reviews, Green and Severs, 1993; Severs et al., 1993, 1996, 2001; Severs, 1998, 1999). This chapter briefly reviews selected aspects of our current understanding of disease-related gap-junction remodelling in the human heart, set in the context of recent findings in experimental animal models.

GAP JUNCTIONS AND CONNEXIN EXPRESSION IN CARDIOMYOCYTES OF THE NORMAL HEART

A thorough understanding of gap junction organization and connexin expression in the normal heart is a prerequisite to the interpretation of any remodeling that may occur in disease. As noted at the outset, connexins 43, 40 and 45 are the principal connexin isoforms of cardiomyocytes and will thus be the focus of the summary that follows. An additional isoform, connexin37, is expressed in vascular endothelial cells, including those of the coronary arterial system (Yeh et al., 1997a, 1998). As discussed elsewhere, gap-junctional intercellular communication and connexin expression in vascular endothelial and smooth muscle cells may play an important part in the response of the arterial wall to injury and in the pathogenesis of atherosclerosis, the underlying cause of ischemic heart disease (Severs, 1998; Severs, 1999; Yeh et al., 1997b; Yeh et al., 2000).

Of the three principal connexins expressed by cardiomyocytes, connexin43 predominates, occurring in abundance in adult working ventricular and atrial cardiomyocytes of all mammalian species, including humans (Beyer et al., 1989; review, Severs, 2000). Connexins 40 and 45 are additionally expressed in specific anatomical locations within the heart (Coppen et al., 1998; Gourdie et al., 1993; Vozzi et al., 1999). Apart from distinctive connexin expression profiles, differences in overall size, distribution and abundance of gap junctions are also observed in the various cardiomyocyte subtypes and regions of the heart (Saffitz et al., 1997; Severs, 1989, 1999; Severs et al., 2001).

The cardiomyocytes of the working ventricles are elongated, branching cells, extensively interconnected by clusters of connexin43-containing gap junctions. The gap junctions are co-organized in intercalated disks with two types of anchoring junction, the fascia adherens and the desmosome, which act in concert with the gap junctions to integrate cardiac electromechanical function. In the intercalated disks of working ventricular myocardium, the gap junctions occur principally in lateral-facing segments of the disk membrane, often with particularly large gap junctions circumscribing the periphery (Gourdie et al., 1991). This and other aspects of gap junction organization, together with features of tissue architecture such as the size and shape of the cells, combine to encourage preferential propagation of the impulse in the longitudinal axis, thereby contributing to the normal pattern of anisotropic spread of the impulse of healthy ventricular myocardium.

Atrial cardiomyocytes are slender cells compared with their ventricular counterparts and so their intercalated disks are typically less extensive. The gap junctions of atrial myocytes, though aggregated into disks, are also found situated along interacting lateral borders of the cells. Connexin40 is abundant in the atrial myocytes of many mammalian species, including humans (Dupont et al., 2001a; Vozzi et al., 1999), co-organized with connexin43 in the same gap-junctional plaques (Severs et al., 2001). Working ventricular myocytes, by contrast, normally lack connexin40. In both ventricular and atrial working myocardium, connexin45 is present in very low quantities, though slightly higher levels are present in the atria than the ventricles (Coppen et al., 1998; Dupont et al., 2001a; Vozzi et al., 1999).

Apart from the working ventricular and atrial cells responsible for the contraction of the cardiac chambers, discrete populations of cardiomyocyte are specialized for generation and conduction of the cardiac impulse (review, Severs, 1989). The myocytes of the sinoatrial node, the site of impulse generation, and the atrioventricular node, where the impulse is slowed en route to the ventricles to ensure sequential contraction of the chambers, are equipped with small, sparse, dispersed gap junctions containing connexin45 (Coppen et al., 1999a, 1999b; Honjo et al., 2002), a connexin that forms low conductance channels *in vitro* (Moreno et al., 1995). These gap junction features suggest relatively poor coupling which, in the atrioventricular node, may contribute to the slowing of conduction, and in the sinoatrial node, to the ability to drive the large mass of surrounding atrial tissue while remaining protected from its hyperpolarizing influence. In the rabbit, the sinoatrial node is connexin43 negative, clearly delineated from the surrounding atrial myocardium by a connective tissue layer except at a restricted zone of connexin45/connexin43 co-expression at the nodal/crista terminalis border. This zone of co-expression has been hypothesized as a candidate pathway for directed exit of the impulse from the node into the atrial tissue (Coppen et al., 1999a). Although connexin45 is the predominant atrioventricular nodal connexin, common to all mammalian species so far examined, some species variation involving limited co-expression of connexins 40 and 45 may occur. In the rodent, the spatial pattern of expression of connexin45 reveals that the atrioventricular node and His bundle form part of an elaborately extended central conduction system circumscribing the atrioventricular and outflow junctional regions (Coppen et al., 1999b). Information on the extent to which these features are present in the human impulse generation and conduction system remains limited, and is currently under further investigation.

In addition to connexin45, cardiomyocytes of the His-Purkinje conduction system in most mammals, including man, express connexin40, a connexin associated with high conductance channels (Bukauskas et al., 1995; Coppen et al., 1998, 2001; Gourdie et al., 1993;

Gros et al., 1994; Severs et al., 2001). Prominent immunolabeling for this connexin, in the form of large, abundant gap junctions, correlates with the fast conduction properties of the bundle branches and Purkinje fiber system which facilitate rapid distribution of the impulse throughout the working ventricular myocardium, (Bastide et al., 1993; Gourdie et al., 1993; Gros et al., 1994). In rodents, connexin45 is co-expressed with connexin40 in a central zone of the bundle branches and Purkinje fibers, enveloped by an outer zone in which only connexin45 is found. In contrast to connexin40, connexin45 is distributed from beginning to end of the entire atrioventricular conduction system (Coppen et al., 1999b). In the connexin40 knock-out mouse, deficiency of connexin40 leads to reduced conduction velocity through the conduction system and right bundle branch block (Hagendorff et al., 1999; Kirchhoff et al., 1998; Simon et al., 1998; Tamaddon et al., 2000; van Rijen et al., 2001). Any residual ability of the His-Purkinje system to support conduction in the absence of connexin40 is attributable to the presence of connexin45 (Coppen et al., 1999b).

ALTERED GAP JUNCTION AND CONNEXIN EXPRESSION IN HUMAN HEART DISEASE

From the established role of gap junctions as pathways for the orderly spread of electrical excitation in the healthy heart, we first hypothesized, from observations made in the early 1990s, that alterations in gap junction organization and expression might potentially contribute to abnormal conduction and arrhythmogenesis in the diseased human heart (Green and Severs, 1993; Smith et al., 1991). Such a concept does not attribute arrhythmia exclusively to gap junction-related alterations; computer and cell culture models emphasize that arrhythmogenesis is multifactorial in origin, involving interplay between gap-junctional coupling, membrane excitability and features of cell and tissue architecture (Rohr et al., 1997; Shaw and Rudy, 1997; Spach et al., 2000). Moreover, altered gap-junctional coupling itself may be multifactorial in origin, involving, for example, regulation of channel gating and assembly/disassembly of functional gap junction plaques, as well as alterations in the overall expression levels of connexins and gap junctions (remodelling). Ethical considerations constrain the scope of experimental studies in human heart tissue, but the magnitude of the global cardiovascular disease burden has driven interest in attempting to determine the relevance of gap junctions to the patient afflicted with heart disease. To this end, research on gap junction and connexin remodelling in human heart tissue offers one practicable handle on the problem, in full recognition that this represents but one facet of the overall perspective to be achieved by integration of data from multiple experimental approaches.

Gap junction and connexin remodelling may take the form of structural remodelling and/or remodelling of connexin expression. These two types of remodelling are not mutually exclusive, but provide a convenient framework for discussion.

Structural Remodelling of Gap Junctions

Structural remodelling involves alteration in the arrangement and organization of gap junctions. A notable example is the loss of the normal ordered distribution of connexin43 gap junctions that occurs in the myocardial zone bordering infarct scar tissue in the ventricles of patients with ischemic heart disease (Smith et al., 1991). Connexin43 immunolabeling in these zones is scattered in disordered fashion over the cells, while that more distant from the infarct remains organized in typical intercalated disk arrays. Both laterally-disposed gap junctions that maintain contact between cells, and internalized and hence non-functional gap-junctional membrane, contribute to the dispersed connexin43 labelling patterns (Smith et al., 1991). Such gap junction remodelling is not due solely to late changes associated with fibrosis, but has been shown in experimental animals to be initiated rapidly after myocardial infarction (Matsushita et al., 1999). Similar alterations in gap junction distribution occur in ventricular hypertrophy in the rat (Emdad et al., 2001; Uzzaman et al., 2000), and in right ventricular hypertrophy induced by monocrotaline have been shown to be accompanied by reduction in longitudinal conduction velocity (Uzzaman et al., 2000).

Disordered arrangements of ventricular connexin43 gap junctions are also prominent in human hypertrophic cardiomyopathy, the most common cause of sudden cardiac death due to arrhythmia in young adults (Sepp et al., 1996). Another form of structural remodelling is apparent in human hibernating myocardium. The term "hibernating myocardium" refers to regions of myocardium that fail to contract properly in the ischemic heart, but which recover contractile function after restoration of normal blood flow by coronary by-pass operation. In hibernating myocardium, the normally large connexin43 gap junctions at the periphery of the intercalated disk become markedly reduced in size compared with those of reversibly ischemic and those of normally perfused (and contracting) regions within the same diseased heart (Kaprielian et al., 1998). In this instance, structural remodelling occurs hand-in-hand with remodelling of connexin expression, as the overall amount of connexin43 immunolabeling is reduced in reversibly ischemic and hibernating myocardium.

Structural remodelling inevitably results in disorganization of the normal ordered pattern of the microconduction pathways. Heterogeneity of distribution, involving focal reduction of connexin43 gap junctions as observed in ischemic and hibernating hearts, was thus hypothesized to lead to localized, potentially arrhythmogenic conduction defects and contraction abnormalities (Dupont et al., 2001b; Kaprielian et al., 1998; Smith et al., 1991). Experimental evidence in favor of this hypothesis has come from optical mapping and echocardiographic studies on chimeric mice created from connexin43-deficient embryonic stem cells and blastocysts of different strains, designed specifically to achieve heterogeneous expression of cardiac connexin43 (Gutstein et al., 2001b).

Remodelling of Connexin Expression

Remodelling of connexin expression may involve quantitative changes, qualitative changes or both. The most extensively documented quantitative alteration in connexin expression in human heart disease involves connexin43. Northern and western blot analyses demonstrate markedly decreased levels of connexin43 transcript and protein in the left ventricle of transplant patients with end-stage congestive heart failure whether due to ischemic heart disease or idiopathic dilated cardiomyopathy (Dupont et al., 2001b). It should be emphasized that measures of total connexin levels, while serving as indicators of the potential capacity for cell-to-cell communication, do not provide information on the quantity of functional (open) channels; hence, a reduction of connexin43 may not, *per se*, be detrimental or indeed have any effect at all. Indeed, computer modelling studies predict that reductions of up to 40% in connexin43 levels would be unlikely to have a major effect on conduction velocity and altered anisotropy ratio (Jongsma and Wilders, 2000). However, in view of the complex relationship between passive and active membrane properties (Rudy and Shaw, 1997; Shaw and Rudy, 1997; Viswanathan et al., 1999) and the assumptions inherent in computer modelling, the precise consequences of reduced connexin43 levels are difficult to predict *in vivo*. From this perspective, it is relevant to take heed of what is actually observed in models of reduced connexin43 expression in the intact heart. Of particular note is the marked increase in incidence, frequency and duration of ventricular tachycardias reported in the intact isolated hearts of transgenic mice expressing half the normal level of connexin43 (Lerner et al., 2000). Furthermore, transgenic mice generated to give cardiac specific loss of connexin43 (86-95% reduction at 4 weeks) develop sudden cardiac death due to arrhythmia by 2 months of age (Gutstein et al., 2001a). Bearing in mind that the extent of connexin43 reduction in the diseased human ventricle varies considerably from one patient to the next, in some regions of some diseased hearts reaching a reduction of >90% of control values, and that the reduction observed is often superimposed on heterogeneity of connexin43 distribution (Dupont et al., 2001b), it remains valid to envisage a possible contribution from gap junction and connexin remodelling to the development of arrhythmia in at least some patients.

Apart from reduced connexin43, the overall level of connexin40 transcript is increased in the ventricles of patients with congestive heart failure due to ischemic heart disease but not that due to idiopathic dilated cardiomyopathy (Dupont et al., 2001b). Immunoconfocal microscopy localizes the site of increased connexin40 expression to a band of myocytes at the endocardial surface associated with and adjacent to the Purkinje fibers. The significance of this expanded zone of connexin40 expression is unclear; one speculation is that it could represent a compensatory response that might improve the spread of depolarization from the conduction tissues in the face of declining connexin43 levels in the ischemic ventricle.

Connexin40 may also have a contributory part to play in an atrial arrhythmia, post-operative atrial fibrillation. Atrial fibrillation has many interacting causes, but a higher than average pre-existing level of atrial connexin40 has been found to correlate with increased incidence of atrial fibrillation after coronary artery by-pass grafting in a small series of patients (Dupont et al., 2001a). At first sight, this correlation might appear paradoxical. However, connexin40 immunolabeling in the human atrium, in contrast to connexin43, typically shows a markedly heterogeneous distribution. This heterogeneity might conceivably give rise to different resistive properties and conduction velocities in spatially adjacent regions of tissue which become enhanced, and hence pro-arrhythmic, the higher the overall levels of connexin40.

CONCLUDING COMMENT

In view of the role of gap junctions in mediating the patterns of current flow that underlie normal heart contraction, gap junction/connexin remodelling in heart disease was proposed as a candidate contributor to cardiac arrhythmogenesis. From where we now stand, remodelling of gap junctions – in particular, disorganization in the distribution pattern of connexin43 gap junctions and reduced levels of connexin43 in the ventricle – has been demonstrated in defined categories of human heart disease and has been correlated with electrophysiologically-identified arrhythmic changes in animal models. While such correlations do not prove cause and effect, and other factors (membrane excitability, cell size, regulation of channel gating etc) certainly come into play, recent work on genetically engineered mice (Gutstein et al., 2001b; Gutstein et al., 2001a; Hagendorff et al., 1999; Kirchhoff et al., 1998; Krüger et al., 2000; Lerner et al., 2000; Plum et al., 2000; Simon et al., 1998; Tamaddon et al., 2000; van Rijen et al., 2001) reinforces the case for further research on gap junction and connexin remodelling in cardiac arrhythmogenesis and contractile dysfunction in the human disease setting.

Acknowledgments

Work in the author's laboratory is supported by the European Commission (QLRT-1999-00516) and the British Heart Foundation. I thank all members of my group who, over the last 10 years, have contributed to the work discussed in this review.

REFERENCE

Bastide, B., Neyses, L., Ganten, D., Paul, M., Willecke, K., and Traub, O. 1993. Gap junction protein connexin40 is preferentially expressed in vascular endothelium and conductive bundles of rat myocardium and is increased under hypertensive conditions. Circ Res 73, 1138-49.

Beyer, E., Seul, K. H., and Larson, D. M. 1997. Cardiovascular gap junction proteins: molecular characterization and biochemical regulation. In Heart Cell Communication in Health and Disease. De Mello, W. C., Janse, M. J., and Norwell, M. A., editors. (Kluwer Academic Publications New York), pp. 45-51.

Beyer, E.C., Kistler, J., Paul, D. L., and Goodenough, D. A. 1989. Antisera directed against connexin43 peptides react with a 43-kd protein localized to gap junctions in myocardium and other tissues. J Cell Biol 108, 595-605.

Bruzzone, R., White, T. W., and Paul, D. L. 1996. Connections with connexins: The molecular basis of direct intercellular signaling. Eur J Biochem 238, 1-27.

Bukauskas, F.F., Elfgang, C., Willecke, K., and Weingart, R. 1995. Biophysical properties of gap junction channels formed by mouse connexin40 in induced pairs of transfected human HeLa cells. Biophys J 68, 2289-98.

Cohn, E.S., and Kelley, P. M. 1999. Clinical phenotype and mutations in connexin 26 (DFNB1/GJB2), the most common cause of childhood hearing loss. Am J Med Genet 89, 130-6.

Coppen, S.R., Dupont, E., Rothery, S., and Severs, N. J. 1998. Connexin45 expression is preferentially associated with the ventricular conduction system in mouse and rat heart. Circ Res 82, 232-43.

Coppen, S.R., Gourdie, R. G., and Severs, N. J. 2001. Connexin45 is the first connexin to be expressed in the central conduction system of the mouse heart. Exp Clin Cardiol 6, 17-23.

Coppen, S.R., Kodama, I., Boyett, M. R., Dobrzynski, H., Takagishi, Y., Honjo, H., Yeh, H.-I., and Severs, N. J. 1999a. Connexin45, a major connexin of the rabbit sinoatrial node, is co-expressed with connexin43 in a restricted zone at the nodal-crista terminalis border. J Histochem Cytochem 47, 907-18.

Coppen, S.R., Severs, N. J., and Gourdie, R. G. 1999b. Connexin45 (α6) expression delineates an extended conduction system in the embryonic and mature rodent heart. Dev Genet 24, 82-90.

Dasgupta, C., Escobar-Poni, B., Shah, M., Duncan, J., and Fletcher, W. H. 1999. Misregulation of connexin43 gap junction channels and congenital heart defects. In Gap Junction-Mediated Intercellular Signalling in Health and Disease. Cardew, G., editor. (John Wiley & Sons Ltd. New York), pp. 212-21.

Dupont, E., Ko, Y. S., Rothery, S., Coppen, S. R., Baghai, M., Haw, M., and Severs, N. J. 2001a. The gap-junctional protein, connexin40, is elevated in patients susceptible to post-operative atrial fibrillation. Circulation 103, 842-9.

Dupont, E., Matsushita, T., Kaba, R., Vozzi, C., Coppen, S. R., Khan, N., Kaprielian, R., Yacoub, M. H., and Severs, N. J. 2001b. Altered connexin expression in human congestive heart failure. J Mol Cell Cardiol 33, 359-71.

Emdad, L., Uzzaman, M., Takagishi, Y., Honjo, H., Uchida, T., Severs, N. J., Kodama, I., and Murata, Y. 2001. Gap junction remodelling in hypertrophied left ventricles of aortic-banded rats: prevention by angiotensin II type1 receptor blockade. J Mol Cell Cardiol 33, 219-31.

Gourdie, R.G., Green, C. R., and Severs, N. J. 1991. Gap junction distribution in adult mammalian myocardium revealed by an antipeptide antibody and laser scanning confocal microscopy. J Cell Sci 99, 41-55.

Gourdie, R.G., Severs, N. J., Green, C. R., Rothery, S., Germroth, P., and Thompson, R. P. 1993. The spatial distribution and relative abundance of gap-junctional connexin40 and connexin43 correlate to functional properties of the cardiac atrioventricular conduction system. J Cell Sci 105, 985-91.

Green, C.R., and Severs, N. J. 1993. Distribution and role of gap junctions in normal myocardium and human ischaemic heart disease. Histochemistry 99, 105-20.

Gros, D., Jarry-Guichard, T., ten Velde, I., De Mazière, A. M. G. L., Van Kempen, M. J. A., Davoust, J., Briand, J. P., Moorman, A. F. M., and Jongsma, H. J. 1994. Restricted distribution of connexin40, a gap junctional protein, in mammalian heart. Circ Res 74, 839-51.

Gutstein, D.E., Morley, G. E., Tamaddon, H., Vaidya, D., Schneider, M. D., Chen, J., Chien, K. R., Stuhlmann, H., and Fishman, G. I. 2001a. Conduction slowing and sudden arrhythmic death in mice with cardiac-restricted inactivitation of connexin43. Circ Res 88, 333-9.

Gutstein, D.E., Morley, G. E., Vaidya, D., Liu, F., Chen, F. L., Stuhlmann, H., and Fishman, G. I. 2001b. Heterogeneous expression of gap junction channels in the heart leads to conduction defects and ventricular dysfunction. Circulation 104, 1194-9.

Hagendorff, A., Schumacher, B., Kirchhoff, S., Lüderitz, B., and Willecke, K. 1999. Conduction disturbances and increased atrial vulnerability in connexin40-defficient mice analyzed by transesophageal stimilation. Circulation 99, 1508-15.

Honjo, H., Boyett, M. R., Coppen, S. R., Takagishi, Y., Severs, N. J., and Kodama, I. 2002. Heterogeneous expression of connexins in rabbit sinoatrial node cells: correlation between connexin isoform and cell size. Cardiovasc Res in press..

Jongsma, H.J., and Wilders, R. 2000. Gap junctions in cardiovascular disease. Circ Res 86, 1193-7.

Kaprielian, R.R., Gunning, M., Dupont, E., Sheppard, M. N., Rothery, S. M., Underwood, R., Pennell, D. J., Fox, K., Pepper, J., Poole-Wilson, P. A., and Severs, N. J. 1998. Down-regulation of immunodetectable connexin43 and decreased gap junction size in the pathogenesis of chronic hibernation in the human left ventricle. Circulation 97, 651-60.

Kirchhoff, S., Kim, J. S., Hagendorff, A., Thonnissen, E., Kruger, O., Lamers, W. H., and Willecke, K. 2000. Abnormal cardiac conduction and morphogenesis in connexin40 and connexin43 double-deficient mice. Circ Res 87, 399-405.

Kirchhoff, S., Nelles, E., Hagendorff, A., Krüger, O., Traub, O., and Willecke, K. 1998. Reduced cardiac conduction velocity and predisposition to arrhythmias in connexin40-deficient mice. Curr Biol 8, 299-302.

Krüger, O., Plum, A., Kim, J.-S., Winterhager, E., Maxeiner, S., Hallas, G., Kirchhoff, S., Traub, O., Lamers, W. H., and Willecke, K. 2000. Defective vascular development in connexin 45-deficient mice. Development 127, 4179-93.

Lerner, D.L., Yamada, K. A., Schuessler, R. B., and Saffitz, J. E. 2000 Accelerated onset and increased incidence of ventricular arrhythmias induced by ischaemia in Cx43-deficient mice. Circulation 101, 547-52.

Mackay, D., Ionides, A., Kibar, Z., Rouleau, G., Berry, V., Moore, A., Shiels, A., and Bhattacharya, S. 1999. Connexin46 mutations in autosomal dominant congenital cataract. Am J Hum Genet 64, 1357-64.

Manthey, D., Bukauskas, F., Lee, C. G., Kozak, C. A., and Willecke, K. 1999. Molecular cloning and functional expression of the mouse gap junction gene connexin-57 in human HeLa cells. J Biol Chem 274, 14716-23.

Matsushita, T., Oyamada, M., Fujimoto, K., Yasuda, Y., Masuda, S., Wada, Y., Oka, T., and Takamatsu, T. 1999. Remodelling of cell-cell and cell-extracellular matrix interactions at the border zone of rat myocardial infarcts. Circ Res 85, 1046-55.

Moreno, A.L., Laing, J. G., Beyer, E. C., and Spray, D. C. 1995. Properties of gap junction channels formed of connexin 45 endogenously expressed in human hepatoma (SKHep1) cells. Am J Physiol 268, C356-C365.

Paul, D.L., Ebihara, L., Takemoto, L. J., Swenson, K. I., and Goodenough, D. A. 1991 Connexin46, a novel lens gap junction protein, induces voltage- gated currents in nonjunctional plasma membrane of Xenopus oocytes. J Cell Biol 115, 1077-89.

Plum, A., Hallas, G., Magin, T., Dombrowski, F., Hagendorff, A., Schumacher, B., Wolpert, C., Kim, J.-S., Lamers, W. H., Evert, M., Meda, P., Traub, O., and Willecke, K. 2000. Unique and shared functions of different connexins in mice. Curr Biol 10, 1083-91.

Rohr, S., Kucera, J. P., Fast, V. G., and Kleber, A. G. 1997. Paradoxical improvement of impulse conduction in cardiac tissue by partial cellular uncoupling. Science 275, 841-4.

Rudy, Y., and Shaw, R. M. 1997. Cardiac excitation: an interactive process of ion channels and gap junctions. Adv Exp Med Biol 430, 269-79.

Saffitz, J. E., Beyer, E. C., Darrow, B. J., Guerrero, P. A., Beardslee, M. A., and Dodge, S. M. 1997. Gap junction structure, conduction, and arrhhythmogenesis: direction for future research. In Discontinuous Conduction in the Heart. Spooner, P. M., Joyner, R. W., and Jalife, J., editors. (Futura Publishing Company New York) , pp. 89-105.

Scherer, S.S., Bone, L. J., Deschenes, S. M., Abel, A., Balice-Gordon, R. J., and Fischbeck, K. H. 1999. The role of the gap junction protein connexin32 in the pathogenesis of X-linked Charcot-Marie-Tooth disease. Novartis Found Symp 219, 175-85.

Sepp, R., Severs, N.J., and Gourdie, R.G. 1996 Altered patterns of intercellular junction distribution in hypertrophic cardiomyopathy. Heart 76, 412-417.

Severs, N. J. 1989. Constituent cells of the heart and isolated cell models in cardiovascular research. In Isolated Adult Cardiomyocytes. volume 1. Piper, H. M., and Isenberg, G., editors. (CRC Press Inc. Boca Raton) , pp. 3-41.

Severs, N. J. 1998. Gap junctions and coronary heart disease. In Heart Cell Communication in Health and Disease. De Mello, W. C., and Janse, M. J., editors. (Kluwer Boston), pp. 175-94.

Severs, N. J. 1999. Cardiovascular disease. In Gap Junction-Mediated Intercellular Signalling in Health and Disease. Cardew, G., editor. (John Wiley & Sons Ltd. New York), pp. 188-206.

Severs, N.J. 2000. The cardiac muscle cell. BioEssays 22, 188-99.

Severs, N. J., Dupont, E., Kaprielian, R. R., Yeh, H.-I., and Rothery, S. 1996. Gap junctions and connexins in the cardiovascular system. In Annual of Cardiac Surgery 1996: 9th edition. Yacoub, M. H., Carpentier, A., Pepper, J., and Fabiani, J.-N., editors. (Current Science London), pp. 31-44.

Severs, N.J., Gourdie, R. G., Harfst, E., Peters, N. S., and Green, C. R. 1993. Review. Intercellular junctions and the application of microscopical techniques: the cardiac gap junction as a case model. J Microsc 169, 299-328.

Severs, N.J., Rothery, S., Dupont, E., Coppen, S. R., Yeh, H.-I., Ko, Y.-S., Matsushita, T., Kaba, R., and Halliday, D. 2001 Immunocytochemical analysis of connexin expression in the healthy and diseased cardiovascular system. Microsc Res Tech 52, 301-22.

Shaw, R.M., and Rudy, Y. 1997 Ionic mechanisms of propagation in cardiac tissue - Roles of the sodium and L-type calcium currents during reduced excitability and decreased gap junction coupling. Circ Res 81, 727-41.

Simon, A.M., Goodenough, D. A., and Paul, D. L. 1998. Mice lacking connexin40 have cardiac conduction abnormalities characteristic of atrioventricular block and bundle branch block. Curr Biol 8, 295-8.

Smith, J.H., Green, C. R., Peters, N. S., Rothery, S., and Severs, N. J. 1991. Altered patterns of gap junction distribution in ischemic heart disease. An immunohistochemical study of human myocardium using laser scanning confocal microscopy. Am J Pathol 139, 801-21.

Spach MS, Heidlage JF, Dolber PC, Barr RC. 2000. Electrophysiological effects of remodelling cardiac gap junctions and cell size. Circ Res 86: 302-311.

Tamaddon, H.S., Vaidya, D., Simon, A. M., Paul, D. L., Jalife, J., and Morley, G. E. 2000 High-resolution optical mapping of the right bundle branch in connexin40 knockout mice reveals slow conduction in the specialized conduction system. Circ Res 87, 929-36.

Uzzaman, M., Honjo, H., Takagishi, Y., Emdad, L., Magee, A. I., Severs, N. J., and Kodama, I. 2000. Remodeling of gap-junctional coupling in hypertrophied right ventricles of rats with monocrotaline-induced pulmonary hypertension. Circ Res 86, 871-8.

van Rijen, H.V.M., Van Veen, T. A. B., Van Kempen, M. J. A., Wilms-Schopman, F. J. G., Poste, M., Krueger, O., Willecke, K., Opthof, T., Jongsma, H. J., and de Bakker, J. M. T. 2001 Impaired conduction in the bundle branches of mouse hearts lacking the gap junction protein connexin40. Circulation 103, 1591-8.

Viswanathan, P.C., Shaw, R. M., and Rudy, Y. 1999. Effects of IKr and IKs heterogeneity on action potential duration and its rate dependence: a simulation study. Circulation 99, 2466-74.

Vozzi, C., Dupont, E., Coppen, S. R., Yeh, H.-I., and Severs, N. J. 1999. Chamber-related differences in connexin expression in the human heart. J Mol Cell Cardiol 31, 991-1003.

Willecke K, Eiberger J, Degen J, Eckardt D, Romualdi A, Gueldenagel M, Deutsch U, Soehl G. 2001. Structural and functional diversity of connexin genes in the mouse and human genome. Biol Chem in press.

Yeh, H.-I., Dupont, E., Coppen, S., Rothery, S., and Severs, N. J. 1997a. Gap junction localization and connexin expression in cytochemically identified endothelial cells from arterial tissue. J Histochem Cytochem 45, 539-50.

Yeh, H.-I., Dupont, E., Rothery, S., Coppen, S. R., and Severs, N. J. (1998). Individual gap junction plaques contain multiple connexins in arterial endothelium. Circ Res 83, 1248-63.

Yeh, H.-I., Lai, Y.-J., Chang, H.-M., Ko, Y.-S., Severs, N. J., and Tsai, C.-H. (2000). Multiple connexin expression in regenerating arterial endothelial gap junctions. Arterioscler Thromb Vasc Biol 20, 1753-62.

Yeh, H.-I., Lupu, F., Dupont, E., and Severs, N. J. (1997b). Upregulation of connexin43 gap junctions between smooth muscle cells after balloon catheter injury in the rat carotid artery. Arterioscler Thromb Vasc Biol 17, 3174-84.

13

IONIC CHANNELS AND FIBRILLATION

Justus M.B. Anumonwo, Omer Berenfeld, Amit Dhamoon,
José Jalife
Dept. of Pharmacology, SUNY Upstate Medical University, Syracuse NY

INTRODUCTION

Cardiac fibrillation is a major health problem in industrialized society today. In the United States alone, ventricular fibrillation (VF) is responsible for approximately 300,000 sudden cardiac deaths (Myerburg,Catellanos,1997). On the other hand, atrial fibrillation (AF) afflicts over 2 million Americans, (Feinberg et al,1995) which makes it the most prevalent cardiac arrhythmia in clinical practice. While AF in and of itself does not usually lead to death, it is the most important cause of stroke. (Wolf et al,1991). Because of the alarming nature of these statistics, understanding the mechanisms underlying fibrillation of the heart is very critical.

Fibrillation is diagnosed on the electrocardiogram (ECG) by ventricular (or atrial) electrical complexes that seem completely aperiodic and show irregular beat-to-beat changes in amplitude and morphology. During VF, the ventricular rate is exceedingly high (>500 beats/min) and disorganized. This leads to a severely depressed cardiac pump function, with adverse consequences on systolic tension and on arterial pressure. Because vital organs are deprived of oxygen, death usually occurs within ten minutes. In the case of AF, while the atrial activation frequency is also very high, the AV node filters most of the atrial impulses, which results in an "irregularly irregular" (Barilla et al,1996) but relatively slow ventricular rate.

The first visual description of fibrillation was provided as far back as the late 1800s. (McWilliam,1887). However, our understanding of the underlying electrical events that result in fibrillation remains incomplete. The ECG manifestations of fibrillation conjure up very complex and haphazard activation sequences of the atria or ventricles. Accordingly, it has become traditional to conceptualize fibrillation as resulting from the co-existence of numerous wavefronts of electrical excitation that meander randomly throughout the myocardium. This idea was the basis of the multiple wavelet hypothesis for atrial fibrillation of Moe and colleagues.(Moe,1962;Moe et al,1964). Recent studies employing sophisticated analytical tools, however, have provided new and important insight into fibrillation both in the atria and the ventricles. (Skanes et al,1998;Mandapati et al,2000; Chen et al,2000;Zaitsev et al 2000;Samie et al,2001) Such investigations have used high-resolution optical mapping with a combination of spectral and nonlinear methods to study the fibrillating myocardium. It is now postulated that electrical waves in the form of functional "rotors" are the main organizing centers of wave propagation during fibrillation. Based on this concept, two divergent mechanisms have emerged that depend on the stability of the rotor. As will be considered in a later section, these are the multiple-circuit hypothesis (Moe et al,1964) of excitation and the single reentrant source hypothesis (Gray et al,1965; Gray et al,1968; Jalife et al,1998). More recently also, cellular electrophysiology and computer simulations have provided additional insight into ionic channel mechanism for the localization of the rotors (Samie et al,2001;Beaumont, Jalife,2000). This chapter discusses our recent ideas on the mechanisms of initiation and maintenance of fibrillation. Emphasis is placed on experimental and theoretical evidence for the role of individual ionic channels in the mechanisms underlying the functional reentrant activity.

MECHANISMS OF FIBRILLATION

The Multiple Wavelets Hypothesis

In the early 20th century, fibrillation was thought to result from multiple foci that rapidly generated electrical impulses, (Winterberg et al,1907;Sherf et al,1958) i.e., ectopic foci, or from single (Lewis,1925) or multiple reentrant circuits in the myocardium.(Mines,1914;Garrey,1914).Later, a combination of experimental and numerical simulation studies led Moe and his co-workers (Moe,1962;Moe et al,1964) to develop the multiple wavelet hypothesis to explain atrial fibrillation. It was proposed that during fibrillatory activity, several (multiple) independent wave fronts meander randomly in the myocardium around strands or "islands" of refractory tissue. As these wavelets wander in the tissue, propagation may speed up or slow down in different regions, depending on the extent to which excitability has recovered in these regions. Thus, central in the hypothesis is randomness in temporal and spatial distribution of membrane properties in the fibrillating tissue. In such underlying substrate, the fibrillation is maintained by the wondering wavelets that may collide, become extinguished, divide, or combine in ever changing sizes, propagation directions and activation patterns. Although the multiple wavelet hypothesis was originally proposed to explain atrial fibrillation, subsequent studies assumed that a similar mechanism was also applicable to VF(Garfinkel et al,2000).

A major advancement in our thinking about the underlying mechanisms of fibrillation came from theoretical (Krinsky, 1978) and experimental (Davidenko et al,1990) evidence demonstrating that the myocardium can sustain electrical activity that rotated around a *functional* obstacle. Weiner and Rosenblueth (1946) carried out the first numerical investigation of reentry and developed a completely new approach to the study of wave propagation in excitable tissues. They demonstrated that when a wave rotates around a small anatomical obstacle in a two-dimensional medium, the wavefront acquires a spiral shape. In addition, they showed that the wave can circulate if the perimeter of the obstacle is larger than the wavelength, which was defined as the product of the refractory period and the conduction velocity. Weiner and Rosenblueth (1946) suggested that rotation around a closed pathway was also possible in the absence of an obstacle. However, it was not until 1965 when Balakhovskii (1965) predicted that appropriate conditions leading to fragmentation of a wavefront ("i.e., a wavebreak") may result in spiral wave rotation in an obstacle-free medium (see also Krinsky,1966;1984;Pertsov et al,1984).Subsequently, in 1977, Allessie et al (1977) developed the "leading circle concept", by showing functional reentry in isolated rabbit atrial preparations, without the involvement of an anatomical obstacle. Given the results of these investigations, there has been a focus on such rotating waves or 'rotors' as the main mechanism underlying fibrillation.

A variety of theoretical and experimental studies have examined the phenomenon of "turbulence" which is associated with fibrillation, (Rogers, Ideker, 2000; Karma, 2000) and it has been argued that the turbulence is a result of a single spiral wave or a pair of counter-rotating spiral waves breaking up into a multispiral disorganized state(Karma,1994).Two possibilities have been advanced to explain break up of spiral waves. The first explanation is based on the restitution hypothesis, (Karma,1994;Gilmour et al,1997) and suggests that oscillations in action potential duration (APD) may be significantly large such that a block of conduction occurs along the wave front. It had been demonstrated previously that when APD was plotted against the preceding diastolic interval, (i.e., the action potential restitution curve), and if the slope of the curve was >1, there was a possibility for APD alternans and destabilization of activity (Chialvo et al,1990) According to such a scenario, spiral wave breakup occurs when the slope of APD restitution exceeds 1(Qu et al,1999). The curvature of the wavefront changes both conduction velocity and APD (Cabo et al,1994). It also changes their restitution properties, thereby modulating local stability, (Beaumont et al,1998) resulting in distinct spiral wave behaviors (Qu et al,2000) Furthermore, APD alternans are hypothesized to be involved in the initiation of complex dynamics that ultimately lead to wavefront destabilization and formation of rotors (Garfinkel et al, 2000). The second explanation for break up is that intramural rotation of muscle fibers confers a high degree of anisotropy to the myocardium, resulting in the twisting and instability of the organizing center or "filament" (Fenton, Karma, 1998; Qu et al, 2000).

The "Mother Rotor" Hypothesis of Fibrillation

Since a decade ago, work from our laboratory has also focused on rotors as the underlying mechanism for fibrillation (Samie et al, 2000; Gray et al,1998; Davidenko et al,1991;Jalife,2000). In contrast to the breakup hypothesis, however, we have proposed that cardiac fibrillation is a consequence of self-organization of non-linear electrical waves with both stochastic and deterministic components (Gray et al,1995). Such a point of view is consistent with the hypothesis that there is spatio-temporal organization during fibrillation in a structurally normal heart, even though there is a wide spectrum of behavior during fibrillatory activity. Thus, as an example, Gray et al,(1995) demonstrated that a single drifting rotor can generate complex patterns of excitation such as is seen in fibrillation. Alternatively, it is hypothesized that fibrillation results from a single or a small number of high-frequency stable "mother" rotors, and that the complex activation patterns are consequent to the fragmentation of the waves emanating from such rotors (Jalife et al,1998) Indeed, more recent experiments from our laboratory (Saitsev et al,2000;Samie et al,2001;Gray et al,1998;Berenfeld et al,2000) and others (Damle et al,1992;Bayly et al,1993;Witkowski et al,1975) have provided evidence that requires a reexamination of the prevailing idea that multiple-circuit reentrant activity is the sole determinant of fibrillatory activity in the myocardium. Some of our studies have implicated a small number of rotors (sometimes single rotors) in the AF recorded in isolated sheep hearts (Skanes et al,1998; Mndapari et al,2000;Chen et al,2000) In these studies, an intriguing peculiarity of the rotor is that it frequently resides in the left atrium (Skanes et al,1998;Mandapari et al,2000;Mansour et al,2001) Possible explanations for this include properties of cells around the pulmonary veins (the rotors are usually found around these veins), or the left-right differences in atrial refractoriness (Barenfeld et al,2000) attributable to differences in ion channel densities and expression patterns(Li et al,2001). In a more recent study (Samie et al,2001) we presented new evidence in the isolated Langendorff-perfused guinea pig heart that strongly supports the hypothesis that fibrillatory conduction from a stable high frequency reentrant source is the underlying mechanism of VF in this species. Moreover, using the whole-cell patch-clamp technique and computer simulations, we demonstrated, for the first time, that regional differences in the distribution of an inward rectifier channel may provide an ionic mechanism for the localization of the source in the LV and the establishment of a consistent gradient of excitation frequency between the left and the right ventricles during VF. In the remainder of this chapter, the focus will be shifted to the role of the ionic channels that have been implicated in rotors dynamics, and how the channel proteins are altered during electrical remodeling, a widely observed phenomenon that is attendant to chronic AF.

IONIC CHANNELS AND VENTRICULAR FIBRILLATION

In the current thinking of mechanisms underlying fibrillation, i.e., the involvement of reentrant circuits, experimental and theoretical studies have shown that the stability of rotors depends on the ability to abbreviate the APD, as well as to reduce wavefront-wavetail interactions (Samie et al, 2001; Beaumont et al, 1998; Starmer et al, 1995). As far back as forty years ago (see Moe et al, 1964), there was evidence that heterogeneity in refractoriness of the atrial myocardium was an important determinant of whether fibrillation can be sustained or not. Clearly, refractoriness and all other electrophysiological properties are determined by the biophysical properties of sarcolemmal membrane ionic channels, including their voltage-dependence and kinetics of activation. The issue of the specific ionic channels involved in fibrillation is currently an area of active research. Such studies have significantly increased our understanding of ionic channels in atrial and ventricular myocardium(Nattel,2002), cell membrane receptors (Sharikov et al, 2001; Dhein, Train, 2001; Wellner-Kienitz, Pott, 2001; Fields et al,1978; Corey, Clapham, 2001) and gap junctional channels (Gros et al,1994) and their roles in fibrillation. A few theoretical and animal models studies will now be considered.

In numerical studies of polymorphic tachyarrhythmias, Starmer et al (1995) investigated the proarrhythmic response to potassium channel blockade. The investigators examined the responses of spiral wave activity to parameter changes mimicking drug effects in a two-dimensional array of excitable cells modeled using the FitzHugh-Nagumo equations. For simplicity, a single excitation current (similar to the sodium current) and a single repolarizing (i.e., potassium current) were used. It was found that the evolution of the spiral wave was insensitive to changes in the delayed rectifier current but was sensitive to changes in the sodium conductance as well as the inward rectifier conductance. In more recent studies from our laboratory, (Beaumont, Jalife, 2000; Beaumont et al,1998) we have used an ionic model to characterize rotors and spiral waves in two dimensions. In one such analysis, we examined the ionic mechanism underlying the formation of an unexcited core. APD distribution around the spiral core was also examined (Figure 1). The central premise here was that although the axial current flow ahead of the activation front was large enough, the central core remained unexcited. In figure 1, Panel A shows wave shape on a cardiac fiber 20, 60 and 100 ms after the application of an electrical stimulation that results in premature repolarization. Panel B illustrates the current-voltage (I-V) plots for three formulations of the inward rectifier current (I_{K1}). In panel C are shown the APD distributions as a consequence of the premature repolarization. Panels D and E are the spirals about

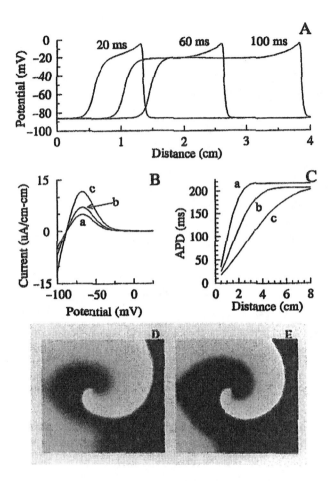

Figure 1. I_{K1} and APD abbreviation.[16] A, Wave shape on a cardiac fiber 20, 60, and 100 msec after application of an external electrical stimulation causing premature repolarization. B, I-V relations for three different formulations (a,b,c) of the inward rectifier current (I_{K1}). C, APD distribution following premature repolarization on a cardiac fiber (as illustrated in A) when the respective I_{K1} formulations of B were used in the ionic numerical model. D and E, Spiral wave reentry about 100 msec after application of the initiating stimulus when the I_{K1} formulation a and c were used in the ionic model of D and E, respectively. With permission from W.B. Saunders.

100 ms after the application of an initiating stimulus, when I_{K1} formulations *a* and *c* (panel B) were used in the ionic model. The results of this simulation demonstrated that the formation of the unexcited core was produced by block of conduction that occurred in a thin rim around the center of rotation. Also, it showed that the

large spatial distribution of APD was produced by the fact that APD was prematurely abbreviated close to the core because of an electrotonic interaction between cells in the core and cells in its immediate surroundings. After such an interaction, the wave tail moves away from the core, propagating independently from the wave front. The spatial extent of the excited state (i.e., the wavelength) is determined by the differences in the propagation velocity of the wave front and the wave tail.

In addition to these theoretical studies, experimental work from our laboratory (Samie et al,2000) and others (Garfinkel et al,2000;Li et al,2001;van Wagoner, Pond 1999) has investigated the role of these and other ionic currents in fibrillation. In one study, we investigated the mechanisms of transition from VF to tachycardias in isolated rabbit hearts, using a combination of tools including high-resolution video imaging with a fluorescent dye and 2-dimensional phase analysis, as well as computer simulations. In the study, we examined the effect of inhibiting the L-type calcium channel on the dynamics of rotating waves (Samie et al, 2000). Specifically, our objectives were to demonstrate functional reentry as a mechanism of VF and monomorphic ventricular tachycardia (MVT), and to elucidate the mechanism of verapamil-induced conversion of VF to MVT. Our results clearly demonstrated that, indeed, rotating waves are the basis of VF and MVT in the isolated rabbit heart. Furthermore, in the presence of verapamil, the dominant frequency of VF decreased from 16.2 to 13.5 Hz. The VF to VT conversion was most likely the result of a decrease in rotor frequency and a decrease in wave front fragmentation that reduced the fibrillatory propagation away from the rotor. We found that the verapamil-induced block of the calcium (L-type) current caused a conduction block at a smaller curvature resulting in a larger core size. This effect was also confirmed in the computer simulations by blocking the slow inward current (I_{si}) in a modified Luo & Rudy model (Beaumont et al,1998) to reproduce the effect of verapamil. The involvement of the calcium current and the core size is therefore clear.

Very recently, we used a combination of high-resolution optical mapping and the patch-clamp technique to present evidence for an ionic mechanism for rotor stabilization and wave front fragmentation (Samie et al,2001). As discussed above, our study showed that VF in the guinea-pig is the result of a highly periodic reentrant source, and that regional (left ventricle>right ventricle) differences in the inward rectifier background current, presumably I_{K1}, may provide an ionic mechanism for the stabilization of the high-frequency source and the establishment of a consistent gradient in frequencies of excitation during VF. Figure 2 shows frequency analysis in the guinea pig heart. Panel A shows ECG typical for VF. Panel B shows that there is a clustering of dominant frequencies (DFs) in well defined domains. Note that a large region on the anterior wall of the LV activates at the extremely high frequency of 26 Hz, whereas the RV only reaches frequencies of about 14 Hz. Panel C shows action potentials recorded from the RV and LV using intracellular microelectrodes. As an initial approach to understand the ionic and molecular mechanism of such a large and very consistent frequency gradient, we used the whole-cell patch-clamp technique to analyze the background current in the RV and the LV and to relate the spatial distribution of the current density to the excitation frequencies and stability. Panel A of figure 3 shows representative I-V curves from two cells isolated from LV and the RV in the same heart. Note the larger outward current in the LV compared to the RV. Similar results were obtained in a total of 10 hearts (19 LV cells and 18 RV cells) (panel B). Overall, the outward current (measured at −50 mV) was

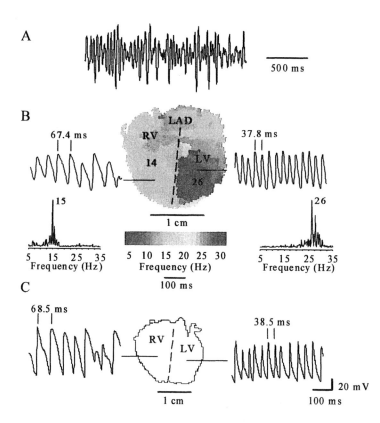

Figure 2. Frequency analysis of VF in the isolated guinea-pig heart.[12] A, ECG trace of VF. B, DF map. DFs in RV range between 10 and 16 Hz; DFs in LV range between 14 and 26 Hz. The highest frequency (26 Hz) is found on the LV anterior free wall. Single pixel recordings and frequency spectra corroborate the DF map findings. C. Microelectrode recordings. APs recorded from the RV and the LV during VF. With permission from the American Heart Association

significantly larger in the LV than in the RV (7.4 ± 0.6 versus 5.3 ± 0.4 pA/pF, p=0.009). To have a better understanding of the effect of the RV and LV differences in rotor dynamics, we used the mean values of the background current shown in figure 3B in a 2-dimensional computer model (see Samie et al ,2001). Results from the simulations are shown in figure 4. Panel A illustrates the simulated steady-state I-V plots for the RV and the LV. The experimental data (from figure 3) have been superimposed. The

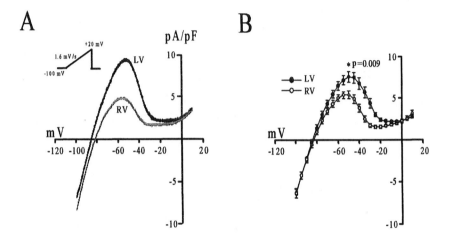

Figure 3. I-V relations of I_B from the guinea-pig ventricular myocytes.[12] A, current-density voltage relation of I_B for sample cells from the RV and LV of the same heart. The inset shows the voltage-clamp protocol. B, Mean I-V relation for I_B (n_{RV}=18 and n_{LV}=19). Currents were normalized to cell capacitance and averaged. Mean RV and LV capacitance, 165 and 167 pF, respectively. With permission from the American Heart Association.

panel also shows simulated single cell action potentials obtained at a stimulus frequency of 1 Hz. The reduced outward current in RV resulted in a longer RV action potential duration than for the LV. Panel B are snapshots of the simulations ($3x3$-cm^2 sheets) in which a smaller (for RV; top) or larger outward background current (for LV; bottom) has been used. The strong rectification in the RV model yielded unstable reentry that self-terminated. In sharp contrast to the RV, the LV showed a stable, high frequency rotor (33 Hz, cycle length = 30 ms) that remained stable for more than 100 rotations. Thus, this experimental and theoretical work in the isolated heart of the guinea pig demonstrates a robust ionic (I_{K1}) mechanism for rotor stabilization and wave front fragmentation.

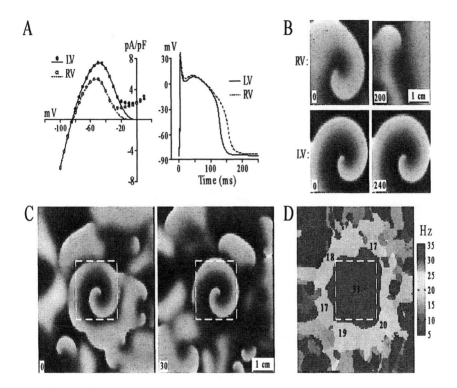

Figure 4. Computer simulations with I_{K1} from the RV and the LV of the guinea-pig.[12] A, Formulation of I_{K1}-V used in the model (solid and broken lines) with corresponding action potentials. Mean experimental data from figure. 6B (circles) are superimposed. B, snapshots of numerical data; 3×3 cm² sheets simulating the RV (top) and LV (bottom). C, snapshots of numerical data in the combined RV-LV model of 6×6 cm². D, DF map obtained from the model in panel C. Numbers in B and C are in ms, and in D in Hz. Broken lines in C and D show the perimeter of the LV model (area, 2×2 cm²). With permission from the American Heart Association.

ION CHANNELS AND ATRIAL FIBRILLATION

It remains to be determined whether chamber specific differences in ion channel density similar to those observed in the guinea pig heart are responsible for the single rotor mechanism of AF. Clearly demarcated gradients in LA-to-RA frequencies have been demonstrated during AF in both dog (Morillo et al,1995) and sheep (Skanes et al,1998;Mandapati et al,2000; Mansour et al,2001) atrial. Similarly, studies in humans suggest that at least some cases of AF may be explained by a mother-rotor mechanism. For example, Horvath et al (2000) reported on human cases of simultaneous LA flutter and RA fibrillation in which the mean LA cycle length of 173 ms (5.8 Hz) was nevertheless shorter than the mean RA cycle length of 236 ms (4.2 Hz). Other studies have shown that refractoriness is shorter in the LA than in the RA. (Papageorgiou et al,1996;Sih et al,1997;Power et al,1998). Very recent experiments by Li et al (2001) strongly suggest that LA-to-RA differences in refractoriness at low frequencies correlate strongly with intrinsic differences in the APD recorded from cells obtained from the two atria. A larger density of the rapid delayed rectifier current (I_{Kr}) in the LA seems to explain nicely such chamber specific differences in APD during pacing at relatively low frequencies (Li et al,2001). However, the kinetics of activation and deactivation of I_{Kr} are too slow to explain the ability of the LA to activate at frequencies as high as 18 Hz, (Zhou et al,1998; Anumonwo et al,1999) so it seems unlikely that such differences could explain the LA-to-RA gradient of frequencies during AF (Mansour et al,2001).

In the experimental setting, acute AF is usually induced by burst pacing and maintained in the continuous presence of acetylcholine (ACh) (Skanes et al,1998; Schuessler et al,1992) or vagal stimulation (Rozenshtraukh et al,1988). ACh is pro-fibrillatory in the atrium because it is capable of abbreviating atrial APD to extreme values, which is an essential factor for the establishment and maintenance of AF. Traditionally, the ability of cholinergic input to promote AF in the normal heart has been attributed to the heterogeneous distribution of vagal innervation and muscarinic ACh receptors throughout the atria, which increases spatial dispersion of refractory periods and results in complex patterns of activation and wavelet formation (Sharifov et al,2001).

Recently published data from our laboratory in the Langendorff-perfused sheep heart (Mansour et al,2001) showed that increasing the ACh concentration from 0.2 to 0.5 µM, increased the frequency of the dominant source in the LA, as well as the LA-to-RA frequency gradient, suggesting that the LA and RA are indeed different in their response to ACh in this species. As such, the hypothesis of a heterogeneous response to vagal innervation must take a more specific form; that is, that stimulation of the ACh-activated inward rectifier potassium current, $I_{K,ACh}$, is somehow stronger in the LA than in the RA, which should set the stage for the development of AF by internal or external triggers through two distinct mutually complementary mechanisms: first, it should greatly abbreviate APD, and thus lead to an increase in frequency of rotation of microreentrant sources in the LA; second, it should increase resting membrane conductance and threshold current, thus reducing excitability. This should allow stabilization of the rotor in the region of greatest APD abbreviation (e.g., the LA). Outside this region, the highly complex atrial structure would contribute to intermittent block in the face of high-frequency excitation emanating from the rotor. As such, ACh should enhance sink-to-source mismatch at branching sites and other areas of changing cell-to-cell coupling and/or geometry and facilitate the development of spatially distributed delays and intermittent block, the hallmark of fibrillatory conduction.

Thus, it is possible that left-to-right differences in AF frequency in the acute sheep heart experiments may result from chamber specific differences in muscarinic receptor density (Fields et al,1978) and/or G protein-coupled Kir3.x channels (Dobrev et al,2001), which are responsible for the ACh-activated inward rectifying current $I_{K,ACh}$. However, it is important to note that several studies have shown that parasympathetic signaling is altered in human atrial myocytes from chronic AF patients. In fact, there is some controversy as to whether the current is increased (Bosch et al,1999) or decreased (Dobrev et al,2001;Brundel et al,2001). In the study of Bosch et al,[70] the presence of AF was associated with a marked shortening of the AP duration and a decreased rate response of atrial repolarization, which correlated with a decrease in $I_{Ca,L}$ and increases in I_{KI} and $I_{K,ACh}$ at hyperpolarizing potentials. These authors concluded that changes in atrial potassium and calcium currents contribute to electrical remodeling in AF and are therefore important factors for the perpetuation of the arrhythmia. More recently, Dobrev et al (2001) also found that chronic AF induces a transcriptionally mediated increase in I_{K1}. However, unlike Bosch et al (1999), these authors found that myocytes from patients with chronic AF showed a downregulation of $I_{K,ACh}$, and concluded that this change was an adaptive response to the continuously high excitation frequency to counteract the shortening of the effective refractory period due to electrical remodeling. Thus, while important information about the underlying mechanisms of rate adaptation and electrical remodeling has been obtained in the last several years of study both in humans and experimental animals (see below), the issue of the molecular mechanisms of AF maintenance and perpetuation is by no means settled.

REMODELING OF ION CHANNELS IN FIBRILLATION

It is widely known that there are compensatory changes in the handling of ions across the cell membrane in response to cardiac diseases (see review by Nattel et al, 2001). The role of ion channels in the substrate changes attendant to myocardial electrical remodeling is a very important, and currently has generated a lot of interest in several laboratories. Thus the phenomenon of atrial tachycardia-induced electrical remodeling, by which "atrial fibrillation begets atrial fibrillation" (Wijfels et al,1995) is now well accepted. A variety of ionic current changes have now been described which likely account for the functional electrophysiological changes caused in experimental models by atrial tachycardia (Nattel,2002). Decreases are observed in I_{to}, $I_{Ca,L}$ and I_{Na} (Gaspo et al,1997). The decreases in $I_{Ca,L}$ seem to be particularly important in explaining action potential abbreviation and loss of rate-adaptation seen in AF. In the rapidly paced canine atrial model of AF, there is downregulation of $I_{Ca,L}$ (Gasppo et al,1999) and several studies have reported that the electrophysiological remodeling accompanying AF could be prevented by pretreatment with calcium channel blockers(Tieleman et al,1997;Daoud et al,1997) which implies that calcium overload is a key factor in the remodeling process. Thus, it has been suggested that calcium overload might trigger the intracellular signaling cascade, altering gene expression and eventually resulting in downregulation of atrial K^+ and Ca^{2+} current densities(van Wagoner ,Pond 1999).

In human atrial myocytes, reductions in I_{to} and reduced gene expression of several potassium currents (Kv1.5, Kv4.3, GIRK1 (Kir3.1), GIRK4 (Kir3.4) and Kir6.2 have been observed (Brundel et al,1999;van Wagoner et al,1997). More recently, Brundel et al (2001) have shown that AF in patients is accompanied by decreases in protein content of the L-type Ca^{2+} channel as well as several potassium channels, including Kv4.3, HERG, Kv1.5, KvLQT1/minK, and Kir3.4/Kir3.1. Altogether, these results suggest that atrial myocytes adapt to chronic rapid excitation by downregulating several potassium channels to counteract the observed changes of the atrial refractory period due to electrical remodeling(Dobrev et al,2001).

Alterations in channel properties attendant to electrical remodeling may provide some opportunity for therapy. The channels present in remodeled, diseased atria often have a different pharmacologic profile than that of "normal" ion channels (Tieleman et al,1997) which may enable specific targeting of the remodeled atria by pharmacologic agents to more rationally modify the new and/or remaining ion channels that underlie the action potentials. A variety of interventions have been applied in an attempt to prevent electrophysiologic remodeling (Tieleman et al,1997). L-type Ca^{2+}

channel blockers prevent the short-term changes caused by <1 hour of atrial tachycardia or AF (Workman et al,2001). Longer-term changes (over 24 hours) are partly inhibited by L-type Ca^{2+} channel blockers, but AF promotion still occurs. T-type Ca^{2+} channel blockers may attenuate the functional and AF-promoting effects of 7 days of atrial tachycardia (ref). Atrial tachyarrhythmias are known to be more common in the setting of heart failure. Heart failure alters adrenergic receptor density and function, as well as G-protein mediated signaling(Rockman et al,1997). In the ventricles, the densities of I_{to}, I_{K1} and possibly $I_{Ca,L}$ are reduced (Kaab et al,1996). Recent work indicates that atrial ion channel function is also altered by ventricular failure (ref) and I_{to}, $I_{Ca,L}$ and I_{Ks} are down-regulated (Kaab et al,1996). Heart failure is associated with increased plasma catecholamine concentration (Cohn et al,1984). This raises the possibility that increased local and circulating catecholamines contribute to the downregulation of ion channels caused by heart failure (Zhang et al,2002). In some models of AF, a slow adaptive hypertrophy of the myocyte occurs secondary to pressure/volume overload (Ausma et al,1997). In a model of spontaneous AF in dogs(Gaspo,1997) it appears that the myocyte adapts to these signals by increasing cell size and promoting formation of a t-tubular network. As discussed above, recent studies have shown that, while $I_{K,ACh}$ is reduced(Dobrev et al,2001), I_{K1} is increased in patients with chronic AF (van Wagoner et al,1997), which raises the interesting question of whether such upregulation is chamber specific and whether it correlates with predictable frequency gradients of frequency in the setting of chronic AF(Dobrev et al,2001;Bosch et al,1999).

CONCLUSIONS

Recent experimental and theoretical findings from several laboratories (Samie et al,2001; Mansour et al,2001;Nattel,2002; Horvath et al,2000;Gerstenfeld et al,1992) have provided compelling evidence for the need to reexamine long-held hypotheses underlying fibrillation in both the atria and the ventricles. Clearly, given the complexity of fibrillation, several competing hypotheses should be expected. Newly developed high resolution imaging tools are making it possible to clarify the specific roles of ectopic activity, single and multiple reentrant circuits in the mechanisms of initiation as well as the dynamics of both AF and VF. The next frontier is to link such global behaviors to underlying ionic and molecular mechanisms. In this regard, the role of chamber specific differences in the density of inward rectifying channels in the mechanism of VF in one animal species is now becoming clear (Samie et al, 2001). Whether such differences will explain the mechanism of VF in other species requires investigation. Also, the underlying ionic determinants of the maintenance of acute AF have not been explored in any detail. The hypothesis that chamber-specific differences in cholinergic receptors or G-protein coupled channels explains the different excitation frequencies normally observed in the LA and RA of certain species is very intriguing and deserves exploration. Finally, the mechanisms linking electrical remodeling to AF perpetuation in chronic AF patients have not been settled. Chronic AF in man is associated with reductions in $I_{K,ACh}$ and $I_{Ca,L}$ but normal or increased I_{K1}. However, the consequences of such a reduced response to parasympathetic activity and altered channel densities on wave propagation dynamics in the spontaneously fibrillating atria have never been studied. Answers to these questions are critically important given the prevalence and the economic consequences of both forms of cardiac fibrillation in the society.

REFERENCE

Allessie MA, Bonke FI, Schopman FJ 1977. Circus movement in rabbit atrial muscle as a mechanism of tachycardia. III. The "leading circle" concept: a new model of circus movement in cardiac tissue without the involvement of an anatomical obstacle. Circ.Res. 41:9-18.

Anumonwo JM, Horta J, Delmar M, Taffet SM, Jalife J 1999. Proton and zinc effects on HERG currents. Biophysical Journal 77:282-298.

Ausma J, Wijffels M, Thone F, Wouters L, Allessie M, Borgers M 1997 Structural changes of atrial myocardium due to sustained atrial fibrillation in the goat. Circulation 96:3157-3163.

Balakhovskii IS 1965. Several modes of excitation movement in ideal excitable tissue. Biophysics 10:1175-1179.

Barilla F, Mangieri E, Critelli G 1996. An irregularly irregular rhythm. Pacing Clin.Electrophysiol. 19:861-862.

Bayly PV, Johnson EE, Wolf PD, Greenside HS, Smith WM, Ideker RE 1993 A quantitative measurement of spatial order in ventricular fibrillation. J.Cardiovasc.Electrophysiol. 4:533-546.

Beaumont J, Davidenko N, Davidenko JM, Jalife J 1998. Spiral waves in two-dimensional models of ventricular muscle: formation of a stationary core. Biophys.J. 75:1-14.

Beaumont,J, Jalife,J. Rotors and spiral waves in two dimensions. In: Cardiac Electrophysiology From Cell to Bedside. Zipes,DP, Jalife,J, eds. 2000. W.B. Saunders, Philadelphia, PA.

Berenfeld O, Mandapati R, Dixit S, Skanes AC, Chen J, Mansour M, Jalife J 2000. Spatially distributed dominant excitation frequencies reveal hidden organization in atrial fibrillation in the Langendorff-perfused sheep heart. J.Cardiovasc.Electrophysiol. 11:869-879.

Bosch RF, Zeng X, Grammer JB, Popovic K, Mewis C, Kühlkamp V 1999. Ionic mechanisms of electrical remodeling in human atrial fibrillation. Cardiovasc.Res. 44:121-131.

Brundel BJ, Van Gelder IC, Henning RH, Tieleman RG, Tuinenburg AE, Wietses M, Grandjean JG, Van Gilst WH, Crijns HJ 2001. Ion channel remodeling is related to intraoperative atrial effective refractory periods in patients with paroxysmal and persistent atrial fibrillation. Circulation 103:684-690.

Brundel BJ, Van Gelder IC, Henning RH, Tuinenburg AE, Deelman LE, Tieleman RG, Grandjean JG, Van Gilst WH, Crijns HJ 1999 Gene expression of proteins influencing the calcium homeostasis in patients with persistent and paroxysmal atrial fibrillation. Cardiovasc.Res. 42:443-454.

Cabo C, Pertsov AM, Baxter WT, Davidenko JM, Gray RA, Jalife J 1994 Wave-front curvature as a cause of slow conduction and block in isolated cardiac muscle. Circ.Res. 75:1014-1028.

Chen J, Mandapati R, Berenfeld O, Skanes AC, Gray RA, Jalife J 2000 Dynamics of wavelets and their role in atrial fibrillation in the isolated sheep heart. Cardiovasc.Res. 48:220-232.

Chialvo DR, Gilmour RF, Jr., Jalife J 1990. Low dimensional chaos in cardiac tissue. Nature 343:653-657.

Cohn JN, Levine TB, Olivari MT, Garberg V, Lura D, Francis GS, Simon AB, Rector T 1984 Plasma norepinephrine as a guide to prognosis in patients with chronic congestive heart failure. N.Engl.J Med. 311:819-823.

Corey S, Clapham DE 2001. The Stoichiometry of Gbeta gamma binding to G-protein-regulated inwardlyrectifying K+ channels (GIRKs). J Biol. Chem. 276:11409-11413.

Damle RS, Kanaan NM, Robinson NS, Ge YZ, Goldberger JJ, Kadish AH 1992. Spatial and temporal linking of epicardial activation directions during ventricular fibrillation in dogs. Evidence for underlying organization. Circulation 86:1547-1558.

Daoud EG, Knight BP, Weiss R, Bahu M, Paladino W, Goyal R, Man KC, Strickberger SA, Morady F 1997   Effect of verapamil and procainamide on atrial fibrillation-induced electrical remodeling in humans. Circulation 96:1542-1550.

Davidenko JM, Kent PF, Chialvo DR, Michaels DC, Jalife J 1990. Sustained vortex-like waves in normal isolated ventricular muscle. Proc. Natl. Acad. Sci. U.S.A. 87:8785-8789.

Davidenko JM, Pertsov AM, Salomonsz R, Baxter WT, Jalife J 1991 Stationary and drifting spiral waves of excitation in isolated cardiac muscle. Nature 355:349-351.

Dhein S, Van Train KF 2001. Muscarinic receptors in the mammalian heart. Pharmacol.Ther. 44:161-82.

Dobrev D, Graf E, Wettwer E, Himmel HM, Hala O, Doerfel C, Christ T, Schuler S, Ravens U 2001. Molecular basis of downregulation of G-protein-coupled inward rectifying K(+) current (I(K,ACh) in chronic human atrial fibrillation: decrease in GIRK4 mRNA correlates with reduced I(K,ACh) and muscarinic receptor-mediated shortening of action potentials. Circulation 104:2551-2557.

Feinberg WM, Blackshear JL, Laupacis A, Kronmal R, Hart RG 1995. Prevalence, age distribution, and gender of patients with atrial fibrillation. Arch. Intern. Med. 155:469-473.

Fenton F, Karma A 1998. Vortex dynamics in three-dimensional continuous myocardium with fiber rotation: Filament instability and fibrillation. Chaos 8:20-47.

Fields JZ, Roeske WR, Morkin E, Yamamura HI 1978. Cardiac muscarinic cholinergic receptors. Biochemical identification and characterization. J.Biol.Chem. 253:3251-3258.

Garfinkel A, Kim YH, Voroshilovsky O, Qu ZL, Kil JR, Lee MH, Karagueuzian HS, Weiss JN, Chen PS 2000. Preventing ventricular fibrillation by flattening cardiac restitution. Proc. Natl. Acad. Sci. U.S.A. 97:6061-6066.

Garrey WE 1914. The nature of fibrillatory contraction of the heart. Its relation to tissue mass and form. Am. J. Physiol. 30:397-414.

Gaspo R, Bosch RF, Bou-Abboud E, Nattel S 1997. Tachycardia-induced changes in Na+ current in a chronic dog model of atrial fibrillation. Circ.Res. 81:1045-1052.

Gaspo R, Sun H, Fareh S, Levi M, Yue L, Allen BG, Hebert TE, Nattel S 1999
    Dihydropyridine and beta adrenergic receptor binding in dogs with
    tachycardia-induced atrial fibrillation. Cardiovasc.Res. 42:434-442.
Gerstenfeld EP, Sahakian AV, Swiryn S 1992 Evidence for transient linking of
    atrial excitation during atrial fibrillation in humans. Circulation 86:375-
    382.
Gilmour RF, Jr., Otani NF, Watanabe MA   1997. Memory and complex
    dynamics in cardiac Purkinje fibers. Am.J.Physiol. 272:H1826-H1832.
Gray RA, Jalife J, Panfilov AV, Baxter WT, Cabo C, Davidenko JM, Pertsov
    AM 1995. Mechanisms of cardiac fibrillation. Science 270:1222-1223.
Gray RA, Pertsov AM, Jalife J 1998. Spatial and temporal organization during
    cardiac fibrillation. Nature 392:75-78.
Gros D, Jarry-Guichard T, ten V, I, de Maziere A, van Kempen MJ, Davoust J,
    Briand JP, Moorman AF, Jongsma HJ 1994. Restricted distribution of
    connexin40, a gap junctional protein, in mammalian heart. Circ.Res.
    74:839-851.
Horvath G, Goldberger JJ, Kadish AH 2000 Simultaneous occurrence of atrial
    fibrillation and atrial flutter. J.Cardiovasc.Electrophysiol. 11:849-858.
Jalife J, Morley GE, Tallini NY, Vaidya D 1998. A fungal metabolite that
    eliminates motion artifacts. J.Cardiovasc.Electrophysiol. 9:1358-1362.
Jalife J. 2000 Ventricular fibrillation: mechanisms of initiation and maintenance.
    Annual Review of Physiology 62:25-50.
Kaab S, Nuss HB, Chiamvimonvat N, O'Rourke B, Pak PH, Kass DA, Marban
    E, Tomaselli GF 1996   Ionic mechanism of action potential
    prolongation in ventricular myocytes from dogs with pacing-induced
    heart failure. Circ.Res.78:262-273.
Karma A 1994. Electrical alternans and spiral wave breakup in cardiac tissue.
    Chaos 4:461-472.
Karma A 2000. New paradigm for drug therapies of cardiac fibrillation.
    Proc.Natl.Acad.Sci.U.S.A. 97:5687-5689.
Krinskii VI 1966 Excitation propagation in nonhomogenous medium (actions
    analogous to heart fibrillation). Biofizika 11:676-683.
Krinsky VI 1978. Mathematical models of cardiac arrhythmias (spiral waves).
    Pharmacology & Therapeutics - Part B: General & Systematic
    Pharmacology 3:539-555.
Krinsky,VI. 1984. Self-Organization: Autowaves and Structures Far from
    Equilibrium. Springer, Berlin.
Lewis, T (1925). The mechanism and graphic registration of the heart beat.
    Shaw & Sons, London.
Li D, Zhang L, Kneller J, Nattel S 2001. Potential ionic mechanism for
    repolarization differences between canine right and left atrium. Circ
    Res 88:1168-1175.

Mandapati R, Skanes A, Chen J, Berenfeld O, Jalife J 2000. Stable microreentrant sources as a mechanism of atrial fibrillation in the isolated sheep heart. Circulation 101:194-199.

Mansour MC, Mandapati R, Berenfeld O, Chen J, Samie FH, Jalife J. 2001 Left-to-right gradient of atrial frequencies during acute atrial fibrillation in the isolated sheep heart. Circulation 103:2631-2636.

McWilliam JA 1887. Fibrillar contraction of the heart. Journal of Physiology 8:296-310.

Mines GR 1914. On circulating excitation on heart muscles and their possible relation to tachycardia and fibrillation. Trans.R.Soc.Can 4:43-53.

Moe GK 1962. On the multiple wavelet hypothesis of atrial fibrillation. Archives Internationales de Pharmacodynamie et de Therapie CXL:183-188.

Moe GK, Rheinboldt WC, Abildskov JA 1964. A computer model of atrial fibrillation. American Heart Journal 67:200-220.

Morillo CA, Klein GJ, Jones DL, Guiraudon CM 1995 Chronic rapid atrial pacing: Structural, functional, and electrophysiological characteristics of a new model of sustained atrial fibrillation. Circulation 91:1588-1595.

Myerburg,RJ, Castellanos,A 1997. Cardiac arrest and sudden cardiac death. In: Heart Disease: A Textbook of Cardiovascular Medicine. Braunwald,E, ed. W.B. Saunders, Philadelphia, PA.

Nattel S 2002 New ideas about atrial fibrillation 50 years on. Nature 415:219-226.

Nattel S, Khairy P, Schram G 2001. Arrhythmogenic ionic remodeling: adaptive responses with maladaptive consequences. Trends Cardiovasc.Med. 11:295-301.

Papageorgiou P, Monahan K, Boyle NG, Seifert MJ, Beswick P, Zebede J, Epstein LM, Josephson ME 1996. Site-dependent intra-atrial conduction delay. Relationship to initiation of atrial fibrillation. Circulation 94:384-389.

Pertsov AM, Emarkova EA, Panfilov AV 1984. Rotating spiral waves in modified FitzHugh-Nagumo model. Physica D 14:117-124.

Power JM, Beacom GA, Alferness CA, Raman J, Wijffels M, Farish SJ, Burrell LM, Tonkin AM 1998. Susceptibility to atrial fibrillation: a study in an ovine model of pacing-induced early heart failure. J Cardiovasc. Electrophysiol. 9:423-435.

Qu Z, Kil J, Xie F, Garfinkel A, Weiss JN 2000. Scroll wave dynamics in a three-dimensional cardiac tissue model: roles of restitution, thickness, and fiber rotation. Biophys.J 78:2761-2775.

Qu Z, Weiss JN, Garfinkel A 1999. Cardiac electrical restitution properties and stability of reentrant spiral waves: a simulation study. Am.J Physiol 276:H269-H283.

Qu Z, Xie F, Garfinkel A, Weiss JN 2000. Origins of spiral wave meander and breakup in a two-dimensional cardiac tissue model. Ann.Biomed.Eng 28:755-771.

Rockman HA, Koch WJ, Lefkowitz RJ 1997 Cardiac function in genetically engineered mice with altered adrenergic receptor signaling. Am.J Physiol 272:H1553-H1559.

Rogers JM, Ideker RE 2000. Fibrillating myocardium : rabbit warren or beehive? Circ.Res. 86:369-370.

Rozenshtraukh LV, Zaitsev AV, Pertsov AM, Fast VG, Krinskii VI 1988. The mechanism of the development of atrial tachyarrhythmia after stimulation of the vagus nerve. Kardiologiia 28:79-84.

Samie FH, Berenfeld O, Anumonwo J, Mironov SF, Udassi S, Beaumont J, Taffet S, Jalife J 2001. Rectification of the Background Potassium Current: A Determinant of Rotor Dynamics in Ventricular Fibrillation. Circ Res 89:1216-1223.

Samie FH, Mandapati R, Gray RA, Watanabe Y, Zuur C, Beaumont J, Jalife J 2000. A mechanism of transition from ventricular fibrillation to tachycardia: Effect of calcium channel blockade on the dynamics of rotating waves. Circ.Res. 86:684-691.

Scherf D, Romano FJ, Terranova R 1958. Experimental Studies on auricular flutter and auricular fibrillation. Am. Heart J 36:241-255.

Schuessler RB, Grayson TM, Bromberg BI, Cox JL, Boineau JP 1992. Cholinergically mediated tachyarrhythmias induced by a single extrastimulus in the isolated canine right atrium. Circ.Res. 71:1254-1267.

Sharifov OF, Fedorov VV, Beloshapko GG, Yushmanova AV, Rosenshtraukh LV 2001. Effects of E047/1, a new antiarrhythmic drug, on experimental atrial fibrillation in anesthetized dogs. J Cardiovasc. Pharmacol. 38:706-714.

Sih HJ, Berbari EJ, Zipes DP 1997. Epicardial maps of atrial fibrillation after linear ablation lesions. J.Cardiovasc.Electrophysiol. 8:1046-1054.

Skanes AC, Mandapati R, Berenfeld O, Davidenko JM, Jalife J 1998. Spatiotemporal periodicity during atrial fibrillation in the isolated sheep heart. Circulation 98:1236-1248.

Starmer CF, Romashko DN, Reddy RS, Zilberter YI, Starobin J, Grant AO, Krinsky VI 1995. Proarrhythmic response to potassium channel blockade. Numerical studies of polymorphic tachyarrhythmias. Circulation 92:595-605.

Tieleman RG, De Langen C, Van Gelder IC, de Kam PJ, Grandjean J, Bel KJ, Wijffels MC, Allessie MA, Crijns HJ 1997 Verapamil reduces tachycardia-induced electrical remodeling of the atria. Circulation 95:1945-1953.

Van Wagoner DR, Pond AL, Lamorgese M, Rossie SS, McCarthy PM, Nerbonne JM 1999. Atrial L-type Ca2+ currents and human atrial fibrillation. Circ.Res. 85:428-436.

Van Wagoner DR, Pond AL, McCarthy PM, Trimmer JS, Nerbonne JM 1997 Outward K^+ current densities and Kv1.5 expression are reduced in chronic human atrial fibrillation. Circ.Res. 80:772-781.

Weiner N, Rosenblueth A 1946. The mathematical formulation of the problem of conduction of impulses in a network of connected excitable elements, specifically in cardiac muscle. Arch. Inst. Cardiol. Mex 16:205-265.

Wellner-Kienitz MC, Bender K, Pott L 2001. Overexpression of beta 1 and beta 2 adrenergic receptors in rat atrial myocytes. Differential coupling to G protein-gated inward rectifier K(+) channels via G(s) and G(i)/o. J Biol.Chem.276:37347-37354.

Wijffels MC, Kirchhof CJ, Dorland R, Allessie MA 1995. Atrial fibrillation begets atrial fibrillation. A study in awake chronically instrumented goats. Circulation 92:1954-1968.

Winterberg H. Studien über Herzflimmern 1907. I. Über die Wirkung des N. vagus und accelerans auf das Flimmern des Herzens. Pflügers Arch. Physiol. 117:223-256.

Witkowski FX, Kavanagh KM, Penkoske PA, Plonsey R, Spano ML, Ditto WL, Kaplan DT 1995. Evidence for determinism in ventricular fibrillation. Phys.Rev.Lett. 75:1230-1233.

Wolf PA, Abbot RD, Kannel WB 1991. Atrial fibrillation as an independent risk factor for stroke: the Framingham Study. Stroke 22:983-988.

Workman AJ, Kane KA, Rankin AC 2001 The contribution of ionic currents to changes in refractoriness of human atrial myocytes associated with chronic atrial fibrillation. Cardiovasc.Res 52:226-235.

Zaitsev AV, Berenfeld O, Mironov SF, Jalife J, Pertsov AM 2000. Distribution of excitation frequencies on the epicardial and endocardial surfaces of fibrillating ventricular wall of the sheep heart. Circ.Res. 86:408-417.

Zhang LM, Wang Z, Nattel S 2002 Effects of sustained beta-adrenergic stimulation on ionic currents of cultured adult guinea pig cardiomyocytes. Am.J Physiol Heart Circ.Physiol 282:H880-H889.

Zhou Z, Gong Q, Ye B, Fan Z, Makielski JC, Robertson GA, January CT 1998. Properties of HERG channels stably expressed in HEK 293 cells studied at physiological temperature. Biophys.J 74:230-241.

14

GAP JUNCTIONS, CARDIAC EXCITABILITY AND CLINICAL ARRHYTHMIAS

Morton F. Arnsdorf, M.D.[1] **and Peter J. Lee, M.D., Ph.D.**[2]
Prtizker School of Medicine, University of Chicago and Section of Cardiology, University of Illinois Chicago

INTRODUCTION

The explosive growth in our understanding of cellular electrophysiology and the relationship to clinical arrhythmias continues, and much of the basic science that concerns the role of gap junctions in arrhythmias has been reviewed in other chapters in this book. The purpose of this chapter is to create an intellectual framework for the clinician that is based on biophysical theory, and to allow the researcher who is not a physician an insight into clinical thought processes.

The concept of cardiac excitability is vague to most clinicians. Intuitively, cardiac excitability brings to mind the ability of heart cells regeneratively to depolarize and repolarize during the action potential and to activate the heart in a sequence that assures a proper cardiac output. The next level of understanding includes cellular characteristics such as ionic channels, the manner in which cells communicate with each other through gap junctions, and anisotropy of conduction that results from a difference in physical properties of the heart that preferentially favors conduction in one direction over another.

The interplay of biophysical theory, prediction experiment and refined theory has been a successful paradigm for the advancement of our understanding. In an earlier and more technical publication, we stressed that the practical use of biophysical theory is to support predictions of how a system under study might respond to new contingencies (Ginsburg, Anrsdorf, 1995). Examples were that these predictions could be long term, for instance, of the risk for sudden cardiac death, or short term, as in the reconstruction of the action potential from currents identified and manipulated by voltage-clamping. The results derived from these predictions themselves become new hypotheses for experimental testing. Faster computers have allowed the development, testing, modification and application of increasingly more refined theoretical models, as in the fascinating application of nonlinear dynamics (Kovacs, 1991) and the development of models, such as that provided by Dr. Rudy in his chapter in this book. Increasingly, such models will be used to create and test hypotheses.

Physicians, who often lack the background to develop and even understand such models, are the experts in developing questions that deal with clinical problems and, therefore, are a necessary link to the researcher. The relationship between gap junctions and cardiac arrhythmias is *terra incognita* for most physicians. The physician, then, needs an intellectual framework for discussing complex topics that can be translated by the latter into hypotheses, experiments, and finally clinical application. The non-physician researcher, in turn, needs a bridge to the bedside.

ELECTROPHYSIOLOGIC MATRICAL CONCEPT OF CARDIAC EXCITABILITY

Inputs and Outputs: Linearities and Nonlinearities

Biophysical systems have inputs (stimuli) and outputs (Reponses), which exist in time and are organized in space and are subject to controlling or influencing feedback systems. The relationship between inputs and outputs may be linear or nonlinear, continuous or discontinuous. The relationship is linear when a stimulus produces a proportional output. For example, a step change in voltage across a resistor as described by Ohm's Law ($V = IR$, where V is voltage, I is current and R is resistance) results in proportional current output; 1 volt changes over a 1 ohm resister produces a continuous set of 1 ampere responses. Even a more complex function such as decremental conduction through cable-like tissues can be described using linear differential equations. The response of a linear system to periodic inputs always has the same periodicities as the input.

Most biological systems, however, are *nonlinear* in that a stimulus produces a disproportional response; for example, the explosive regenerative response of the action potential on the attainment of threshold in response to a small step increase in intracellular current. The subthreshold responses in transmembrane voltage to steps in intracellular current injection may be fairly continuous until threshold is attained when there is a sudden *discontinuous* response to the same magnitude stimulus.

The nonlinear nature of a system is frequently evident. The response may have features inconsistent with the idea of proportional responses to stimuli (Goldberger, Rigney, 1991) including, for example, bifurcations (Denton et al, 1990), bistability (Landau et al, 1990) and hysteresis (Lorente, Davidenko, 1990). In bifurcations, the character of the response evolves in time, or as a parameter is changed, in a specific sequence; and one of us has suggested that bifurcations, particularly those assisted by conditions, occur commonly in clinical electrophysiology, and that this is an important principle in arrhythmogenesis and in the actions of antiarrhythmic drugs (Arnsdorf et al 1985, Arnsdorf, Sawicki 1996, among others, reviewed in Arnsdorf, Makielki 2001). Bistable systems are characterized by a given stimulus leading to two or more kinds of response; for example, a propagated response and the initiation of triggered activity. In hysteresis, the response after a stimulus has reached some fixed amplitude differs, depending on how fast and/or in what direction the stimulus had been changed previously in the course of reaching that amplitude. The response of a nonlinear system to a periodic input the response may include harmonic and/or subharmonic frequencies, or can fall in arbitrary ratios (N:M) of integers, with respect to the input period.

Gap Junctions, The Electrophysiologic Matrix, and Assisted Bifurcations

Cardiac excitability has a certain intuitive meaning suggesting the ease with which cardiac cells undergo individual and sequential regenerative depolarization and repolarization, communicate with each other, and propagate electrical activity in a normal and abnormal manner. The heart beat arises from a highly organized control of ionic flow through channels in the cardiac membrane, the myoplasm, the gap junctions between cells and the extracellular space. These bioelectric events are regulated within very tight limits to allow the coordinated propagation of excitation and contraction of the heart that is necessary for an efficient cardiac output. In theory, the relationship between the cellular organization of gap junctions and the conduction of impulses importantly determines the activation pattern of the myocardium. This has been demonstrated for impulse propagation in the postnatal terminal crest of neonatal, weanling, and adult rabbits (Spach, Heidlage 1995) and in neonatal and adult canine ventricular muscle (Spach et al, 2000). Abnormalities in the regulatory mechanisms often accompany cardiac disease.

Conceptually, cardiac excitability can be thought of as resulting from the action and interactions of an electrophysiologic matrix of cellular properties. The normal matrix must be altered by arrhythmogenic influences which affect one or more components of excitability to produce abnormal excitability, and the interaction between the matrix altered by an arrhythmogenic influence and an antiarrhythmic drug creates yet another matrix that hopefully is antiarrhythmic or antifibrillatory, but which may be proarrhythmic. The matrical antifibrillatory, but which may be proarrhythmic. The matrical concept we have proposed previously (Arnsdorf et al 1985, Arnsdorf, Sawicki 1996, among others, reviewed in Arnsdorf, Makielki 2001) describes the essentially nonlinear character of cardiac excitability and propagation in a way that is intuitive to the physiologist and hopefully the clinician without requiring explicit mathematical equations, but since they are system parameters, also have mathematical relationships.

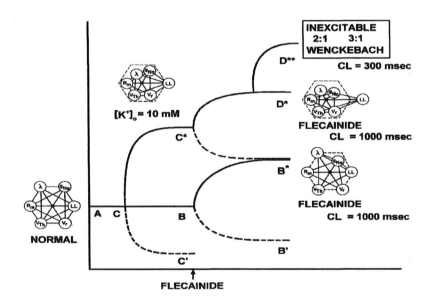

Figure 1 Bifurcation diagram of the electrophysiologic matrices obtained from data in this study. The major points made in the text are that electrophysiologic changes occur as a system, such change may be antiarrhythmic or proarrhythmic, often there is little difference in the antiarrhythmic and proarrhythmic matrix, and the predominant effect of a drug depends on the matrix encountered. See text for discussion. Reproduced with permission from Arnsdorf and Sawicki (1996).

Figure 1 is a bifurcation diagram of the electrophysiologic matrices obtained from data in a recent cellular electrophysiologic study on the interactions between changes in extracellular potassium concentration, $[K^+]_o$, and flecainide (Arnsdorf, Sawicki 1996). The matrix, labeled "Normal" is at a physiologic $[K^+]_o$ and has a regular hexagonal shape indicative of a normal state. In subsequent examples, abnormal states, presumably the arrhythmogenic matrical configurations, are represented by matrices of irregular polygonal shape. The bonds between the matrix elements show the interactions and mutual dependencies. This matrix includes the resting potential (V_r), threshold voltage (V_{th}), Na^+ conductance (g_{Na}), membrane resistance (R_m), the length constant (λ), and, as a measure of overall excitability, the liminal length (LL), all of which will be defined below. There are many other determinants that could have been included in this depiction, but these have been chosen for simplicity. The matrix is a shorthand way of delineating complex interactions. The interactions, however, are dynamic. The interactions, then, are not constant but vary between homeostatic limits.

The interaction between the antiarrhythmic drug flecainide and the normal matrix at point B results in a new matrix at B^*, which in this experiment was largely unchanged except for a slight decrease in sodium conductance indicated by g_{Na} moving towards the center of the hexagon. Hyperkalemia alone, in contrast, caused multiple electrophysiologic changes in both active and passive properties and drove the equilibrium from C to a new equilibrium at point C^* characterized by decreases in R_m, λ, V_{th}, V_r, and g_{Na}. Hyperkalemia consistently produced this type of matrical configuration and was responsible for what is termed an *assisted bifurcation* that consistently moved the system from point A to point C^*.

If the tissue with the electrophysiologic matrix created by hyperkalemia at C^* was exposed to flecainide, a second bifurcation occurred leading to the equilibrium at D^*. Further bifurcations occur that depended on the rate of stimulation resulting in a situation at point D^{**} in which the liminal length requirements were either not met resulting in inexcitability or were met intermittently resulting in a 2:1

or some other excitable response. Note how similar the matrical configurations are after the "arrhythmogenic" intervention of increasing $[K^+]_o$ and after the application of flecainide, suggesting a narrow toxic to therapeutic ratio. The dashed lines represent paths that might be taken were another drug used (B'), were $[K^+]_o$ lowered below 5.4 mM (C'), or were $[K^+]_o$ returned from 10 mM to 5.4 mM in the presence of flecainide (C^* to B^*). The matrix has many more dimensions than are shown here, as there are many more ionic channels including gap junctions and each element, in turn, is determined by underlying properties, such as ion channel conductances. The active (source) and passive (sink) properties, which form the elements of the matrix, are not usually independent of each other. For

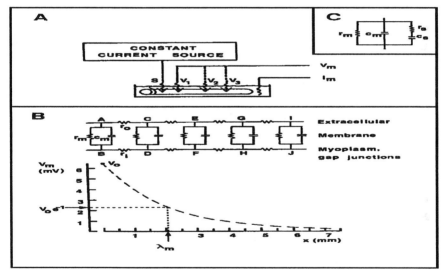

Figure 2. A. Experimental arrangement for cable analysis. The stimulus is the stepwise application of a constant current that is injected intracellularly through a microelectrode located near the ligated end of a cardiac Purkinje fiber (S). The response is a change in the transmembrane voltage (V_m) recorded by microelectrodes at several points along the preparation (V_1, V_2, V_3, etc.). The transmembrane stimulating current (I_m) is monitored via the bath ground. B, an electrical analogue for a cable-like preparation is shown at the top of this panel and includes membrane resistance (r_m), membrane capacitance (c_m), internal longitudinal resistance (r_i) due to the effects of the myoplasm and gap junctions and external resistance (r_o) due to the extracellular space. At the bottom of the panel, transmembrane voltage is plotted as a function of distance (x) in the steady state after intracellular current application.

depicted parameters. For the sake of discussion, let us focus on two of these parameters, the length or space constant (λ) and the liminal length (LL).

The *length* or *space* constant (λ) is a measure that expresses the extent of influence of the electrotonic wavefront that precedes the action potential. Figure 2A shows the experimental arrangement for cable analysis. The stimulus consists of a sudden injection of intracellular current (S) through a microelectrode near the ligated end of a cardiac Purkinje fiber, and the response to the change in transmembrane voltage (V_m) is recorded at several points along the preparation. The stimulating current, I_m, is monitored via the bath ground. An electrical analog for a cable-like preparation, showing membrane resistance (r_m), membrane capacitance (c_m), internal longitudinal resistance (r_i) due to the myoplasm and gap junctions, and external resistance (r_o) due to the extracellular space, is shown in the upper portion of Figure 2B. Panel C is an analog that represents membrane behavior more accurately by inclusion of series elements r_s and c_s in addition to r_m and c_m. Returning to panel B, below the electrical analog is plotted V_m as a function of distance between the stimulating and the recording microelectrodes (x) in steady state after intracellular current application. The arrow marks length constant, λ, which is defined as $V_o e^{-1}$, where V_o is the voltage at the point of stimulation. Note again, the exponential fall of the voltage. It is this electrotonic voltage that fulfils or fails to fulfill the requirements for the next patch of membrane to attain threshold and produce a regenerative action potential.

$\lambda = \sqrt{r_m/(r_i+r_o)}$ or, when r_o can be neglected, $\lambda = \sqrt{r_m/r_i}$. R_m depends on the integrity of the cell membrane, and r_i depends primarily on the state of the gap junctions linking the cell. An increase in r_i, then, as may occur with the closing of gap junctions secondary to injury will decrease λ.

Liminal length (LL) is the amount of tissue that must be raised above threshold so that the inward depolarizing current from that patch of membrane exceeds the repolarizing influences of adjacent tissues and results in an action potential. If the local electrotonic currents are sufficient to fulfill the liminal length requirements of the neighboring patch or patches of membrane, these patches will also produce action potentials. These events repeat and the sequential depolarization of patches of membrane results. If the liminal length of a patch is not fulfilled, this patch and its neighboring tissue will not be activated. The concept of liminal length was first proposed by Hodgkin and Rushton in nerve (Hodgkin, Rushton, 1946), and subsequently by Fozzard and his coworkers in cardiac Purkinje fibers (Dominguez. Fozzard, 1970; Fozzard, 1972). Liminal length can be well-approximated by the relation:

$$\frac{0.855 Q_{th}}{2 \left(\pi \right)^{3/2} a \, C_m \, \lambda \, V_{th}}$$

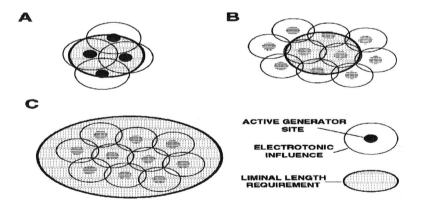

Figure 3 Schematic representation of the liminal length concept. Panel A: The black circles represent active generator sites, the circle surrounding each is the electrotonic influence of the generator, the stippled area is the amount of tissue required to be raised above threshold to provide activation current sufficient to overcome the repolarizing currents of neighboring cells, and the white areas represent the excess in source of sink. B. The strength of the active generator site (grey circles) and the distance of the electrotonic currents (smaller circles) are decreased. More active generator sites must be recruited to attain the liminal length requirements (white area), and the excess of source to sink is less than in panel A. A further increase in the liminal length from whatever cause will render the tissue inexcitable. See text for discussion. Reproduced with permission from Arnsdorf and Sawicki (1996).

where Q_{th} is the charge threshold, a is the radius, C_m is the membrane capacitance, λ is the length constant and V_{th} is the voltage threshold. As discussed in the previous paragraph, an increase in r_i will decrease λ which, in turn, will increase the liminal length thereby decreasing cardiac excitability. A decrease in r_i will have the opposite effect on liminal length and cardiac excitability. As we have discussed in some detail, the action potential can be considered a local membrane event and the fulfillment of the liminal length requirement by the local circuit currents can be considered the propagated event (Arnsdorf, Sawicki, 1996).

A schematic representation of the liminal length concept and the interplay between the active generator properties and the electronic influence is shown in Figure 3. In panel A, the black circles represent active generator sites (e.g., sodium channels), the circle surrounding each is the electrotonic influence of the generator, the stippled area is the amount of tissue required to be raised above threshold to provide activation current sufficient to overcome the repolarizing currents of neighboring cells, and the white areas represent the excess in source over sink. In panel B, the strength of the active generator site (gray circles) and the distance of the electrotonic currents (smaller circles) are decreased. More active generator sites must be recruited to attain the liminal length requirements (stippled area), and the excess of source to sink is less than in panel A. A further increase in the liminal length from whatever cause will render the tissue inexcitable (panel C).

Returning again to Figure 1, the idea of the bifurcation diagram is that it shows the transition from one equilibrium to another. If conditions favor taking one path to a new equilibrium rather than another, this is called an *assisted* bifurcation. The bifurcations depicted reflect a set of experiments in which $[K]_0$ was varied in controls and after exposure of cardiac Purkinje fibers to flecainide (Arnsdorf, Sawicki, 1996). Point A is the normal dynamic equilibrium shown as a normal matrix. The interaction between flecainide and the normal matrix at point B resulted in a new matrix at B*, which in this experiment was largely unchanged except for a slight decrease in sodium conductance. Hyperkalemia alone drove the equilibrium primarily upward from C to a new equilibrium at point C*. Hyperkalemia, then, was responsible for an *assisted bifurcation* that consistently drove the system from point A to point C*.

If the tissue with the electrophysiologic matrix created by hyperkalemia at C* was exposed to flecainide, a second bifurcation occurs led to the equilibrium at D*. Further bifurcations occurred that depended on the rate of stimulation resulting in a situation at point D** in which the liminal length requirements were not met resulting in inexcitability or were met intermittently resulting in a 2:1 or some other response. Note how similar the matrical configurations were after the "arrhythmogenic" intervention of increasing $[K^+]_o$ and after the application of flecainide, suggesting a narrow toxic to therapeutic ratio. The dashed lines represent paths that might be taken were another drug used (B'), were $[K^+]_o$ lowered below 5.4 mM (C'), or were $[K^+]_o$ returned from 10 mM to 5.4 mM in the presence of flecainide (C* to B*).Changes in gap junctional conductance that would increase liminal length and decrease □ as discussed above would result in a matrical configuration similar to that seen at D*, except that g_{Na} would not be reduced and V_r would likely remain unaffected. Although not experimentally tested, our presumption is that a decrease in gap junctional conductance would produce an assisted bifurcation that routinely would result in a matrical configuration. Complete closure of the gap junctions would tend to render the tissue inexcitable unless some other type of cell-cell communication were present (e.g., some type of capacitative coupling).

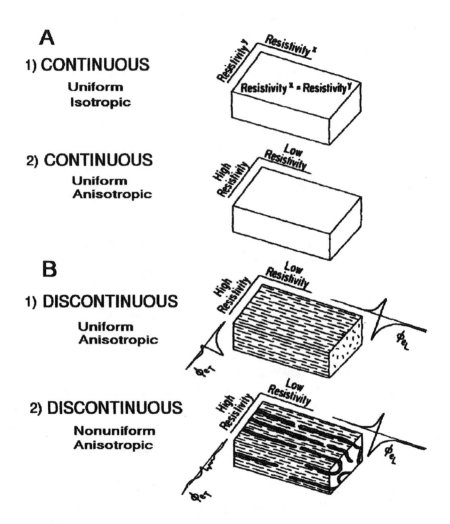

A

1) CONTINUOUS

**Uniform
Isotropic**

2) CONTINUOUS

**Uniform
Anisotropic**

B

1) DISCONTINUOUS

**Uniform
Anisotropic**

2) DISCONTINUOUS

**Nonuniform
Anisotropic**

Figure 4 Characteristics of tissues viewed as conductive media supporting propagation. A1: Medium whose resistivity is constant and the same in all directions. A2: Medium whose resistivity is constant in a given direction but differs in different directions. B1: Medium with discrete impedances, such as high-resistance junctions, in the transverse direction. The resistivity is not constant, but the distribution of these impedances is similar throughout the medium. B2: Medium with irregularly arranged discrete transverse barriers. Transverse propagation can occur simultaneously via multiple paths. ϕ_e symbolizes extracellularly recorded potentials (Spach et al 1990).

THE CONTROL OF GAP JUNCTIONS

The control of gap junctions has been an important part of many Chapters in this book. A few points, however, are particularly important to provide the bridge between basic science and the clinical domain. The work of Heidenheim around the turn of the century (Heidenheim, 1901) led to the idea that the heart was an anatomical and electrical syncytium. This conflicted with the earlier physiologic observations of Engelmann (1875,1877} who noted a decline in injury current and a sealing off of cells after injury to the frog heart. When Engelmann cut the heart with scissors, the cells at the cut surface became inexcitable while those at a short distance remained excitable. Moreover, the injury current after the cut decreased with time. Small myocardial segments, connected by bridges of intact tissue, could be stimulated at any point, and stimulation at any point caused contraction throughout the entire preparation. Microscopically, Engelmann could not detect nerves connecting the cells and concluded that the impulse was conducted from one cell to the next. Cells in health tissue were connected electrically with others, but cell injury and death resulted in a sealing off of the normal from the injured or dead cells. This led to Engelmann's famous dictum that "Cells live together but die singly".

The electron microscopic studies of Sjöstrand and Anderson (1954) described the intercalated disk and showed that cardiac cells were bound by membranes without any direct cytoplasmic connection between cells. The structure responsible for intercellular communication is the gap junction. Connexins group to form a hexameric structure containing a central pore. This structure is termed a connexon or hemichannel. A working gap junctional channel is formed when a connexon in one cell becomes localized in a cell membrane and matches sterically with a connexon from a neighboring cell. How this coupling of hemichannels is driven to occur is unknown.

Aspects of gap junctional control were summarized in our review (Ginsburg, Anrsdorf, 1995) and are considered in depth in this book. To briefly summarize, gap junctional conductance may be nearly ohmic or, under some conditions, can be voltage-dependent. We have suggested that voltage-dependency may be important in poorly coupled cells, and perhaps this voltage-dependency "fine-tunes" cell-cell communication in injury (Lal, Arnsdorf, 1992). Gap junctional conductance can be modified by transients in internal calcium concentration and/or pH, the presence of lipophiles, arachidonic acid pathway intermediates, hypoxia, strophanthidin, hypertonicity and other changes that may be part of the ischemic process or therapeutic intervention. Many other factors are likely involved in cell-cell communication. For example, the angiotensin renal system seems to be important in regulating cell-cell communication (see review (De Mello, Danser, 2000). Angiotensin II can decrease gap junctional conductance within seconds (De Mello, Altieri, 1992; De Mello, 1996), an action that can be countered by the ARII blocker losartan and ACE inhibitors such as enalapril. The specific distribution of gap junctions becomes less organized in injury. There may also be tissue specific differences in the density and distribution of gap junctions. The distribution in SA nodal tissue, atria, the AV node, Purkinje fibers, and ventricular muscle differs and may well play an important role in physiologic regulation. We are only beginning to learn about the assembly of connexins into channels and the degradation of these structures (see review (Saffitz et al, 2000). The turnover of cardiac connexins is surprisingly rapid with half-lives of 1 to 5 hours. This has led to some work studying the intracellular pathways responsible for degradation of gap junction proteins, and the proteasome and lysosome both are involved in Cx43 degradation. It is interesting to speculate that synthesis and perhaps as or more importantly, degradation, adjust cardiac cell-cell coupling in health and disease. As will be discussed below, the distribution of gap junctions seem to be important in creating the substrate for reentrant arrhythmias.

CLINICAL EXTRAPOLATIONS

Gap junctions play a number of roles in health and disease. Although often characterized as a "passive" cellular property, as discussed, gap junctions close in response to a number of stimuli, environmental changes and, in poorly communicating cells, to voltage. We will consider clinical extrapolations of gap junctional function in three areas related to arrhythmogenesis and the actions of certain drugs: (1) integrative functions, (2) anisotropy, and (3) the isolation of injured cells.

Integrative Functions

Excitability

The concept of liminal length has been introduced earlier as has the contribution of gap junctions to the determinants of the liminal length. An intuitive definition is the liminal length amount of tissue that must be raised above threshold so that the inward depolarizing current from that patch of membrane exceeds the repolarizing influences of adjacent tissues and results in an action potential.

Although the term is not often used, liminal length and excitability is critically important in the design and use of cardiac pacemakers. Only one publication has attempted to relate current thresholds and liminal length using disc electrodes of various sizes, the experimental findings corresponded closely to the theoretical calculations (Lindemans et al, 1978).

If our argument is correct that the action potential is the local event and the fulfillment of the liminal length requires is the propagated event, the clinical importance of this concept becomes apparent. Quite possibly the dysfunction or failure of normal pacemakers (e.g., SA nodal arrest or SA nodal block), deviations from preferential conduction, abnormalities of impulse propagation and other electrophysiologic events that relate to excitability are determined, in part, by abnormalities of the gap junctions.

Excitability depends importantly on cell-cell communication. A number of the regulatory mechanisms of cell-cell communication are discussed in this and in other chapters. Without doubt, connexin synthesis, degradation, assembly into channels, distribution, conductances, and open-probability times are important determinants of excitability in normal and pathophysiolgic situations. Partial and complete cellular uncoupling occurs in ischemia. Disease states may cause a redistribution of gap junctions. This will be discussed in more detail later in this Chapter, but, as an example, disturbed Cx43 gap junction distribution correlates with the location of reentrant circuits at the border of infarct zones in the dog (Peters et al, 1997), and down-regulation of Cx43 expression and loss of the largest gap junctions have been noted in the hibernating myocardium of patients with chronic heart failure (Keprielan et al, 1998).

Automaticity

The mechanism of automaticity in the SA node is not fully understood, but it seems to arise from a changing balance between positive inward currents which favor depolarization and positive outward currents which favor repolarization: the depolarizing inward current being primarily a calcium current and the outward repolarizing currents primarily potassium currents.

Entrainment can be defined as the coupling of a self-sustaining oscillatory system to an external forcing oscillation with the result that either both oscillations have the same frequency or the frequencies are related in a harmonic fashion (Michaels et al, 1993). The concept of electrotonic interactions and entrainment among cells is difficult, but will is very important to our thinking about clinical arrhythmias. As will be discussed below, entrainment is used clinically to interrupt reentrant rhythms. In this case, the self-sustaining oscillatory system is the cycle length of the applied extrastimuli that forces the circus movement to assume the same cycle length.

Cardiac pacemaker rhythms may be synchronized to a variety of external periodicities including cellular and vagal stimulation (Guevara et al, 1981;Jalife, Moe, 1979;Jalife et al 1983;levy et al, 1969). Brief nature of perturbations in cardiac pacemaker activity indicates that the sensitivity to the perturbation varies periodically (see review (Michaels et al, 1983)). A periodic perturbing input, such as a pacemaker cell of electrical stimulation, can influence a second pacemaker to discharge at rates that are faster or slower than its intrinsic rate.

Bleeker et al (1980) used correlative morphologic and electrophysiologic approaches to assess the functional and morphological organization of the rabbit SA node. They found that there is a dominant pacemaker region rather than a dominant cell that is responsible for the automatic activity of the SA node. The compact portion of the SA node contains several thousand cells that depolarize and production action potentials almost synchronously. All these cells seem to be influencing each other through cell-to-cell coupling, a process that has been called *mutual entrainment* (Winfree, 1980). The entrainment may be 1:1 or some harmonic of the underlying, basic frequency. Jalife and Michaels (1985) list the requisites for mutual entrainment as follows: (1) there must be some form of communication that allows for mutual interaction between pacemakers; (2) the response of any given pacemaker to perturbations by its neighbor(s) must be phase-dependent; and (3) this phase-dependent response must have an advancing or delaying influence on its neighbor(s) so equality of periods can results. Jalife and his coworkers (Jalife, 1984) further suggested that the synchronization of cells is due not to the influence of a "dominant" pacemaker cell, but from the mutual interaction of many individual pacemaker cells that represented a "democratic consensus" as to when the cells should discharge.

The interactions between the vagus and the SA node have been reviewed recently (Jalife, Michaels, 1985). Brown and Eccles (1934) observed that the effects of brief bursts of vagal stimuli on the rate of the sinus pacemaker depended on the intensity and timing of the train Experimental and simulation studies suggest that the vagal control of the SA nodal rate can be explained by vagal input entraining the already mutually entrained pacemaker cells that are responsible for SA nodal pacemaker (Jalife, 1984; Michaels et al 1984;Mobley, Page, 1972;Michaels et al, 1989). In these studies and simulations, phase-locking, period-doubling bifurcations, and other characteristics were observed that suggested nonlinear or chaotic dynamics.

Normally, the integrated activity of pacemaker cells in the compact region of the SA node has the fastest rate and the most consistent pacemaker. This initiates the sequential depolarization of the atria, AV node, His-bundle branch-terminal Purkinje system, and ventricular muscle. The propagating impulse will activate the latent pacemaker cells before they can spontaneously depolarize sufficiently to produce an action potential. The latent pacemaker is then reset, and repetitive excitation of the pacemaker cell will actually inhibit spontaneous phase 4 depolarization. So long as the SA node remains the fastest pacemaker and conduction throughout the heart is intact, subsidiary pacemakers will be suppressed and the SA node will control the overall heart rate.

The electrotonic interaction between pacemaker and nonpacemaker cells due to current flow among cells through gap junctions favors the suppression of subsidiary or abnormal pacemakers. Wit and Rosen suggest that this mechanism may be important in suppressing automaticity in the AV node where atrial cells, which normally do not have pacemaker activity and which have resting potentials that are more negative than those of the AV nodal cells, creates a circuit with current flow between AV nodal and atrial cells that suppresses nodal automaticity. Similar interactions may occur where latent pacemaker cells are next to non-pacemaker cells such as in the atria or perhaps in areas where the terminal Purkinje fibers, which normally possess pacemaker activity, may be modulated by the greater mass of ventricular tissue that normally does not have pacemaker activity. It is interesting to speculate that normal non-pacemaker cells may suppress areas of abnormal automaticity as well.

Chronic or inappropriate nonparoxysmal sinus tachycardia occurs is an unusual condition that occurs in individuals without apparent heart disease or other causes for sinus tachycardia such as thyrotoxicosis, heart failure, anemia, fever, and infection (Bauernfeind et al 1979; Yee et al, 1984). Its cause is unknown, but it is thought to reflect a disorder of autonomic control. Some individuals, however, are quite resistant to pharmacologic interventions, and one might speculate that perhaps part of the "democratic" entrainment and subsequent modulation of the sinus rate is lost, the result being that more rapid pacemakers control the heart rate. The sinus node is a long complex distributed along the crista terminalis. Intracardiac echocardiography was used in dogs to define the crista terminalis and to localize the position of an ablation catheter relative to the sinus node, following which radiofrequency ablation could modify sinus pacemaker function (Kalman et al 1995). The same group then used the same approach to modify sinus node function in individuals with "inappropriate" sinus tachycardia (Lee et al, 1995). The region ablated was that showing the earliest atrial activation which, presumably, is the area of the SA node containing the fastest pacemakers. The result was a 25% reduction in the sinus heart rate, and it seems likely that that the fastest pacemaker cells were either ablated or otherwise physically separated from the remainder of the pacemaker complex and the atria. The remaining SA nodal cells then mutually entrained at a slower rate.

Parasystole can be modulated or at times annihilated by electronic interactions through gap junctions (see review (Castellanos et al, 1990). The rate of the parasystolic pacemaker will be slowed by entrainment with early non-parasystolic beats, while the rate of the pacemaker will be increased by entrainment with late non-parasystolic beats. Phase-response curves can be generated in some individuals. The modifying beats may result from a normal sinus rhythm or from any other type of rhythm. If there is an area of conduction block around the parasystolic focus, self-modulation can occur depending on the degree of block. Self-entrainment can also occur which may be responsible for alternating short-long cycles sometimes seen in ectopic ventricular tachycardia. In the laboratory, critically timed subthreshold depolarizations can annihilate an automatic focus, and possibly this type of pacemaker annihilation occurs clinically.

Integrated and Fragmented Wave-fronts in Impulse propagation

Normally, gap junctions allow electrotonic interactions that importantly integrate the wavefront. Given two neighboring cell columns in which one column conducts more rapidly than the other, the faster fiber through electrotonic interaction will speed up the slower fiber, and the slower fiber will slow down the faster fiber. The result is a unit of two columns, travelling at a uniform, intermediate speed. In the heart, many such interactions produce a smooth, integrated wavefront of activation that is responsible for the highly controlled and efficient contraction of the heart needed to maximize cardiac output. An integrated wavefront, moreover, is unlikely to produce reentry.

In the 8-week canine infarct, fractionated electrograms can be recorded from the surface of the infarct zone, yet action potentials recorded from myocytes within these zones are normal (Gardner et al, 1985;Urcell et al 1985). Pathological studies showed that the muscle fibers were widely separated and disoriented by connective tissues. The slow, fragmented activation that gave rise to the fractionated electrograms, therefore, was not due to changes in the active generator, but rather to disruption in the integrative electrotonic interaction between cells caused by fibrosis that physically disconnected the cells. This type of fragmented conduction is thought to be an important substrate for reentrant arrhythmias. It is these signals that are recorded by the signal-averaged electrocardiogram and are sought during ablation studies, so they are very important markers diagnostically and clinically.

Drifting and stationary electrical spiral waves are likely involved in arrhythmogenesis. Electrotonic interactions seems to be importantly involved in the genesis of such phenomenon. Using computer simulations based on a membrane model of the ventricular cell, the core of the rotating activity exerts a strong electrotonic influence that abbreviates the duration of the action potential and thereby the wave length in neighboring tissues which, in turn, stabilizes and perpetuates the spiral wave (Beaumont et al, 1998).

Anisotropy in Integrating Wavefronts and in Arrhythmogenesis

The concept of anisotropy has been considered in substantial detail in other Chapters in this book as well as in reviews (Ginsbner, Arnsdorf, 1995;Lesh et al, 1990; Spach, 1995; Keener, Panfilov 1995; Wikswo, 1995; Wit et al, 1995). In essence, anisotropy is a measured difference of a physical property related to the direction in which the measurement is made. Structural anisotropy is intrinsic to the structure of the myocardial tissue. This anisotropy can be a normal characteristic of tissues depending on the fiber axis and the normal distribution and functionality of gap junctions linking cells longitudinally and transversely. Anisotropy can be the result of disease; or, at times, it can be created with a therapeutic intention as is the case with radiofrequency ablation. Functional anisotropy can result from the establishment of lines of functional block. Much of what follows is speculation since it is difficult to study cellular coupling in man.

A few comments on what underlies anisotropy are in order. As a general statement, the velocity of impulse propagation is faster parallel to fiber orientation than perpendicular to orientation, and these velocities are termed longitudinal and transverse, respectively. Passive resistivity within and between cells depends on gap junctional connections and on geometry including tapering shape and bifurcations, and several of these influences have been elegantly modeled. Some studies have found a rough relationship between diameter and conduction velocity (Draper ,Mya-Tu, 1959), but others have found conduction velocity to be quite constant regardless of diameter, as in Purkinje fibers (Schoenberg et al 1995). Anisotropy within a fiber may explain in part the failure of conduction velocity to correlate with diameter in the Purkinje fiber (Pressler, 1984). In this situation, the local circuit currents at the edge of the propagating wave front preferentially flow longitudinally within a column of cells, and conduction velocity, then, would be independent of diameter if the "fiber size" was determined not by the size of the individual cells, but rather by the number of cells. The extracellular space also influences conduction. Another possible interpretation of the failure of conduction velocity to correlate with diameter in Purkinje fibers assumes that the extracellular clefts are more important in larger cells so that the effects of $(r_o + r_i)$ may be counter the influence of diameter. Goldstein and Rall (1974) modeled the change in conduction velocity in situations of changing fiber and geometry and found that with a step reduction in diameter, conduction velocity increases, with a step increase in diameter, conduction velocity decreases. This follows from the amount of current lost downstream in the sink. When branching was considered, the impulse approaching the branching site first decreased in velocity since the branches provided a larger sink, and, once beyond the junction and into a smaller branch, the conduction velocity increased. Interestingly, extracellular space anisotropy may be discordant directionally with intracellular anisotropy (Sepulveda et al, 1983).

Propagation through three-dimensional tissues is far more complex than one-dimensional propagation along cable-like fibers such as Purkinje fibers. To describe anisotropic propagation empirically on a macroscopic scale, Madison Spach and his colleagues proposed measurement of the effective axial resistivity, $\overline{R_a}$, which is the value of internal resistivity, in order to account for the observed speed of propagation along any direction, not just along the long axis of muscle fibers (Spach 1995; Spach et al, 1981; Spach et al, 1982). Unlike R_i in linear continuous cable theory, which incorporates only axial cytoplasmic resistivity and end-to-end GJ conductivity, $\overline{R_a}$ also includes implicitly the influences of cellular geometry and packing, extracellular resistivities, side-to-side couplings, and other features. Equations based on axial resistivity have successfully predicted propagation on a macroscopic scale (several mm or more), even along pathways of complex or heterogeneous structure. Excitation in young hearts spreads along smooth contours in directions off the long axis, indicating uniform anisotropy, but, in older preparations, the fast longitudinal path was narrow and had abrupt borders (Spach, Dolber, 1986;Spach et al, 1990). Off the long axis, excitation spread very slowly and in irregular or zig-zag fashion and often reached a trans-verse site multiphasically. This dissociation or fractionation indicates propagation by multiple paths, which could not occur in uniformly anisotropic tissue. Propagation with these features has been called discontinuous, dissociated microscopic, or fractionated (Spach, Dolber, 1986;Spach et al, 1988), and is seen frequently in the electrophysiology laboratory where fractionated potentials serve as a marker for ablation. Figures 4 through 6 summarize some of these concepts. Figure 4 shows the characteristics of tissue when viewed as a conductive medium supporting propagation. Figure 5 shows anisotropy of the action potential waveform and propagation velocity in the crista terminalis. Figure 6 shows nonuniform anisotropic propagation.

Anisotropic activation and propagation originate in large part with structural features of cardiac muscle. The fine structure of normal cardiac muscle suggest that myocytes form "unit" bundles of 2-15 cells that have connections every 0.1 mm to 0.2 mm which are

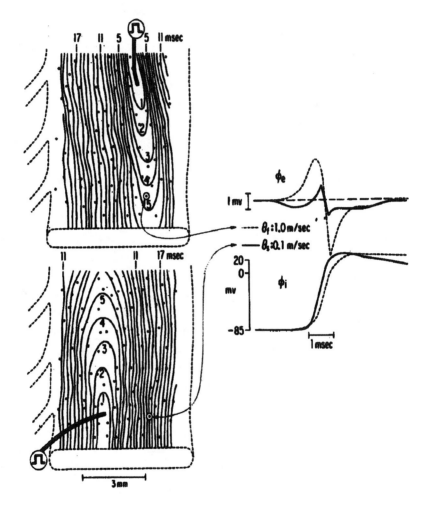

Figure 5 Anisotropy of AP waveform and propagation velocity Θ in the crista terminalis. Left: Points of stimulation are indicated by square pulses; dots indicate sites of extracellular recording. Right: Extracellular (ϕ_e) and intracellular (ϕ_i) potentials at the right were recorded at points (circled and arrowed) longitudinal (dotted traces) and transverse (solid traces) to a point of stimulation. dV/dt_{max} was higher and τ_{foot} was longer in the transverse direction. Isochrone maps (left), constructed from the extracellular recordings, indicate uniform anisotropy; conduction velocity, calculated as the distance traveled normal to an isochrone per unit time, was lower transversely, despite higher dV_m/dt_{max} (Spach et al 1981).

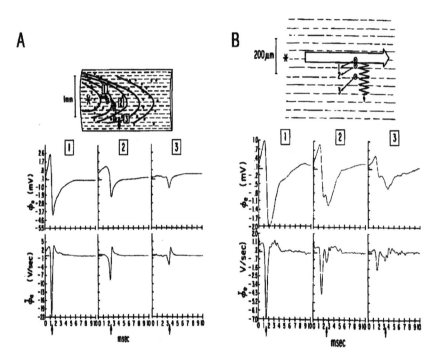

Figure 6 Nonuniform anisotropic propagation in atrial tissue. A: Preparation from 2-year-old male. Excitation spread smoothly from site of initiation (*), as shown by the continuous isochrones (top). Smooth extracellular voltage waveforms (ϕ_e) and their time derivatives, recorded from circled points numbered (1,2,3), indicate monophasic excitation (bottom). The thin dashed lines show the orientation of the fibers. Arrows at the bottom of each panel mark the times of dV_m/dt_{max} of the underlying action potentials, which were used to construct the isochrones. Isochrones are separated by 1 msec. B: Preparation from 42-year-old male. The prominent open arrow on the preparation (top) indicates that in a narrow longitudinal region, propagation was fast and uniform as shown in trace (1) at bottom. The saw-tooth indicates that, in directions not collinear with the fiber axis, excitation spread along an irregular zig-zag course. The corresponding extracellular waveforms and derivatives, seen in traces (2) and (3) at bottom, are multiply peaked, indicating that excitation spread nonuniformly by multiple paths (Spach, Dolber, 1986).

arranged into separate fascicles that connect with each other at longer distances, possibly related to diameter (Sommer, Johnson, 1979). The fascicles group into macroscopic bundles that have complex and varying interconnections.   The localization of gap junctions, particularly in adult tissues, is dominantly in end-to-end connections, leaving transverse electrical coupling with a smaller magnitude and less uniformity than longitudinal coupling, consistent with slower and more indirect propagation off the long axis (Gourdie et a; 1991; Gourdie et al 1992; Hoyt et al 1989; Sommer Scherer 1985; Pressler et al 1995). The density of immunostained Cx43 per cell is less in the AV node than in either atrial or ventricular myocardium with a punctate distribution within and along the borders of the nodal cells as well as variation in intensity of Cx43 staining in different portions of the AV node (Pressler et al 1995).   Recent studies (Hagendorf et al, 1989; Verheule et al, 1999) suggest that Cx40 instead of Cx43 play major role in atrial conduction while Cx43 is more important in ventricular conduction (Eloff et al 2001;Gutstein et al 2001).   While the heterogeneous expression of gap junctions might contribute to the conduction characteristics of specific tissues, but it is the predominantly end-to-end distribution in atrial, Purkinje and ventricular tissues that favors anisotropic conduction, while the punctate distribution in the AV node would favor current distribution in all directions.

Cellular anisotropy may also be important both in normal and abnormal activation. In presence of normal intercellular coupling and normal kinetics of I_{Na}, cellular anisotropy provides a major intrinsic protective mechanism against arrhythmias (Spach, Heidlage, 1995; Wolk et al 1999). This is based on the argument that the architecture of the myocardium creates varying electrical loads at a cellular level which, in turn, results in varying delays and excitatory events between and among cells. There is a feedback effect of cellular loading on the subcellular sodium current and the kinetics of the sodium channels, which integrates the propagation of the wave front. The myocardial architecture becomes pro-arrhythmic, either when there is a decrease in diversity at a microscopic cellular level (allowing large fluctuation of load to develop and be distributed) or when the loss of side-to-side connections produces gross nonuniform anisotropy, facilitating unidirectional block in the absence of repolarization inhomogeneities. According to this theory, the myocardial architecture becomes proarrhythmic when there is either a decrease in diversity at a microscopic cellular level which can result in large fluctuations of load, or when there is a loss of side-to-side gap junctional connection producing gross nonuniform anisotropy which, in turn, creates areas of unidirectional block even in the absence of any inhomogeneities of repolarization (Spach, Boineau, 1997).

Recent experiments in swine have demonstrated that reentry and wave splitting tend to occur around the papillary muscles or in anisotropic areas with abrupt changes in fiber orientation and provide further evidence that the intramyocardial Purkinje system may be important to the genesis of reentry (Valderrabano et al 2001). The concept of Purkinje muscle reentrant excitation is venerable (Sasyniuk, Mendez, 1971), and simulation studies now suggest it is involved in polymorphic ventricular arrhythmias (Barenfeld, Jalife, 1998).

The distribution of gap junctions are thought important in the genesis of reentrant arrhythmias (Spooner et al 1997). Aging (Spach, Dolber, 1986) and disease (Luke, Safitz, 1991;Peters et al 1993; Severs 1994; Smith et al 1991) alter the distribution and number of gap junctions. After myocardial infarction, diffusely distributed gap junctions reappear along the side of cells (Luke, Safitz, 1991; Smith et al 1991), and, such remodeling of gap junctions occurs in the border zone that is involved in reentrant circuits (Peters, Wit, 1998; Peters et al, 1997). Electrical coupling between cell pairs from he border zone also seems to be decreased. Cellular scaling (that is, the consequences of difference in cell size) seems to be important in determining the delay of impulse transfer between cells and of mean V_{max}, and the suggestion has been made that the maintenance of the size of mature cells during pathological remodeling of gap junctions also plays an important role in sustaining at a maximum level for a given state of the sodium current (Spach et al 2000).

As mentioned, some anisotropic structure may change in the chronic phase after injury. For example, it has been observed in experimental animals that damaged longitudinal pathways can be supplanted by intact transverse-longitudinal-transverse alternates which may be very long and have less than the normal strength of coupling (Wit, Rosen, 1989; Wit et al 1995;Kootsey 1991). Propagation through such re-structured tissue should become substantially slower and more variable than normal, and electrotonic coupling may become more prominent (Luke, Safitz, 1991;Smith et al 1991), features that can support stable arrhythmogenic patterns of propagation (Wit et al 1995; Spach, 1991). There has been some interest in the material properties of the ventricle during remodeling after myocardial infarction. Stress extension curves demonstrate directional anisotropy of both infarcted and remote myocardium (Gupta et al 1994), which, we suspect, will have electrophysiologic consequences. Recently, left venrticular hypertrophy in the guinea pig was fond to reduce anisotropy of conduction (Carey et al 2001). The ratio between longitudinal and transverse conduction velocity declined in papillary muscle as left ventricular hypertrophy developed, primarily due to a decrease of longitudinal conduction velocity. This would decrease the length constant and might, therefore, also decrease the safety factor (below) and conduction in the affected tissues.

The cellular contribution to the dispersion of refractoriness and to the modification of anisotropic properties can also occur during repolarization, and this is considered in great detail in a recent book (Gussak et al, in press). An interesting example given the increasing recognition of the importance of potassium channels was the demonstration that potassium-channel openers could produce in the left ventricle of the rabbit functional conduction block that facilitated reentry and by the dispersion of refractoriness (Robert et al 1989).

Anisotropic conduction, then, can cause the slow conduction, the area of unidirectional conduction block, or both involved in reentry. Anatomical pathways may be involved, but anisotropy can also occur without an anatomical pathway. Wit et al (1995) distinguish between functional and anisotropic reentry. They suggest that the functional characteristic that causes the leading circle type of reentry is a difference in refractory periods in adjacent areas caused by inhomogeneous conduction. In reentry caused by anisotropy, the essential feature is a difference in effective axial resistance to impulse propagation dependent on fiber direction. Clearly, the two overlap.

Safety Factor

Another concept that should understood by the clinicians is that of the safety factor. As discussed above, liminal length (LL) is the amount of tissue that must be raised above threshold so that the inward depolarizing current from that patch of membrane exceeds the repolarizing influences of adjacent tissues and results in an action potential. If the local electrotonic currents are sufficient to fulfill the liminal length requirements of the neighboring patch or patches of membrane, these patches will also produce action potentials. These events repeat and the sequential depolarization of patches of membrane results. The term safety factor is the excess in the activating current or charge over that just required to produce a regenerative propagated response, or, more succinctly, the excess of source over sink.

Clinicians are well aware that propagation can fail more readily in certain tissues such as the AV node, while propagation rarely fails in the His-Purkinje system or in atrial and ventricular muscle. Fast response tissues that depend on the rapid inward sodium current for regenerative depolarization (atria, bundle of His, fascicles and bundle branches, terminal Purkinje fibers, ventricular muscle, and certain accessory pathways) have a higher safety factor than slow response tissues that depend on the kinetically slow inward calcium current for regenerative depolarization (AV node). Fast response tissues that are depolarized during injury have a lower safety factor than normal because of partial inactivation of the sodium current or, at times, because the tissue now becomes dependent on the calcium current for phase 0 depolarization.

Passive properties of the sink also determine the safety factor. Failure of conduction can occur at points where passive properties change discontinuously, for example at points of branching. If the cross-sectional area and length of a segment are constant, membrane surface area will increase and R_m will decrease at a branch point. As mentioned, conduction velocity will change when fibers change their diameter or branch (Goldstein, Rall, 1974). In general, increased diameter or more branching led to a slower conduction velocity as the sinking of current downstream was greater. Critically slowed conduction at times resulted in the failure of propagation and, at other times, in an echo beat, reflections, and other signs of mismatch (see also (Lewis, Grindrod, 1991;Mendez et al 1970;Veenstra et al 1984)). Extensive branching, as found in the AV node, is associated with lower safety.

Although longitudinal propagation is faster than transverse propagation, it may not be safer. Heptanol uncoupling of gap junctions (Balke et al 1988; Delgado et al 1990;Delmar et al 1987) and injury (Kleeber, Janse, 1995) blocked slow transverse propagation earlier than fast longitudinal propagation. Increasingly premature extrastimuli which encroach upon the relative refractory period of the myocardial tissue has been observed to block longitudinal propagation earlier than transverse (Spach et al 1981;Spach et al 1982;Spach et al 1990). In these studies, fast longitudinal propagation became first decremental and then ceased, while transverse propagation, though fractionated, continued. The underlying reason for disparate observations with respect to safety or failure of propagation is most likely differences in the microscopic nonuniform anisotropy of tissue structure (Spach et al 1990).

Gap junctions also play an important role in determining the safety factor, and we have previously considered this in some technical detail (Ginsburg, Arndforf 1995). Gap junctional conductances have been studied using voltage-clamp, and the same type of source over sink relationship applies. Most simply, the safety factor of the transfer of current from one cell to another can be considered in terms of the number of open gap junctions which in turn translates as the conductance (reciprocal of resistance) between cells. When the input resistance is high, as in the SA node, junctional conductance can be sufficient to allow synchronization of cells when there are only a few channels (Anumonwo et al 1991;Weingart, Maurer1988). When input resistance is low, as in ventricular muscle, rapid conduction requires tens or hundreds of active channels (Weingart Maurer, 1988; 1990). The differential expression of connexins in different tissues influences the "source-to-sink" relationships. For example, although the conduction is rapid, the "sink" is likely to be large in ventricular myocytes, partially due to the large conductance and voltage-insensitivity of Cx43 predominantly responsible for conduction in the ventricle. The tissue-specific differential expression of connexins would suggest functional heteromeric and/or heterotypic gap junctions consisting of multiple connexin isoforms. The properties of such gap junctions likely determine the safety factor in conduction between two areas of the heart (for example, SA node and atrial tissue). Recent studies on feasibility and properties of the heteromeric and heterotypic gap junctions are discussed in other chapters.

Injury affects the spatial distribution and overall density of gap junctions (Luke, Safitz, 1991; Smith Cohe 1984). Injury decreases cellular coupling and, therefore, makes properties that are dependent on coupling, such as conduction velocity, more susceptible to modification by rate-dependent factors such as intracellular calcium concentration and pH (Pressler et al 1995; Buchanan Gettes 1990;Hiramatsu et a; 1988;Maurer Weingart 1987) or transjunctional voltage (Lal, Arnsdorf 1992; Jongsma et al 1991; Veenstra 1991) than in normal tissue (Veenstra, 1991; Spacn et al 1982). These influences may be exquisitely sensitive to beat-to-beat changes in rate.

Animal and human studies have shown that circulating wavefronts often make a sharp turn around an anatomic or functional barrier. Studies in Langendorff-perfused rabbit hearts utilizing a thin layer of anisotropic ventricular myocardium made using a cryoprocedure indicate that decreasing the safety factor by lowering the excitatory current by perfusing the tissue with increased potassium or the Class I drug, flecainide, preferentially impairs U-turn conduction as compared to transverse or longitudinal conduction (Danse et al 2000).

Excitable Gap and Entrainment

An *excitable gap* in a reentrant circuit is a region of the circuit where the cardiac cells have had sufficient time to reactivate and recover their excitability before the return of the reentrant wave. In general, the excitable gap is larger in areas of slow conduction and smaller or nonexistent in areas of rapid conduction. Once again, anisotropy in which transverse conduction is slower than longitudinal conduction would be expected to produce excitable gaps with differing spatial extents.

A fully excitable gap in an anisotropic reentrant circuit allows termination of a reentrant arrhythmia. A spontaneous extrasystole or an electrically paced beat can enter the circuit in the excitable gap and influence the reentrant circuit in a number of ways. The termination of a reentrant tachycardia by a single extrasystole or a burst of extrasystoles is thought to result from the entry of an impulse into the excitable gap which, in turn, renders a critical portion of the circuit inexcitable.

A fully excitable gap also allows *entrainment,* which, as described earlier, concerns the interaction of two oscillators. Entrainment clinically refers to special interactions between stimulation of the tissue and the reentrant circuit. Waldo and his coworkers in a classic paper published in 1977 described the transient entrainment of type I atrial flutter (Waldo et al 1977). They observed that if the atrium was paced somewhat faster than the rate of the type I atrial flutter, the rate of the tachycardia increased to match that of the faster pacing rate; that is, it was entrained; and, with cessation of the pacing or slowing of the pacing rate, the original rate of the atrial flutter returned or, frequently, the arrhythmia terminated. Studies by Waldo and his colleagues and others followed on transient entrainment in atrial flutter (Waldo 1995; Stevenson et al 1995; Cosio et al 1996), ventricular tachycardia (Stevenson et al 1995; Blanck et al 1994; Jazayeri et al 1994; Stenvenson 1995) among others}, AV nodal reentrant tachycardia or AV reentrant tachycardia using an accessory AV bypass tract (Stenvenson 1995), intraatrial reentrant atrial tachycardia (Stenvenson et al 1995; Poty et al 1996) and even atrial fibrillation (Kalman et al , 1996).

Waldo and his colleagues propose four criteria to establish the presence of transient entrainment (Waldo, 1995; Okumura etal 1987; Henthorn et al 1988). Constant fusion beats must be recorded in the ECG during constant pacing at a rate somewhat faster than the rate of the spontaneous atrial flutter, except for the last paced beat which is entrained but not fused. The last beat, then, will have the morphology of the spontaneous atrial flutter. The fusion beats during rapid pacing will result in morphologically constant atrial deflection on the ECG. At different rates of constant pacing, however, the fusion differs, and the morphology of the atrial recording will also differ. But the morphology will be constant for the new rate. Interruption of the tachycardia is associated with localized conduction block to one or more sites for one beat, followed by subsequent activation of that site or sites from a different direction. The morphology of the atrial electrogram at the blocked site or sites will change, and the conduction time will be shorter. Evidence for progressive fusion can be shown on the electrogram with a demonstration of a change in conduction time and electrogram morphology at one recording site when paced from another site at two different constant pacing rates that are faster than the spontaneous rate of the tachycardia but which do not interrupt the arrhythmia.

Sometimes, pacing at a rate somewhat faster than that of the spontaneous atrial flutter results in capturing the tachycardia without interrupting the tachycardia and without demonstrating any of the criteria for entrainment. This may be due to concealed entrainment in which the antidromic wave of the paced beat blocks in an area of slow conduction due to collision with the wavefront of the preceding beat. The orthodromic wavefront conducts completely around the circuit, traverses the area of slow conduction which allows previously excited tissue to become reactivated, finds no wavefront with which to collide, and so continues in the circuit restoring the atrial flutter. The circuit, however, may be interrupted if the antidromic beat and the orthodromic wave front from the previous beat block in the area of slow conduction. None of the transient entrainment criteria are met, yet the arrhythmia may be terminated. Concealed entrainment can be established only if transient entrainment can be demonstrated by pacing at another site, and they suggest that pacing from sites high in the right atrium should always permit the demonstration of transient entrainment.

The issues involved in entrainment concern all reentrant arrhythmias. Because of the importance in determining the site of reentry and ablation in ventricular tachycardia, most of the discussion of entrainment will be part of the discussion of sustained monomorphic ventricular tachycardia.

Isolation of Injured Cells

Teleologically, the shutdown of gap junctions by increased $[Ca^{++}]_i$, lowered pH or other determinants may isolate cells that have undergone injury from normal cells. The analogy would be the closing watertight doors in a submarine when the integrity of one compartment has been compromised. In cells, this isolation means that normal cells will not lose their cytoplasmic contents by leakage through the injured cell to the other cells. This isolation will prevent toxic metabolites, high concentrations of calcium and hydrogen ions from entering normal cells, thereby creating a chain reaction of cell injury and death. This isolation will also prevent the flow of current between cells having different transmembrane potentials (e.g., normal transmembrane voltage in normal cells and a less negative than usual transmembrane voltage in injured, depolarized cells). Clinically, such mechanisms may be protective of the injured heart. Such mechanisms, however, may also be arrhythmogenic since the cells taken out of the circuit may cause zig-zag activation conducive to reentry.

SELECTED ARRHYTHMIAS

Gap junctional functioning and cell-cell coupling, of course, cannot be studied easily in the human heart. Much of what follows about the relationship between anisotropy and arrhythmias in man is inferred.

Atrial Flutter

Atrial flutter is a reentrant arrhythmia in that it excites an area of the atrium and then travels sufficiently slowly in a pathway that is sufficiently long that the initially excited area recovers its excitability and can be reactivated (Waldo et al, 1977; Watson, Josephson, 1980; Inoue et al 1981; Disertori et al 1983; Klein et al 1986; Cosio et al 1988; Kalman et al 1996; Nakagawa et al 1996; lash et al 1996). A single premature extrastimulus or rapid atrial pacing can both initiate atrial flutter and, because there is an excitable gap, terminate the arrhythmia. The excitable gap is the portion of a reentrant circuit that has recovered its excitability and can again be depolarized. The excitable gap also allows entrainment with overdrive pacing during atrial flutter.

As noted by Lesh et al (1990), an interpretation of the early observations by Watson and Josephson (1980) suggests anisotropy in the mechanism of the atrial flutter given the site dependency of the induction of the arrhythmia in the high right atrium which would be a part of the reentrant tract while coronary sinus stimulation, outside the pathway, rarely induced the arrhythmia. Moreover, Watson and Josephson noted fragmented electrograms in the atrium near the His Bundle suggesting slow, discontinuous propagation transverse to fiber orientation. Whether such slow conduction is necessary for atrial flutter, however, has been debated. Recently, an extrastimulus technique was used to construct conduction curves of the delay following extrastimulation versus the S1-S2 interval, and the observed fractionation of electrograms was much greater in patients with atrial flutter as compared with control which, in turn, suggests that slow and inhomogeneous conduction within the atrium is likely related to the development of the atrial flutter (Tai et al 2001).

Electrophysiologic mapping has been performed in a few patients with atrial flutter in the catheterization laboratory and at surgery. A large macroreentrant circuit in the right atrium is involved in type I atrial flutter. If one begins the cycle at the end of the negative deflection of the F wave in lead II, the impulse at that point exists in the low right atrial septum between the inferior vena cava and the tricuspid valve; it then travels anteriorly through the region of the low septum, then superiorly and anteriorly up the medial surface of the right atrium, and returns over the lateral and posterior free wall. It has been suggested that a narrow portion of right atrial septal myocardium, located between the orifice of the tricuspid valve and the coronary sinus, is a required part of the reentrant circuit in most types of atrial flutter (Klein et al 1986; Kalman et al 1996; Nakagawa et al 1996; Chu et al 1994; Olgin et al 1995).

It has long been known that transverse conduction velocity across the crista terminalis is much slower than the longitudinal conduction velocity, being 0.09 m/sec and 1.05 m/sec in the 1981 investigation by Spach and his colleagues (1981) (see Fig. 5). In a recent compilation, the weighted average in a number of studies was a conduction velocity of 1.23 m/sec for longitudinal and 0.09 m/sec for transverse conduction (Pressler et al 1995; Armen, Frank, 1949; Simonson, 1961; Morady et al 1989). The shape of myocytes in the crista terminalis is elongated, similar to that of ventricular myocytes, but the cells are connected mostly end-to-end (Saffitz et al 1994) with gap junctions distributed densely within the connections. This geometric arrangement is likely responsible for the difficulty of an impulse to cross the crista terminalis and the Eustachian ridge and valve, thus favoring anisotropic propagation around rather than through these structures, providing a localized target for disrupting the arrhythmia. The Eustachian valve and ridge or the inferior vena cava form one border of the isthmus and the tricuspid valve annulus the other. A diagrammatic representation of the circuit involved in atrial flutter is shown in Figure 7. The flutter isthmus was examined pathologically in 50 hearts obtained at autopsy from individuals without atrial tachyarrhythmias (Waki et al 2000). Three quarters of these hearts had a nonuniform trabecular pattern in which there were abundant cross-overs and interlacing trabeculae, especially in the area just inferior to the coronary sinus os. Such anatomy would favor nonuniform conduction and conduction delay. The study raised the question as to what might have changed in individuals with atrial flutter.

Nomenclature for the types of atrial flutter has been confusing. It has been suggested that the classification of atrial flutter be based on the location of these anatomical barriers (Kalman et al 1997). Typical atrial flutter would be rotation around the tricuspid annulus with the crista terminalis and the Eustachian ridge as posterior barriers. Subclassification of typical atrial flutter would depend on the direction of rotation of the wave front. The common form of atrial flutter uses the circuit described above which could be described as "counterclockwise" flutter if one looks from the left ventricle through the tricuspid valve into the right atrium. Atrial flutter may use the

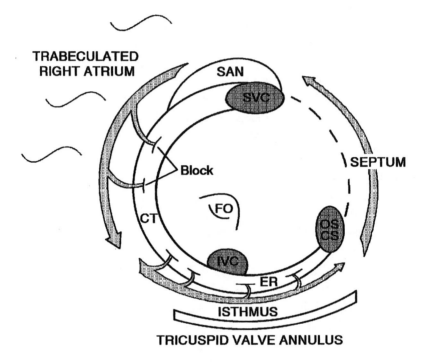

Figure 7 Diagrammatic representation of the circuit used in the common form of atrial flutter. The wave front courses in the trabeculated right atrium and usually fails to cross the crista terminalis (CT) due to poor cell-cell connections in the crista itself (indicated by "block"). The Eustachian ridge (ER) is an extension of this anatomical barrier. The impulse passes through an area called the "isthmus" that is bound on each side by the Eustachian ridge (ER) and the tricuspid valve annulus. The isthmus is an anatomic target for ablation, usually between the inferior vena cava (IVC) and the tricuspid annulus but also between the Eustachian ridge and the tricuspid annulus. The small isthmus between the tricuspid valve annulus and the coronary sinus ostium (OS CS) has also been the target of ablation with some success. Activation continues in the intraatrial septum. SAN, sinoatrial node; SVC, superior vena cava; IVC, inferior vena cava; CT, crista terminalis; ER, Eustachian ridge; FO, foramen ovale; OS CS, os of the coronary sinus

same circuit defined by the same anatomical barrier in a clockwise manner.   In this scheme, "clockwise" flutter would be a subclassification of common flutter.   Experience suggests that although clockwise flutter is the presenting clinical arrhythmia in only a few patients, it can be induced by EPS study in most (Kalman et al 1997). In this classification, a "true" atypical form of atrial flutter uses circuits and barriers other than those of clockwise and counterclockwise flutter (Kalman et al 1997).

Atypical flutter is heterogeneous, tends to be unstable, often converts into atrial fibrillation, and may terminate spontaneously or become a typical clockwise or clockwise atrial flutter (Kalman et al 1997). The mechanisms of atypical atrial flutter are speculative. On the one hand, the transitions between atypical atrial flutter, atrial fibrillation, and common atrial flutter suggest that lines of functional block are involved; while on the other hand, patients tend to develop the same morphology of atypical flutter suggesting that the lines of block may have an anatomic basis (Kalman et al 1997).

Atrial Fibrillation

The genesis and maintenance of atrial fibrillation is a very complex topic that recently has been elegantly reviewed (Nattel et al 2000; Nattel, Li 2000;Falk, 2001;Jahangir et al 2001; Gibbons et al in press). The normal atria are composed of complex trabeculae which would favor heterogeneous conduction. Video imaging and mapping have been used to study reentry and epicardial breakout patterns during atrial fibrillation in the isolated sheep heart, and anisotropy related to the orientation of the atrial fibers and pectinate muscles was found (Gray et al 1996). Further, the atria contain numerous orifices that result in a transition between atrial myocardium and vascular endothelium, which serve as physical barriers to favor reentry. Specialized nodal regions and transitional fibers with differing electrophysiological properties exist in the atria as well. There are regional differences in ion channel distribution and in electrophysiological properties (Wang et al 1996; Feng et al 1998).

Both sympathetic and parasympathetic nerve fibers are distributed nonuniformly throughout the atria, and alterations in autonomic tone have been implicated in the development of atrial fibrillation (see, for example, (Coumel, 1996)).

Disease of the atria often involves fibrosis and the juxtaposition of normal and diseased atrial myocytes (Bharati, Lev, 1992;Guiraudon et al 1992; Frustaci et al 1997) which may affect cell-cell communication and contribute to anisotropy. Heart failure promotes atrial fibrillation in the dog, a process that seems mediated by the development of interstitial fibrosis (Li et al 1999). Inflammation may also play a role in some individuals, and a recent report found 66% of atrial biopsy specimens from patients with lone atrial fibrillation had histological changes consistent with an inflammatory myocarditis (Frustaci et al 1997).

There are contradictory data concerning connexins involved in cell-cell communication. In experimental atrial fibrillation, some studies show up-regulation of Cx43 expression in dogs (Elvan et al 1997) while others found no change in Cx43 mRNA or protein expression in goats (Van der Velden et al 1998). Van der Velden, et al. found patchy areas in the atria in which Cx40 expression was reduced (Van der Velden et al 1998). In a subsequent study, this group found a decrease in the ratio between atrial Cx40 and Cx43 that correlated with cellular myolysis without any change in the Cx40 in a goat model of atrial fibrillation (Van der Velden et al 2000). Transgenic mice that lack Cx40 are more susceptible to the induction of atrial tachyarrhythmias, but mice that are heterozygous for Cx40 are not (Hagendorf et al 1999; Venheule et al 1999). Recently, the expression of Cx40 and Cx43 was studied in the atria of patients with and without chronic atrial fibrillation as well as in an animal model of atrial fibrillation (Polontchouk et al 2001). Cx40, but not Cx43, increased in the human atria and in the rat. In the rat, anisotropy was reduced, perhaps allowing the change in pathways of activation to change and resulting in the appearance of continuously changing pathways.

The arrhythmia can be initiated by several mechanisms that cause rapid, irregular electrical activity. In the landmark demonstration in 1995, Wijffels, Kirchhof, Dorland and Alessie showed atrial fibrillation itself altered atrial electrophysiology in a way that begot atrial fibrillation and changed much of our thinking (Wijffels et al 1995). Since the report, a great deal has been learned about electrical and structural remodeling in atrial fibrillation. The changes may be rapid and include functional electrophysiological changes or may be quite slow such as altered gene expression of ion channels (see reviews (Nattel et al 2000; Nattel, Li, 2000;Van Wagoner, 2001)) or the development of fibrosis (Li et al 1997) .

Moe and his coworkers proposed the multiple wavelet hypothesis as an underlying cause of atrial fibrillation in which multiple independent activation wavelets circled around functionally refractory tissue, some were extinguished while others survived to activate other areas of tissue as daughter wavelets (Moe, Abildskov, 1959). In recent years, more sophisticated models of this type of reentry have been developed (Nattel et al 2000; Allessie et al 1985). High-density mapping of atrial fibrillation in man has confirmed this mechanism (Konings et al 1994). Rather well defined circuits have been defined, and, based on mapping studies during surgery for preexcitation syndrome, three patterns have been proposed involving single or multiple wave fronts (Allessie et al 1998).

Rapidly discharging foci, most commonly located in or near the pulmonary veins, may mimic atrial fibrillation or may initiate multiple-wavelet reentry atrial fibrillation (Jais et al 1997;Haissaguerre et al 1998). Multiple pulmonary foci may exist in an individual, and such sites may be located in the right atrium, the superior vena cava, or the coronary sinus. Histological and electrophysiologic studies indicate that electrophysiologic active cardiac muscle may extend into the pulmonary veins (see review (Gibbons et al, in press)).

It would seem, then, that the structural substrate of the atria, particularly in disease, creates anisotropic conditions conducive to the development of multiple wavelet reentry. To this is added diversity in the distribution of ion channels, physical obstacles, and nonuniform distribution of autonomics. Ectopic activity, whether atrial premature beats, supraventricular arrhythmias, or the discharge of automatic pacemakers in the pulmonary arteries and at other sites, can trigger reentry and atrial fibrillation. Atrial fibrillation, once initiated, causes electrical and structural remodeling that helps maintain atrial fibrillation. While anisotropy seems important in the initiation and maintenance of atrial fibrillation, the role of gap junctional change and redistribution as part of electrophysiologic remodeling remains largely open to speculation.

Therapeutic interventions include traditional pharmacological therapy to prevent ectopic beats, decrease automaticity, and interrupt reentrant circuits by affecting depolarizing and repolarizing currents. Electrophysiologic remodeling, however, possibly provides new approaches, some of which have been reviewed recently (Nattel et al 2000; Nattel, Li, 2000). Rapid conversion of atrial fibrillation to a normal sinus rhythm may obviate some of the electrophysiologic and structural remodeling that favors the recurrence and maintenance of the arrhythmia, and perhaps an implantable atrial defibrillator will be useful in this regard. Perhaps angiotensin converting enzyme inhibitors may prevent the type of structural remodeling that promotes atrial fibrillation in a dog model of atrial fibrillation. Mibefradil, a T-type calcium channel antagonist, but not diltiazem, reduces atrial remodeling caused by atrial tachycardias (Fareh et al 1999; Fareh et al 2001).

Other Atrial Arrhythmias

Spach and his coworkers studied the electrophysiologic properties in human atrial pectinate bundles that had been removed at surgery from aged individuals (Spach et al 1988). Premature beats were introduced in these non-uniformly anisotropic bundles resulting in dissociated zig-zag conduction and anisotropic reentry within regions as small as 50 mm^2. Electrograms were also recorded that were fragmented, analogous to those recorded at the time of open-heart surgery. It is quite likely that this substrate underlies virtually all reentrant atrial arrhythmias by contributing to the formation of the areas of slow conduction and unidirectional block essential for reentry.

Atrioventricular Nodal Reentrant Tachycardia

Atrioventricular nodal reentrant tachycardia (AVNRT) is a common arrhythmia, accounting for approximately two-thirds of cases of paroxysmal supraventricular tachycardia. AVNRT is a reentrant rhythm that utilizes the AV node and, usually, perinodal atrial tissue (McGuire et al 1993; McGuire et al 1993). The term "atrioventricular junctional reentrant tachycardia" is being used increasingly, because more than just the AV node is often involved in the reentrant circuit. The bundle of His is probably not a necessary part of the reentrant circuit, since the arrhythmia is at times associated with 2:1 AV block (i.e., the completion of two complete circuits is evidenced by two retrograde P waves while only one of the impulses traverses the His bundle on the way to the ventricles indicating that the bundle of His is not a necessary component of the circuit). In addition, His bundle electrograms indicate that reentry is proximal to the recording site (Schmitt et al 1988; Weh et al 1990). The topic has been comprehensively reviewed (Jackman et al 1995).

The AV node depends upon the inward calcium current for the regenerative phase of the action potential which, in large part along with anatomical factors, accounts for the slow conduction velocity through the AV node. The simplest concept of AV nodal physiology that allows AV nodal reentry has long been based on the postulated existence of two functionally different AV nodal pathways with differing conduction velocities and refractory periods (Moe et al

1956). The so-called "fast" or β- pathway conducts rapidly and most commonly has a relatively long refractory period; while the "slow" or α- pathway conducts relatively slowly and most commonly has a shorter refractory period. These pathways join and enter a final common pathway in the AV node.

These early studies suggested functional dissociation into a fast and slow pathway (Denes et al 1973), and the two forms of AVNRT based this model were identified: the common slow-fast AVNRT in which antegrade conduction was through the slow pathway and retrograde conduction through the fast pathway and the uncommon fast-slow AVNRT in which antegrade conduction occurred through the fast pathway and retrograde conduction through the slow pathway. A third form of AVNRT utilizes a slow pathway for antegrade conduction and another slow pathway for retrograde conduction.

For a number of years, it was postulated that there was a proximal common pathway within the AV node, but it is now thought that the proximal fast and slow pathways are in perinodal atrial tissue in virtually all patients. The functional dissociation results in a rather reproducible sequence of events. The proposed sequence in the common form of AVNRT, which affects 80% or more of patients, is as follows. The normal sinus beat enters the AV node and the impulse travels down both the fast and slow pathways. The impulse traveling down the fast pathway reaches the His bundle first creating a refractory wake, and the impulse in the slow pathway runs into the refractory wake of the impulse that had traveled down the fast pathway. The impulse traveling down the slow pathway is extinguished when, in the area of the final common pathway, it runs into the refractory wake of the impulse that had traveled down the fast pathway. The fast pathway has a longer refractory period than the slow pathway, so a critically timed premature atrial beat (or less commonly, a premature junctional or ventricular beat with retrograde conduction) may enter the AV node, find the fast pathway refractory, but still be able to conduct via the slow pathway through the final common pathway to the bundle of His. If the fast pathway has recovered its excitability by the time the slow pathway impulse reaches the distal junction of the two pathways, the impulse may be able to conduct retrograde up the fast pathway. The circuit may then become repetitive with antegrade conduction down the slow pathway and retrograde conduction up the fast pathway resulting in a sustained tachycardia, the so-called slow-fast pathway type of AVNRT. The electrocardiogram in this setting shows a supraventricular tachycardia in which the P wave is buried in the QRS complex or occurs slightly before or slightly after the QRS complex, often in fusion with the QRS complex.

In about 10 percent of patients, the reentrant circuit involves antegrade conduction down the fast pathway and retrograde conduction down the slow pathway. This is called the uncommon or fast-slow pathway type of AVNRT. The P wave appears shortly before the QRS complex. In another 9 or 10% of individuals, both antegrade and retrograde conduction occur over slow pathways.

The exact anatomic distribution of these pathways is uncertain. As illustrated in Figure 8, Koch's triangle is bounded by the tricuspid ring and the tendon of Todoro which bracket the coronary sinus at the base of the triangle and are in close proximity forming the apex near the His bundle at the membranous septum. As an approximation, Koch's triangle can be divided into thirds: the anterior, which contains the compact AV node and the fast pathways; the middle; and the posterior, which is associated with the coronary sinus. High resolution electrophysiologic mapping indicates that retrograde fast pathway conduction during the common form of AVNRT causes the earliest atrial activation at the apex of Koch's triangle in the vicinity of the junction between the AV node and the bundle of His (Mc Guire et al 1983). Retrograde slow pathway conduction during the uncommon form of AVNRT activates the atrium earliest in the lower (most frequent) or middle portion of Koch's triangle near the os of the coronary sinus. This localization has allowed the successful ablation of fast and slow pathways to cure recurrent AVNRT. Figure 8 shows the landmarks related to Koch's triangle.

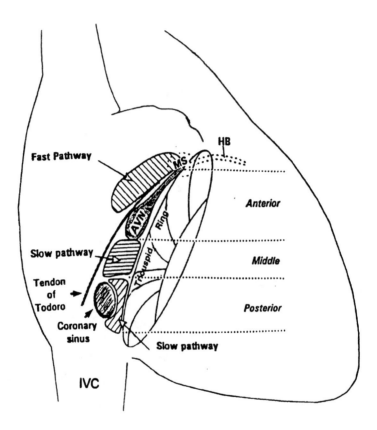

Figure 8 Schematic representation of Koch's triangle which is bounded by the tricuspid ring and the tendon of Todoro. The tendon of Todoro and the tricuspid ring are in close proximity can be divided into thirds: the anterior contains the compact AV node; the posterior contains the coronary sinus; and the middle or mid-septal third is between the anterior and posterior portions. The anterior third is associated with fast pathways, and the middle and posterior thirds with slow pathways.

The microscopic anatomy of the AV node and the perinodal atrial tissues is complex, and the relationship of anatomy to electrophysiology is only poorly understood (Janse et al 1971;Hoe et al 1995;Anderson et al 1995). The AV node appears to be non-uniformly anisotropic from the macroscopic to the microscopic scales. The small, unorganized cells are poorly coupled as indicated by the short space constant recorded by De Mello (1977). The paucity of gap junctions in the AV node is, in part, responsible for the slowing of conduction velocity within the AV node and at its interface with the atria (Pressler et al 1995;DeFelice, Challice, 1969; Kawamura, James 1971; Marino, 1979). The density and distribution of gap junctions in the AV node is of interest. The density of immunostained Cx43 per cell is less in the AV node than in either atrial or ventricular myocardium with a punctate distribution within and along the borders of the nodal cells as well as variation in intensity of Cx43 staining in different portions of the AV node (Pressler et al 1995). Cx43 and Cx45 are found in AV node and may be the major players in conduction through the AV node. It is interesting to speculate that differences in their single-channel conductance might contribute to the difference conduction velocity if differential local expression could be demonstrated. In addition, the characteristic pattern of distribution of gap junctions in the AV node, regardless of the subtypes, might also disperse currents in many directions rather than in a preferred direction. Gordon Moe and his colleagues in their landmark study in 1957 proposed "longitudinal dissociation" as likely underlying the observed dual AV nodal physiology (Moe, Preston 1956), an assumption that has been confirmed subsequently in studies that demonstrated longitudinal dissociation without anatomical evidence of separate pathways (Janse et al 1971; Mendez, Moe 1966). Indeed, the existence of both horizontal and longitudinal dissociation has been demonstrated in man (Roy et al 1983).

Atrioventricular Reentrant Tachycardia

Approximately 30% of cases of paroxysmal supraventricular tachycardias arise from reentry that utilizes both the AV node and an accessory pathway in the reentrant circuit. The features of the AV node of importance to anisotropy have been discussed above.

Atrioventricular accessory pathways can conduct antegrade from the atrium to the ventricle or orthodromically from the ventricle to the atrium. The accessory pathway conducts rapidly than does the AV node since the depolarization phase of the action potential in the former relies on the rapid, transient inward sodium current, rather than on the slow inward calcium current as is true for the AV node. As a result, antegrade conduction results in the ventricles being excited earlier than they would be through normal AV nodal conduction, and this is called preexcitation. Antegrade conduction through the accessory pathway also results in eccentric ventricular activation as compared to normal activation through the AV node. For reasons that are not clear, these accessory pathways result from incomplete isolation of the atria from the ventricles during cardiogenesis.

The characteristics of the active generator properties and cell-cell conduction as well as the electrotonic influence of the ventricles, and, to a lesser extent, of the atria, determine the functional characteristics of these accessory pathways. The speed of conduction and refractoriness of the accessory pathways vary greatly. Some allow conduction at rates of 300 beats/min and even faster; while others conduct very slowly, have long action potentials, and may show various types of atrioventricular block reminiscent of the AV node. Some allow bi-directional conduction, while others allow conduction one way but not the other. Overall, about 95% of atrioventricular accessory pathways conduct rapidly and have the characteristics of sodium dependent phase 0 action potentials that occur in normal "fast response" myocardium. Five percent show decremental conduction, the mechanism of which is uncertain. Possible explanations include geometric factors including those involved in anisotropy, partial inactivation of the sodium channel, and, perhaps, dependence on a calcium channel.

Usually there is no evidence of preexcitation during normal sinus rhythm, but AVRT is a common arrhythmia (perhaps 5%) in individuals with preexcitation, most commonly involving atrioventricular and atrionodal or atriofascicular pathways. AVRT tends to have a faster rate than atrioventricular nodal reentrant tachycardia (AVNRT) and often exceeds 200 beats/min, but there is a great deal of overlap in the rates of the two arrhythmias. The arrhythmia may occur in the absence or presence of other structural heart disease, and the symptoms and importance often depend on the underlying heart disease. Accessory pathways may be multiple (Gallagher et al 1984; Bardy et al 1984; Ward et al 1984), and individuals with AVRT may not infrequently have AVNRT (Pritchett et al 1980;Smith et al 1983).

The reentrant circuit responsible for the AVRT can be of two types: *orthodromic* in that the impulse travels through the AV node, down the infranodal specialized conduction system, to the ventricles, and returns to the atrium through an accessory pathway; or *antidromic* in that it conducts from the atrium to the ventricle through the accessory pathway and returns through the AV node.

In orthrodromic AVRT antegrade conduction is through the AV node and retrograde conduction through an accessory pathway, usually of the atrioventricular type. There is usually no evidence on the routine ECG of an accessory pathway during normal sinus rhythm, that is, there is no evidence of ventricular preexcitation. These accessory pathways cannot conduct antegrade from the atrium to the ventricles, but they can conduct unidirectionally from the ventricle to the atrium (Coumel, Attuel, 1974; Barol, Coumel, 1977;Neus etal 1975;Pritchett et al 1978). These pathways are said to be "concealed" since their existence cannot be ascertained from the ECG during normal sinus rhythm, but demonstrate an electrophysiologic effect during the orthodromic ART. Possibly, some pathways are not "concealed" but cause little preexcitation on antegrade conduction due to location or electrophysiologic properties.

The reasons for this unidirectional conduction are uncertain, but perhaps safety factor is of importance. It seems reasonable to hypothesize that the electrical mass of the ventricle is sufficient to generate electrotonic currents that can activate the accessory pathway, while the mass of the atrium is insufficient to active the ventricular myocardium. Other possibilities include geometric differences or perhaps some type of rectification. Whatever the mechanism, the atrial impulse seems to enter the accessory pathway and blocks near the ventricular insertion site (Kuck et al 1990).

The rate may exceed 200 beats/min. Since antegrade Av conduction is over the normal pathway, the QRS complexes are normal, may show functional aberrant conduction, or, reflect preexisting bundle branch or fascicular block. The reentrant circuit is relatively large, as compared to AV nodal reentrant tachycardia, so the P wave follows the QRS complex and usually appears in the ST segment or the T wave. The RP interval will be less than half the RR interval. Most pathways are eccentric and left-sided, so atrial activation commonly begins in the left atrium resulting in inverted P waves in lead I. Septal pathways and right-sided pathways near the AV node may give rise to the usual type of retrograde atrial activation.

Antidromic AVRT is responsible for perhaps 10% of PSVT in patients with accessory pathways and has a wide complex tachycardia due to antegrade conduction through the accessory pathway and retrograde conduction through the AV node. These patients frequently have several accessory pathways that can support antidromic AVRT (Gallagher et al 1981; Bardy et al 1984; Ward et al 1984). Because of the eccentric antegrade activation of the ventricles and lack of AV nodal conduction, full preexcitation will be displayed with a large delta wave and broadened QRS complex. Because the circuit is relatively long, the retrograde P wave will appear in the ST segment or the T wave. Since retrograde atrial activation arises from the impulse emerging from the AV node, the usual retrograde activation pattern will be observed with the RP interval less than half the RR interval. When present, the resulting P-wave might help distinguishing this arrhythmia with functional bundle-branch block from monomorphic ventricular tachycardia. Functional bundle branch block on the ipsilateral side of the accessory pathway results in a longer circuit length which in turn slows the rate of the tachycardia; lengthening in cycle length by more than 35 msec strongly suggests AVRT. Conversely, the disappearance of bundle branch block may decrease the cycle length. Septal pathways, however, may not result in such changes.

Orthodromic AVRT and AVNRT together form most cases of paroxysmal supraventricular tachycardia. The common form of AVNRT has a shorter circuit than AVRT, so the retrograde P wave in AVNRT is usually buried in the QRS complex (may be slightly before or after the QRS complex) while, as mentioned, the retrograde P wave in AVRT usually appears in the ST segment or the T wave. AVNRT occur in patients with WPW (Pritchett et al 1980;Smith et al 1983;Welens, Durrer 1973).

AVRT often precedes atrial fibrillation in individuals with (Campbell et al 1970;Sung et al 1977; Fujimura) or without (Roark et al 1986) preexcitation. Most patients who have been resuscitated from ventricular fibrillation secondary to preexcitation have inducible AVRT or a previous history of this arrhythmia. In one laboratory, 35% of episodes of atrial fibrillation were preceded by AVRT (Fujimura et al 1990). AVRT seems to be a trigger for atrial fibrillation only in the susceptible patient with preexcitation, and there is some suspicion that there are intrinsic electrophysiologic abnormalities in the right atrium (Fujimura et al 1990) which most likely would be related to conditions that cause anisotropic reentry. Operative ablation of accessory pathways often results in the cure of both AVRT and atrial fibrillation in individuals who have both arrhythmias (Sharma et al 1985). There has also been some success with intracardiac ablation (Wellens et al 1994), and perhaps the accessory pathway is not necessary for atrial fibrillation but it may help perpetuate atrial fibrillation in individuals who have a predisposition to such an arrhythmia (Wathen et al 1993).

Atrioventricular reentrant tachycardia associated with a long RP' interval

The term "incessant" supraventricular tachycardia is applied to a supraventricular tachycardia when it is present for at least 90% of the time a patient is monitored (Sung, 1983). The underlying mechanism may be reentry or enhanced automaticity, and here we will consider only the former. Coumel, et al, in 1967 reported on a "permanent" form of reciprocating supraventricular tachycardia that they considered due to AV nodal reentry that involved antegrade conduction through a functionally fast pathway and retrograde conduction through a functionally slow pathway (Coumel et al 1967). Their finding was subsequently confirmed by others (Sheinman et al 1974). Later investigations indicated that such incessant or permanent forms of junctional reciprocating tachycardia utilized accessory pathways (Sheinman et al 1974;Gallagher, Sealy 1978). There has been some debate as to whether the intranodal mechanism exists, but it is accepted now that both types of mechanisms can produce incessant tachycardia.

Antegrade conduction through the accessory pathway does not occur. Electrophysiologic testing indicates that these pathways are almost always posteroseptal, decrease their ability to conduct as a function of rate, and result in eccentric atrial activation until block occurs in the accessory pathway. The decremental conduction properties have led to speculation that the return pathway may be accessory AV nodal structures (Ward, Camm 1982), but such decremental conduction has been documented in a case of verapamil-sensitive incessant tachycardia utilizing a left lateral accessory pathway (Okumura et al 1986). A complex, tortuous paraseptal pathway has been describe in one patient which may explain, in part, the decremental conduction (Critelli et al 1984). Most commonly, the return pathway is a posteroseptal accessory pathway. Atrial activation, then, begins in the low right atrium or near the coronary sinus. It is intriguing to attribute conduction slowing and unidirectional block to anisotropy, perhaps with a marginal safety factor, to these cases, particularly in the report by Okumura and his colleagues (Critelli et al 1984).

There is no evidence of preexcitation on the ECG during sinus rhythm or atrial pacing since antegrade conduction does not occur over the accessory pathway. Because of slow conduction through the retrograde limb of the circuit, the interval between the QRS complex and the retrograde P wave (the R-P' interval) is long. The retrograde P wave occurs late in the cardiac cycle and the RP' interval is longer than the PR interval. Since atrial activation begins in the low right atrium or near the coronary sinus in the most common form, the P waves are inverted in II, III and aVF. The appearance of ventricular preexcitation has noted in some patients who have undergone ablation therapy, usually with first-degree AV block but at times with a very short PR interval (Critelli et al 1984). Incessant supraventricular tachycardia can lead to a cardiomyopathy which can be reversed if ablation is successful (Wu et al 2000).

Atrioventricular Accessory Pathways

As mentioned, 95% of atrioventricular accessory pathways conduct rapidly and have the characteristics of sodium dependent phase 0 action potentials that occur in normal "fast response" myocardium. Five percent show decremental conduction, the mechanism of which is uncertain. Possible explanations include geometric factors including those involved in anisotropy, partial inactivation of the sodium channel and perhaps dependence on a calcium channel. The last two would decrease the safety factor.

A few comments on the controversial nature of the so-called James and Mahaim fibers are in order as part of the discussion of anisotropy. The Lown-Ganong-Levine syndrome is characterized by palpitations in patients with an ECG that shows a short PR interval and a normal QRS duration (Lown et al 1952). For many years, this disorder was thought to be due to tracts that connected the atrium with the low AV node or the His bundle via the so-called James fibers (James, 1961). An alternative concept is that the short PR interval with a normal QRS pattern results, in most cases, from enhanced or accelerated AV nodal conduction and less often from an accessory pathway (Denes et al 1977;Benditt et al 1978; Bauernfeind etal 1982). A short PR interval appears to be more frequent in patients with concealed accessory pathways (Benditt et al 1978), but has also been associated with dual pathway physiology and AV nodal reentrant tachycardia. However, only patients with symptomatic tachyarrhythmias are studied electrophysiologically; as a result, it is uncertain whether all individuals with a short PR interval and normal QRS complex have enhanced AV nodal conduction or accessory pathways near the AV node. The loss of normal integrative function within the AV node could explain the observation in that a very rapidly conducting bundle, unmodified by the electrotonic interactions from more slowly conducting neighboring tissues, would result in more rapid conduction through the AV node.

The issue of the Mahaim pathways, which arise from the AV node or one of the bundle branches and insert into ventricular tissue, has been reviewed in detail (Klein et al 1994). It was presumed that these pathways could explain patients in whom the PR interval was normal (because the AV node was normally traversed) but the QRS was widened (presumably due to eccentric activation of the ventricles) (Wellens 1971). Some patients also had a prolonged PR interval with eccentric ventricular activation. This could be explained by slowed AV nodal conduction and anomalous connections at the level of or below the AV node. Surgical (Gillette et al 1982;Klein et al 1983) and more recent catheter ablation studies (McClelland et al 1994; Cappato et al; Grogin et al 1994; Li et al 1994), however, suggest that electrophysiologic characteristics attributed to nodoventricular Mahaim fibers are due to atriofascicular accessory connections with decremental conduction. One report, for example, suggests the presence of an atrioventricular connection in the tricuspid ring which has slow and rate-dependent conduction, blocks with adenosine, has intrinsic automaticity, and links to a rapidly conducting insulated pathway that generates a "His-like" potential (McClelland et al 1994). For the reasons discussed earlier, anisotropy and a decreased safety factor could produce the appropriate electrophysiologic environment.

Ventricular Tachycardia

Most ventricular arrhythmias are due to reentry which, as is characteristic of most reentrant circuits, requires an area of conduction sufficiently slow that the tissue to be reentered can be reactivated. An area of unidirectional block plays the role initially of determining the direction of the initiating wave front and then providing an area for the returning wave front to conduct.   The details of the underlying electrophysiology in anisotropic reentry as a cause of ventricular arrhythmias have been reviewed in detail (Wit et al 1995).

Coronary artery disease is the most important cause of sustained monomorphic ventricular tachycardia. The important mechanisms have already been discussed. Those related to gap junctional function include the slowing of conduction due to increased resistance to the axial flow of current which, as discussed above, if thought of in terms of Spach's effective axial resistivity includes the influences of cellular geometry and packing, extracellular resistivities, and side-to-side couplings, and other features), presumably mostly due to a decrease of gap junctional conductance; the extent, distribution and function of the gap junctions; and nonuniform conduction longitudinally and transversely.   In ventricular tissue as in atrial tissue, non-uniform anisotropy due to preserved longitudinal conduction but disturbed lateral cell-cell connections (due to fibrosis or other causes) results in irregular activation, disruption of an integrated wave front, and "zig-zag" conduction, which, in turn, results in slow activation (see, for example, Gardner et al 1985; Spach et al 1982; Spach, Dolber, 1986;Urcell et al 1985). In anisotropic conduction, the safety factor may actually be lower for longitudinal than for transverse conduction.

As mentioned earlier, the underlying reason for disparate observations with respect to safety or failure of propagation is most likely differences in the microscopic nonuniform anisotropy of tissue structure (Spach et al 1990) as well as alterations in the active generator source during injury. The decreased safety factor in the longitudinal as compared to the transverse direction discussed above may also be important in establishing the characteristics of unidirectional conduction in tissues. The important studies from Andrew Wit's laboratory have been mentioned, but deserve reemphasis because they indicate the importance of altered structural properties without significant change in the active generator properties. In these studies, dogs were studied 8 weeks after the induction of a myocardial infarction. Fractionated electrograms were recorded from the surface of the infarct zone, yet action potentials recorded from myocytes within these zones are normal (Gardner et al 1985;Urcell et al 1985). Under the microscope, connective tissue widely separated and distorted the muscle fibers. The conclusion was that the slow, fragmented activation that gave rise to the fractionated electrograms was not due to changes in the active generator which indeed had normal action potentials, but rather to disruption in the integrative electrotonic interaction between cells caused by fibrosis that physically disconnected the cells. These signals that are recorded by the signal-averaged electrocardiogram and are sought during ablation studies, so they are very important markers diagnostically and clinically. The sustained monomorphic tachycardia in these as well as in other similar studies most likely has anisotropic reentry as the primary underlying mechanism although damage to the source may contribute (Dillon et al 1988;Cardinal et al 1988;El-Sherif et al 1981;Kramer et al 1985, among others).

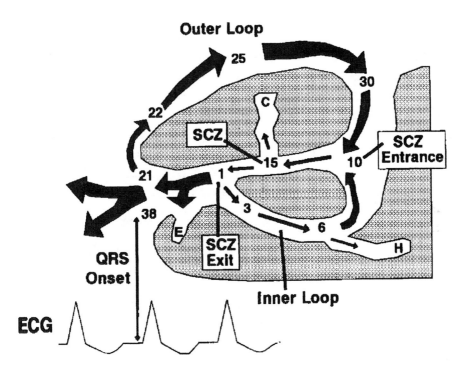

Figure 9 Functional components of reentrant circuits in chronic post-myocardial infarction. The shaded areas are inaccessible. The black arrows are propagating wave fronts. The numbers refer to the points or sites at which recordings were obtained during mapping. The electrocardiogram (ECG) is that of the sustained monomorphic ventricular tachycardia. The slow conduction zone (SCZ) and its entrance and exit are indicated. Two reentrant loops are depicted: an outer loop that includes the myocardium bordering the scarred zone and an inner loop that is determined and defined by the scarring and electrical uncoupling. Sites C, E and H represent dead ends. From Stevenson with permission (1995).

Figure 9 is a simple model of the functional components of the reentrant circuits in chronic post-infarction tissue as conceptualized by Stevenson (Stevenson, 1995). The propagating wave fronts are shown as black arrows, the inexcitable areas are shaded, and the numbers are catheter mapping sites. The wave front enters the slow conduction zone (SCZ) at point 10 in the scar, passes through a zone of slow conduction near point 15 and exits at point 1, producing the onset of the QRS complex near site 38. The impulse may pass through one of two reentrant circuits. The clockwise outer loop extends from point 1 through points 22 and 25 to point 30 in myocardium at the border of the scar and contributes to the QRS complex. An inner loop extends from point 1 through points 3 and 6 to site 10. Depolarization in the inner loop does not contribute to the surface ECG. The inner and out loops meet at point 10, the entrance to the slow conduction zone. If the conduction time through the two loops is similar, the circuit has a figure-of-eight configuration and the region from point 10 to point 1 is a common pathway. If the conduction time in the two loops is not equal, the faster loop determines the cycle length of the tachycardia and is called the dominant loop with the slower, non-dominant loop behaving as a bystander. There may be dead ends (sites C, E, and H), multiple reentrant circuits and more than one entrance or exit site. If there are two areas of exit, the same slow conduction zone may result in two different QRS morphologies. Sometimes, the scar may create a single outer loop with no common pathway, or, the reentrant circuit may be entirely within the scar.

Pacing at or near some reentrant circuit sites may entrain the circuit without altering the QRS complexes of the tachycardia. For example, pacing at point 15 may produce an orthodromic wave front that propagates to the exit as in the spontaneous tachycardia. The stimulated antidromic wave fronts, that is, the wave front from point 15 to point 10, are extinguished by collision with a returning orthodromic wave front. This is an example of entrainment with concealed fusion. With the cessation of pacing, the last stimulated orthodromic wave front passes through the circuit and returns once again to depolarize the pacing site after one complete circuit. As a result, the interval from the last paced stimulus to the next depolarization at the pacing site approximates the ventricular cycle length. This is called the postpacing interval.

Pacing at a site distant from the reentrant circuit, say at the border of the infarct scar in the outer loop, may entrain or reset the tachycardia, but the QRS complexes differ from the spontaneous arrhythmia due to fusion of the stimulated excitation wave fronts with the tachycardia wave fronts in the myocardium. This would be an example of classic entrainment. The postpacing interval in this case would also match the ventricular tachycardia cycle length.

Pacing at bystander sites adjacent to the reentrant circuit, for example site C, may entrain with concealed fusion. The postpacing interval in this case, however, would be the circuit time plus the time it takes to travel from C to point 15, and the cycle length is longer than the cycle length of the tachycardia.

Sustained monomorphic ventricular tachycardia can be initiated electrophysiologically in most patients with ischemic heart disease who have sustained the arrhythmia spontaneously (Di Marco et al 1985 and many others). Sustained monomorphic ventricular tachycardia associated with MI most commonly occurs during the chronic phase (Wellens et al 1976; Joseph et al 1978; Fisher et al 1977, among others). The first episode of sustained monomorphic ventricular tachycardia is often seen within the first year post-MI. However, the median is three years and the onset of the arrhythmia may occur as late as 10 to 15 years, a possible reflection of a ventricular aneurysm (Cohen et al 1983). A left ventricular aneurysm develops in up to 15 percent of patients who experience a myocardial infarction. An aneurysm, of course, is a classical substrate for reentrant arrhythmias.

The relationship between sustained monomorphic ventricular tachycardia and ventricular fibrillation is uncertain. Sustained monomorphic ventricular tachycardia may simply be the company kept by ventricular fibrillation in a number of patients or, in the appropriate setting such as recurrent ischemia; it may provide a rapid wave front that becomes fractionated, leading to ventricular fibrillation.

Nonischemic dilated cardiomyopathy is often accompanied by poor R-wave progression in the precordial leads, reflecting a decrease in anterior forces due either to replacement of muscle with fibrous tissue or perhaps to a change in the activation sequence due to fibrosis affecting the subendocardial Purkinje system (Wilensky et al 1988), conditions favorable to anisotropic reentry. Intraventricular conduction abnormalities, particularly left bundle branch block, and ST-T wave abnormalities are also common. Ventricular arrhythmias are often seen in nonischemic dilated cardiomyopathy. Premature ventricular beats and couplets occur in over 90 percent of patients and nonsustained ventricular tachycardia in up to 60 percent; however, sustained monomorphic ventricular tachycardia is unusual, occurring in five percent or less (Huang et al 1983; Meinertz et al 1984).

Hypertrophic cardiomyopathy is familial disease characterized by myocardial hypertrophy in the absence of precipitating conditions such as hypertension. At a microscopic level, there is extensive myocardial disarray with bundles crossing each other in different directions, whorls of muscle cells, perpendicular branching, and fibrosis. Particularly in the disease caused by troponin T mutation, even in the absence of significant hypertrophy, sudden death is common. Recently, the degree of histological myocardial disarray has been linked to sudden death in the troponin T disease (Varnava et al 2001). It is likely that anisotropic reentry underlies many of these reentrant arrhythmias as a result of the disorganized cardiac muscle architecture, fibrosis and microvascular abnormalities, and in some cases, myocardial thickness. The muscular disarray and fibrosis often results in a "pseudoinfarct" pattern with poor R wave progression across the precordium, and up to one-half have Q-wave abnormalities in the inferior and/or lateral leads. Frequent ventricular arrhythmias and an increase in sudden death have been reported for hypertrophic cardiomyopathy carrying the troponin and other mutations (Brigden,1987;McKenna, Franklin 1988; Fananapazir et al 1989;Spirito et al 1989;Maron et al 1987; Maron et al 1987), among others}. Hypertrophic cardiomyopathy may or may not be obstructive, and both forms have a similar natural history. Ventricular tachycardia has been found in about 25 percent of patients studied with Holter monitoring, and some believe that ventricular tachycardia is associated with a higher risk of sudden death. The incidence of sustained monomorphic ventricular tachycardia varies with the population observed. In a general population with HCM, 20 percent had nonsustained ventricular tachycardia but sustained monomorphic ventricular tachycardia was rare (Shakespeare et al 1982). On the other hand, inducible sustained monomorphic ventricular tachycardia is present in almost 50 percent of patients who have had either cardiac arrest or syncope and who undergo programmed electrical stimulation (Kuck et al 1988; 1987;Kowey et al 1984).

Bundle branch reentrant ventricular tachycardia is a somewhat special category of sustained monomorphic ventricular tachycardia in that its mechanism involves abnormal conduction through structures that are normally present (Lloyd et al 1982;Caceres et al 1989). The bundle branches consist of bundles of Purkinje fibers which are inherently anisotropic to favor rapid conduction. Bundle branch reentrant ventricular tachycardia occurs with both ischemic and nonischemic heart disease and is usually severe with cardiomegaly and a history of congestive heart failure. The associated fibrosis may affect conduction and unidirectional block in a way favorable to the induction of this arrhythmia. Most commonly, antegrade conduction is down the right bundle branch with delayed depolarization of the left ventricle resulting in a ventricular tachycardia with a typical left bundle branch block appearance. In some patients, however, the reverse sequence of conduction occurs, leading to a right bundle branch block appearance. The PR interval may be normal or prolonged. The mean electrical axis is usually about +30 degrees, but a conduction defect in the left anterior fascicle will produce a marked leftward (superior) axis deviation. Recently, the longer HV interval often seen in bundle branch reentrant ventricular tachycardia has been thought due in part to anisotropic conduction (Fisher, 2000). The postulate is that the impulse travels retrogradely in the left bundle branch and continues proximately and at the same velocity in the same fibers as it proceeds through the His bundle. At the same time, the impulse propagates more slowly laterally to the fibers of the right bundle branch and then proceeds down to the ventricle. This combination of normal velocity reaching the His bundle and the delay in reaching the right bundle prior to continuing to the ventricle could account for most of the longer HV interval.

Although sustained monomorphic ventricular tachycardia is most commonly due to organic heart disease, particularly chronic ischemic heart disease, both sustained and nonsustained monomorphic ventricular tachycardia can occur in the absence of any demonstrable heart disease. Most fall into three descriptive categories, namely, repetitive monomorphic ventricular tachycardia, paroxysmal sustained ventricular tachycardia and left ventricular idiopathic ventricular tachycardia. As will be discussed, although triggered activity has been suggested as the underlying mechanism for most of these arrhythmias, anisotropy at a microscopic scale may underlie the arrhythmias as well.

Repetitive monomorphic ventricular tachycardia is characterized by frequent short bursts of monomorphic nonsustained ventricular tachycardia and is also called right ventricular tachycardia, catecholamine sensitive ventricular tachycardia and exercise-induced ventricular tachycardia (Brooks, Burgess, 1988; Parkinson, Papp, 1942; Buxton et al 1983; Coumel et al 1985, among others). The arrhythmia usually arises at the septal aspect of the right ventricular outflow tract, but may arise from the right ventricular inflow tract, the free wall of the right ventricular outflow track and the left ventricle. The electrocardiogram in some 70% of patients shows left bundle branch block and an inferior axis (Brooks, Burgess, 1988). A right bundle branch pattern with a monophasic R wave in V_1 with an inferior axis suggests the origin at the left ventricular outflow tract.

On the basis of electrophysiologic testing, the sensitivity to catecholamines and the response to calcium antagonists, beta-adrenoreceptor blockers and adenosine has led to the supposition that triggered activity rather than reentry has been thought to be the mechanism. While it is true that the signal averaged ECG in the time domain is usually normal, high frequency components are often recorded within the QRS complex using fast Fourier transformation (Kinoshita et al 1995), components not recorded in normal or in patients with arrhythmogenic right ventricular dysplasia. These high frequency components perhaps represent anisotropic reentry on a microscopic scale.

Paroxysmal sustained ventricular tachycardia is considered by some to be a distinct clinical syndrome (Richie et al 1989), but not all investigators agree (Mont et al 1992). It seems to be more commonly induced by electrophysiologic provocation suggesting a reentrant mechanism, although much of the same evidence suggestive of a triggered mechanism exists as well. For example, adenosine and edrophonium rather consistently terminate the arrhythmia, suggesting that cAMP-mediated triggered activity is the underlying mechanism (Lerman et al 1986).

Zipes and his colleagues described Idiopathic left ventricular tachycardia in 1979 (Zipes et al 1979), and Belhassen and his colleagues described the termination of this ventricular tachycardia with intravenous verapamil (Bellassen et al 1981). Electrophysiologic mapping localizes the site of origin to the inferior aspect of the midseptal region. The electrocardiogram characteristically shows a right bundle branch block, a left superior axis, and a QRS duration usually of 120 to 140 msec. A few show right axis deviation. Frequency analysis using fast Fourier transform has shown an abnormal high-frequency component of the terminal portion of the

QRS complex that may distinguish these patients from normals (Kinoshita et al 1995) which, with the ability of electrophysiologic stimulation to provoke, entrain and terminate the arrhythmia, suggests a reentrant mechanism (Okumura et al 1988) despite the verapamil-sensitivity. The arrhythmia has also been called "fascicular" since a distinct Purkinje spike usually precedes the onset of the QRS, but the retrograde His bundle spike can be dissociated from the QRS complex by premature stimulation in the ventricle, atrium, or bundle of His suggesting that the posterior fascicle of the left bundle branch may be involved in or at least in close proximity to the reentrant circuit (Ward et al 1984).

CREATION OF ANISOTROPY WITH THERATEUTIC INTENTION

Anisotropy can be created with a therapeutic intention. In this case, surgery or radiofrequency ablation is used to dissociate and uncouple cells through trauma and subsequent scarring. A few examples will be considered.

Atrial Flutter

Typical atrial flutters is clockwise or counterclockwise rotation around the tricuspid annulus with the crista terminalis and the Eustachian ridge as posterior barriers. The isthmus is a reasonable anatomic target for ablation, usually between the inferior vena cava and the tricuspid annulus but also between the Eustachian ridge and the tricuspid annulus (Klein et al 1986; Cosio et al 1988; Olgin et al 1995; Touboul et al 1989; Olshansky et al 1990).

A smaller isthmus is present between the tricuspid valve annulus and the coronary sinus ostium, and there has been some success in abolishing atrial flutter by ablating this isthmus. The initial success rate for the ablation of atrial flutter, as defined by the termination of the arrhythmia and/or the inability to induce atrial flutter has ranged from 65% to 100%. The recurrence rate is between 7% and 44%. Factors which increase the risk for recurrence include a history of atrial fibrillation, increased right atrial size and perhaps anatomic features (Nath et al 1995). The data suggests that the criteria for successful ablation need to more stringent including, for example, the demonstration of block in the isthmus during proximal coronary sinus and low right atrial pacing (Poty et al 1995). Ablation guided by intracardiac echocardiography may be useful with one study showing that the best site for ablation may be between the tricuspid annulus and the Eustachian ridge rather than the more commonly used area between the tricuspid annulus and the orifice of the inferior vena cava (Olgin et al 1995). Ablation of this site is more difficult, however, and new types of ablation catheters may need to be developed to ablate this area efficiently. Intracardiac echocardiography may also be useful in identifying anatomic variability among patients.

Atrial Fibrillation

Atrial fibrillation is another arrhythmia in which anisotropy may be produced with ntion. Because of the morbidity and mortality associated with atrial fibrillation and the disappointing results of pharmacological therapy in maintaining sinus rhythm after cardioversion, there has been increasing interest in nonpharmacologic strategies, and both surgical and nonsurgical interruption of old pathways with the creation of new pathways of conduction are interesting strategies.

The goals of the ideal procedure for atrial fibrillation have been summarized by Ferguson and Cox (1995) are abolition of atrial fibrillation, restoration of sinus rhythm, reestablishment or maintenance of atrioventricular synchrony, restoration of atrial transport and reduction or elimination of the risk of thromboembolism by eliminating passive stasis of blood in either or both atria.

The first attempts were surgical. One such technique is the "corridor" operation in which the sinus node, a strip of atrial tissue, and the atrioventricular node were isolated from the rest of the atria, thereby allowing sinus rhythm to be sustained. In an initial report, seven of nine patients treated with this procedure maintained sinus rhythm with a mean follow-up of three to 41 months, but four patients required a pacemaker due to postoperative sinus node dysfunction (Leitch et al 1991). In a larger study, the biatrial isolation procedure was found to leave the free wall tissue of the right and left atria fibrillating, while the ventricles were being activated by the SA node through the corridor (van Hemel et al 1994). The corridor procedure, therefore, fails attaining the criteria since long term anticoagulation is required and normal atrial-ventricular synchrony is not restored.

Atrial fibrillation was abolished An alternative is the "maze" operation in which several small incisions are made in the atrium to interrupt the potential reentrant pathways required for atrial fibrillation (Cosio et al 2000). Atrial fibrillation cannot be sustained after this procedure because the impulse is not able to reenter upon itself. Cox in (2000) reported on 346 patients. The perioperative mortality was 2 to 3%. and AV conduction restored in virtually all patients. 93% had left atrial transport return. A small percentage required permanent pacemakers, and some had a blunting of the chronotropic response. The Cleveland Clinic reported that 90.4% of patients were in sinus rhythm or with an atrial pacemaker 3 years after the maze procedure (McCarthy et al 2000). The Mayo Clinic reported similar results and stressed that the restoration of sinus rhythm improved left ventricular ejection fraction in most patients (Shaff et al 2000)}. Kosakai (2000) reported on more than 2500 patients in Japan in which a variety of maze and other procedures were used. Best success was obtained with a maze procedure.

A modified maze procedure, designed to limit myocardial damage, reports in patients undergoing surgery for mitral valve disease or an atrial septal defect reported that the technique was effective in restoring sinus rhythm (85 percent) and atrial contractility (71 percent) (Sandoval e al 1996).

A recent report has used radiofrequency energy to create lines of conduction block in both atria during cardiac surgery as a modification of the maze procedure with a resulting freedom from atrial flutter and fibrillation of over 78% and with documented left atrial transport function in 77% (Sie et al 2001). The Maze III procedure has been adapted to be done by minimally invasive techniques (Cox et al 2000).

The surgical experience inspired interventional electrophysiologists to use radiofrequency catheter ablation for atrial fibrillation. The progress of this approach has been reviewed recently (Gibbons et al in press) with limited success using linear ablation in the right and left atria. Ablation strategies targeting the triggering foci in the pulmonary veins or other sites have been developed, but the recurrence rate remains as high as 55%. The ablative procedures are also complicated by systemic embolization, pulmonary vein stenosis, pericardial effusion and tamponade, and phrenic nerve paralysis.

Hybrid pharmacologic and ablative therapy has been proposed in a select group of patients in which antiarrhythmic drugs, most commonly a class IC drug or amiodarone converts atrial fibrillation to atrial flutter, and atrial flutter then becomes the sole rhythm (Huang et al 1998). In these patients, ablation of the flutter often results in maintenance of sinus rhythm so long as antiarrhythmic therapy is continued to prevent reemergence of the fibrillation.

Another approach has been radiofrequency ablation of the AV node and permanent pacing in symptomatic patients with medically refractory atrial fibrillation. A recent meta-analysis of 1181 patients (Wood et al 2000) significantly reduces cardiac symptoms and increases exercise duration, quality of life and ejection fraction.

Atrioventricular Nodal Reentrant Tachycardia

The most common circuit (over 90 percent) is antegrade down a relatively slowing conducting pathway and retrograde up a more rapidly conducting pathway. Less commonly, the antegrade circuit utilizes the more rapidly conducting pathway with return along the slower pathway. The delineators of Koch's triangle have been discussed, and the triangle itself can be divided into thirds. The anterior third contains the fast pathways and is in close proximity to the compact AV node. The posterior third is associated with the coronary sinus, and the middle third is between the two. The slow pathways are in the middle and posterior thirds.

Radiofrequency ablation can be aimed either at the fast pathway (anterior) or the slow pathway (posterior) (see Fig. 8). The anterior approach to ablation delivers the RF energy in the anterior third of Koch's triangle somewhat anterior and proximal to the His Bundle. The target site is determined either anatomically or by the amplitude of the local atrial electrogram. In about 30 percent of patients with successful ablation, there is still an antegrade gap and retrograde conduction despite elimination of the reentrant arrhythmia. This observation demonstrates that small alterations in the reentrant circuit are often sufficient to prevent the arrhythmia. Complete AV block, as would be expected, is a not uncommon complication of the anterior approach with an incidence of about six percent (range 0 to 21 percent).

The posterior approach delivers the RF energy in the middle or posterior septal region near the coronary sinus ostium with the slow pathway as the target. The target site is determined either by anatomic position or by the morphology of the electrogram. Some electrophysiologists begin ablation in the mid-septal portion, but most begin in the posterior third of Koch's triangle where the risk of AV block is the least. With anatomic targeting, the ablation catheter is placed posterior to the coronary sinus ostium and is then progressively moved anteriorly towards the His bundle. RF energy is applied in each position and provocative electrophysiologic stimulation is used to determine efficacy. With electrogram targeting, the ablation catheter is positioned at the His bundle and then withdrawn posteriorly along the mitral annulus searching for putative slow pathway potentials. Again, the RF energy is titrated. Approximately 80 percent of successful ablation sites are found between the coronary os and the tricuspid valve. The dual pathway physiology is eliminated about one-half to two-thirds of cases. In the remainder, the dual pathway physiology persists even though reentrant arrhythmia is abolished. It is not necessary to eliminate all slow pathway conduction, since it may be possible to induce single atrial echoes even though the sustained arrhythmia has been eliminated. As a technical note, the wide distribution of sites and the fact that slow pathway conduction can be affected by energy application at several sites in the same patient suggests that there may be multiple slow pathways or multiple atrial insertions.

Ventricular Tachycardia

Catheter ablation has been primarily used in three types of ventricular tachycardia: microreentrant, bundle branch block reentrant associated with structural heart disease and idiopathic ventricular tachycardia in which the arrhythmia is not associated with underlying structural heart. The interested reader is referred to the recent review by Stevenson and Delacretaz (Stevenson and Delacretaz, 2000), but a few comments are in order.

The vast majority of microreentrant ventricular tachycardias that have been treated with ablation are of the sustained monomorphic form. A number of recent reports have reviewed the methods that have been advocated to locate the site of ventricular tachycardia (Blanck et al 1994; Stevenson 1995;Stevenson, Delacretaz 2000;Kline et al 1993; Josephson 1993;D'Avila et al 1994;Prytowsky et al 1994; Borggrefe et al 1995). During reentrant types of ventricular tachycardia accompanying ischemic heart disease, low amplitude signals detected by electrophysiology testing usually allow the identification of the orthodromic and antidromic areas of conduction and indicate the area of interest for ablation.   The slow conduction and areas of unidirectional block of anisotropic conduction are often detected by locating areas with isolated mid-diastolic potentials which cannot be dissociated from the tachycardia by pacing and often represent a vulnerable portion of the reentrant circuit and predict a good response to ablation (Fitzgerald et al 1988) . Entrainment has been discussed in detail above, and the best ablation site can, in about 50 percent of cases, be further defined by entrainment, without evidence for fusion, in an area of slow conduction (Fitzgerald et al 1988;Garan, Ruskin 1988; Morady et al 1988; Stevenson et al 1993). This results in a QRS complex that is identical to that of the spontaneous ventricular tachycardia (entrainment with concealed fusion) and that has a long stimulus to QRS duration. If the anisotropic pathways that underlie reentry are constant, pacing from near the site of arrhythmogenesis should have a QRS morphology similar to the spontaneous arrhythmia.   This is called pace mapping in which left and right endocardial ventricular pacing is performed during sinus rhythm in an attempt to mimic the QRS complex of the spontaneous arrhythmia. The correlation between the site of stimulation and the resultant point of epicardial emergence of activation may be poor, however, and there is concern about the frequency of both false negative and false positive results (Stevenson et al 1995;Josephson et al 1982;Kuchar et al 1989).

Figure 10 shows mapping data obtained from an individual who had experienced a myocardial infarction and later developed ventricular tachycardia (from (Stevenson, Delacretaz 2000)). A CARTO™ electrophysiologic navigation system (Biosense Webster) was used that plots the precise catheter position along with color-coded electrophysiologic information (Gepstein, Evans, 1985). Although detail is lost in this black and white depiction of a color image, the upper panels show the left ventricle in the right anterior oblique

Bipolar voltage

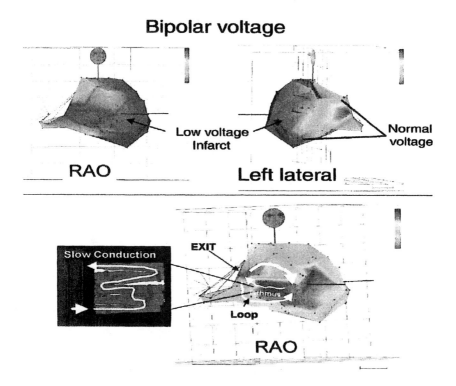

Figure 10 The mapping data are from a patient who developed ventricular tachycardia late after an anterioapical wall myocardial infarction. Mapping was performed using the CARTO™ electrophysiologic mapping system that plots the precise catheter position along with color-coded electrophysiologic information (Biosense Webster, Diamond Bar, CA). Detail is lost in the black and white rendition of the color image, but the reader can get the sense of the power of the technique. The top two panels show the left ventricle in right anterior oblique (RAO) and left lateral views. Details are lost in the black and white rendition of the color image, butthe large anteroapical infarction is indicated by an extensive area of low voltage, the location of which is indicated by the arrows. The lower right panel shows the map of ventriculartachycardia in the same patient. The ventricle is again shown in a right anterior oblique projection with the apex at the right and the base at the left hand side of the image. Colors in the original figure indicate the activation sequence, and again detail is lost in the black and white renditions. Arrows have been drawn to clarify the activation sequence of the circuit. The reentrant circuit is located in the septum. The wave front starts at the area marked "exit" near the base of the septum and splits into two loops that circle around the superior and inferior aspect of the septum toward the apex, re-entering an isthmus in the circuit that is proximal to the exit region. Radiofrequency ablation in the isthmus abolishedtachycardia. The mechanism of slow conduction through the infarct region that has been observed in previous histopathologic studies is illustrated schematically in the inset at lower left. Survivingmyocyte bundles are separated by fibrous tissue that forces the wave front to take a circuitous path through the region. From Stevenson with permission {282}.

lower left schematically shows the mechanism of slow conduction in which muscle bundles are separated by scarring that results in the circuitous path underlying the arrhythmia. Problems are that there may be false isthmuses, the isthmus or circuit may be quite deep and therefore unidentifiable or unable to be ablated from the endocardium, multiple reentrant circuits may exist, and the arrhythmia may be hemodynamically unstable making mapping difficult. The term "clinical tachycardia" refers to ventricular tachycardias that occur spontaneously, while those that are electrophysiologically induced but not observed spontaneously are referred to as "nonclinical tachycardias." Not infrequently, a nonclinical ventricular tachycardia may appear after ablation of the clinical ventricular tachycardia. Another imaging system that may become clinically important is a real-time interactive cardiac magnetic resonance imaging system which can image the ablated tissue (Lardo et al 2000). A variety of newer approaches using "cooled" radiofrequency ablation, epicardial approach via an introducer into the pericardial space, and small catheters that can access the coronary sinus and cardiac veins and other approaches are nicely summarized by Stevenson and Delacretaz (2000).

The long-term success of ablation remains to be determined, and it is difficult to summarize the data because of differences in patient populations, details of the mapping and ablation, and number of patients (see reviews, (Stevenson and Delacretaz ,2000;Borggrefe et al 1995)). The Percutaneous Catheter Mapping and Ablation Registry, in which DC shock ablation was primarily used, reported that only about one-third of subjects remained free of arrhythmia while the mortality rate, including mortality related to the procedure itself, was 25 percent (Evans et al a 1986). Less information is at present available with radiofrequency current ablation, although this procedure is now preferred. Gonska and his colleagues published two reports on the use of radiofrequency ablation for ventricular arrhythmias (Gonska et al 1994;1994). In the larger study, 136 patients with coronary disease who had one configuration of sustained monomorphic ventricular tachycardia underwent either radiofrequency ablation (72 patients) or DC current ablation (64 patients) (Gonska et al 1994). The mapping procedure included pace mapping during sinus rhythm, endocardial activation mapping, identification of isolated mid-diastolic potentials, and pacing interventions during ventricular tachycardia. The success rate (74 versus 77 percent) and complication rate (10 versus 14 percent) were similar with the two procedures. Strickberger et al (1997), Rothman et al (1997), and Stevenson et al (1998) attempted ablation on a total of 108 ablations. An average of 3.6 to 4.7 different ventricular tachycardias were induced in each patient. All inducible monomorphic ventricular tachycardias were abolished in 33% while no effect resulted in 22%. In the remaining, the ventricular tachycardias that had been targeted for ablation were ablated, but other inducible ventricular tachycardias remained. The mean duration of follow-up was 12 to 18 months during which 66% of individuals were free of recurrent ventricular tachycardia, 24% had recurrences, and 2.8% had "sudden death" but fortunately most had an implanted defibrillator.

Bundle branch reentry has been successfully treated using ablation. The site of ablation for ventricular tachycardia due to bundle branch reentry with the most common left bundle branch block pattern is the right bundle branch. Catheter ablation has been very successful in bundle branch reentrant tachycardia that characteristically has a left (rarely a right) bundle branch morphology. In one report, for example, DC current ablation of the right bundle branch in seven patients resulted in abolition of the arrhythmia in all patients; there were no recurrences on follow-up (Tchou et al 1988). Similar findings were noted in a larger study of ablation in 28 patients (Caceres, 1989). These results suggest that ablation therapy is the treatment of choice for this type of ventricular tachycardia.

Idiopathic ventricular tachycardia, thought not associated with structural organic heart disease, usually arises in the right ventricular outflow tract. In the discussion of these arrhythmias above, it was suggested that anisotropic microreentry might underlie at least some of these tachycardias. Triggered activity is also a probably mechanism and arises from a very localized area of myocardium. Pace mapping is a useful means to identify the best sites for ablations in idiopathic ventricular tachycardia arising from the right ventricular outflow tract (Wilber et al 1993). On the other hand, the target for ablation in idiopathic left ventricular tachycardia (which originates in the apicoseptal portion of the left ventricle) is often best defined as site with the earliest local electrogram and identification of a Purkinje potential (Nakagawa et al 1993;Klein et al 1992). A number of ablation studies of modest size have now been reported in idiopathic ventricular tachycardia with initial success rates ranging from 75 to 100 percent for tachycardias that originate in the right ventricular outflow tract, and 50 to 90 percent for those that originate at other sites. There is limited information on long-term follow-up. In one study of 20 patients with idiopathic left ventricular tachycardia, for example, the initial success rate was 85 percent and there were no recurrences at 7-8 months (Wen et al 1994). Six patients underwent a repeat electrophysiologic study; none were inducible. Similar results were reported in another study in which ablation was successful in about 85% of patients with right or left sided idiopathic ventricular tachycardia (Rodriguez et al 1997). Failures resulted usually from the inability to induce the arrhythmia or to map it adequate as well as by location deep within the septum or in the epicardium over the septum.

The data is very limited for other forms of ventricular tachycardia that may have anisotropic reentry as a basis. The role of ablation in arrhythmogenic right ventricular dysplasia and Tetralogy of Fallot remains to be defined. Preliminary evidence suggests that radiofrequency catheter ablation may be successful in some patients with sustained ventricular tachycardia and dilated cardiomyopathy (Evans et al 1986;Kottokamp et al 1995). In a series of 26 patients in patients with ventricular tachycardia caused by non-ischemic cardiomyopathy, the underlying causes were scar and reentry in 62%,

an ectopic focus in 27% and bundle branch reentry in 19% (Delecretaz et al 2000).

Surgery is another way of eliminating pathways by creating barriers and redirecting the wave front of activation, and the topic has been reviewed recently (Lawrie, Pacifico, 1995). The most commonly employed surgical techniques are endocardial resection, myocardial excision and cryoablation. The need for surgery for ventricular tachycardia has decreased given the improvements in acute care of myocardial infarction to prevent the formation of aneurysms and extensive fibrosis, catheter ablation and the use of tiered implantable devices that including pacing and d.c. electroversion. Other types of nonischemic ventricular tachycardia amenable to surgery include cardiomyopathies (dilated and hypertrophic), arrhythmogenic right ventricular dysplasia, cardiac tumors, long QT syndrome, postoperative Tetralogy of Fallot, valvular heart disease and a smattering of other etiologies. The results currently are quite good in the highly selected cases that come to surgery.

SUMMARY AND THE FUTURE

The intention of this Chapter in the previous edition of this book was is to create an intellectual framework for the clinician based on biophysical theory, and to allow the researcher who is not a physician an insight into clinical thought processes. The intention remains the same. A substantial body of new information, basic, clinical, and translational, has arisen since the last edition. Yet the principles remain the same. The role of gap junctions in normal excitability, the synchronization of pacemakers, anisotropic conduction and the maintenance of an integrated wave front through electrotonic interactions among fiber bundles remains central to the discussion. Increasingly, it seems that gap junctional dysfunction frequently

underlies abnormal anisotropic conduction and reentry both in supraventricular and ventricular arrhythmias, particularly in the presence of chronic organic heart disease. Experimental studies in chronic infarction in which fibrosis has separated the myocytes while the myocytes themselves have normal action potentials show that non-uniform anisotropic conduction provides a substrate sufficient for *reentrant tachycardias*. *To make the discussion seemingly less esoteric* for the clinician, the results of surgical procedures and catheter ablation have been considered techniques to create anisotropic conduction with therapeutic intention. In the last edition of this book, we thought that possibly antiarrhythmic drugs will be developed that improve coupling or induce uncoupling specifically in injured cells, but progress has been slow. We also predicted that pacing from multiple sites may normalize non-uniform anisotropy, but little new information is available except perhaps in the use of synchronized pacing in the treatment of heart failure. New approaches to currently inaccessible reentrant circuits are being developed which will increasingly be applied to the ablation of ventricular tachycardias.
  The rapid development of new and better mapping and navigational devices with three-dimensional reconstruction and tracking of radiofrequency ablative lesions will present new diagnostic and therapeutic modalities.

REFERENCE

Allessie M.A., Konings K.T., Kirchhof C.J (1998). Mapping of atrial fibrillation. In: Atrial Fibrillation: Mechanisms and therapeutic Strategies, Olsson S.B., Allessie M.A., Campbell R.W., eds. Armonk,NY: Futura Publishers, pp. 37-49. (N)

Allessie M.A., Lammers W.J.E.P., Bonke F.I.M., et al (1985). Experimental evaluation of Moe's multiple wavelet hypothesis of atrial fibrillation. In: Cardiac Electrophysiology and Arrhythmias, Zipes D.P., Jalife J., eds. Orlando: Grune and Stratton, pp. 265-.

Anderson R.H., Ho S.Y., Wharton J., Becker A.E. (1995) Gross anatomy and microscopy of the conducting system. In: Cardiac Arrhythmias, (ed 3rd) Mandel W.J., ed. Philadelphia: J. B. Lippincott Company , pp. 13-54.

Anumonwo J.M.B., Delmar M., Vinet A., Michaels D.C., Jalife J (1991). Phase resetting and entrainment of pacemaker activity in single sinus nodal cells. Circ Res. 68:1138-53.

Armen R.N., Frank T.V(1949). Electrocardiographic patterns in pneumothorax. Diseases of the Chest. 15:709-.

Arnsdorf M.F., Sawicki G.J (1996). Flecainide and the electrophysiologic matrix: The effects of flecainide acetate on the determinants of cardiac excitability in sheep Purkinje fibers. J Cardiovasc Electrophysiol. 7:1172-82.

Arnsdorf M.F., Schmidt G.A., Sawicki G (1985). The effects of encainide on the determinants of cardiac excitability in sheep Purkinje fibers. J Pharmacol Exp Ther. 223:40-8.

Arnsdorf MF, Makielski JC: Excitability and Impulse Propagation. In: Physiology and Pathophysiology of the Heart. 4th edition, chapter 6. Sperelakis, N (ed). New York: Academic Press, (2001), pp. 99-132.

Balke C.W., Lesh M.D., Spear J.F., Kadish A., Levine J.H., Moore E.N (1988). Effects of cellular uncoupling on conduction in anisotropic canine ventricular myocardium. Circ Res. 63:879-92.

Bardy G.H., Packer D.L., German L.D., Gallagher J.J. (1984) Preexcited reciprocating tachycardia in patients with Wolff-Parkinson-White syndrome: Incidence and mechanisms. Circ. 70:377-91.

Barold S.S., Coumel P. (1977) Mechanisms of atrioventricular junctional tachycardia: Role of reentry and concealed accessory bypass tracts. Am J Cardiol.; 39:97-106.

Bauernfeind R.A., Amat-y-Leon F., Dhingra R.C., et al (1979). Chronic nonparoxysmal sinus tachycardia in otherwise health persons. Ann Intern Med. 91:702-10.

Bauernfeind R.A., Swiryn S., Strasberg B., Palileo E., Wyndham C., Duffy C.E., Rosen K.M. (1982) Analysis of anterograde and retrograde fast pathway properties in patients with dual atrioventricular nodal pathways: observations regarding the pathophysiology of the Lown-Ganong-Levine syndrome. Am J Cardiol.; 49:283-90.

Beaumont J., Davidenko N., Davidenko J.M., Jalife J (1998). Spiral waves in two-dimensionalmodesl of ventricular muscle: Formation of a stationary core. Biophys J. 75:1-14.

Belhassen B., Rotmensch H.H., Laniado S. (1981) Response of recurrent sustained ventricular tachycardia to verapamil. Br Heart J.; 46:679-82.

Benditt D.G., Pritchett L.C., Smith W.M., Wallace A.G., Gallagher J.J. (1978) Characteristics of atrioventricular conduction and the spectrum of arrhythmias in lown-ganong-levine syndrome. Circ. 57:454-65.

Berenfeld O., Jalife J (1998). Purkinje-muscle reentry as a mechanism of polymorphic ventricular arrhythmias in a 3-dimensional model of the ventricles. Circ Res. 82:1063-77.

Bharati S., Lev M (1992). Histology of the normal and diseased atrium. In: Atrial Fibrillation: Mechanism and Management, Fall R.H., Podrid P.J., eds. New York: Raven Press, pp. 15-39.

Blanck Z., Dhala A., Deshpande S., Sra J., Jazayeri M., Akhtar M (1994). Catheter ablation of ventricular tachycardia. [Review]. Am Heart J. 127:1126-33.

Bleeker W.K., MacKay A.J.C., Masson-Pevet M., Bouman L.N., Becker A.E (1980). Functional and morphological organization of the rabbit sinus node. Circ Res.46:11-22.

Borggrefe M., Chen X., Hindricks G., Haverkamp W., Willems S., Kottkamp H., Rotman B., Martinez-Rubio A., Shenasa M., Block M., Breithardt G. (1995) Catheter ablation of ventricular tachycardia in patients with coronary heart disease. In: Cardiac Electrophysiology: From Cell to Bedside, (ed 2nd) Zipes D.P., Jalife J., eds. Philadelphia: W. B. Saunders Company , pp. 1502-17.

Brigden W. (1987) Hypertrophic cardiomyopathy. Brit Heart J.; 58:299-302.

Brooks R., Burgess J.H. (1988) Idiopathic ventricular tachycardia. Medicine.; 67:271-94.

Brown G., Eccles J (1934). The action of a single vagal volley on the rhythm of the heart beat. J Physiol (Lond). 82:211-41.

Buchanan J.W., Gettes L.S (1990). Ionic Environment and Propagation. In: Cardiac Electrophysiology: From Cell to Bedside, Zipes D.P., Jalife J., eds. Philadelphia: Saunders, pp. 149-56.

Buxton A.E., Waxman L.H., Marchlinski F.E., Simson M.B., Cassidy D., Josephson M.E. (1983) Right ventricular tachycardia: Clinical and electrophysiologic characteristics. Circ.; 5:917-27.

Caceres J., Jazayeri M., McKinnie J., Avitall B., Denker S.T., Tchou P., Akhtar M. (1989) Sustained bundle branch reentry as a mechanism of clinical tachycardia. Circ.; 79:256-70.

Campbell R.W., Smith R.A., Gallagher J.J., Pritchett E.L., Wallace A.G. (1977) Atrial fibrillation in the preexcitation syndrome. Am J Cardiol.; 40:514-20.

Cappato R., Schluter M., Mont L., Kuck K.H. (1994) Anatomic, electrical, and mechanical factors affecting bipolar endocardial electrograms. Impact on catheter ablation of manifest left free-wall accessory pathways. Circ. 90:884-94.

Cardinal R., Vermeulen M., Shenasa M., Roberge F., Page P., Helie F., Savard P. (1988) Anisotropic conduction and functional dissociation of ischemic tissue during reentrant ventricular tachycardia in canine myocardial infarction. Circ.; 77:1162-76.

Carey P.A., Turner M., Fry C.H., Sheridan D.J (2001). Reduced anisotropy of action potential conduction in left ventricular hypertrophy. J Cardiovas Electrophys. 12:830-5.

Castellanos A., Moleiro F., Saoudi N.C., Myerburg R.J (1990). Parasystole. In: Cardiac Electrophysiology from Cell to Bedside, Zipes D.P., Jalife J., eds. Philadelphia: W. B. Saunders Company, pp. 619-27.

Cauchemez B., Haissaguerre M., Fischer B., Thomas O., Clementy J., Coumel P. (1996) Electrophysiologic effects of catheter ablation of inferior vena cava-tricuspid annulus isthmus in common atrial flutter. Circ.; 93:284-94.

Chen S.A., Chiang C.E., Wu T.J., Tai C.T., Lee S.H., Cheng C.C., Chiou C.W., Ueng K.C., Wen Z.C., Chang M.S. (1996) Radiofrequency catheter ablation of common atrial flutter: Comparision of electrophysiologically guided focal ablation technique and linear ablation technique. JACC.; 27:860-8.

Chu E., Kalman J.M., Kwasman M.A., Jue J.C., Fitzgerald P.J., Epstein L.M., Schiller N.B., Yock P.G., Lesh M.D(1994). Intracardiac echocardiography during radiofrequency catheter ablation of cardiac arrhythmias in humans. JACC. 24:1351-7.

Cohen M., Wiener I., Pichard A., Holt J., Smith H. Jr., Gorlin R. (1983) Determinants of ventricular tachycardia in patients with coronary artery disease and ventricular aneurysm. Am J Cardiol.; 51:61-4.

Cosio F.G., Arribas F., Barbero M.J(1988). Validation of double-spike electrograms as markers of conduction delay or block in atrial flutter. Am J Cardiol. 61:775-80.

Cosio F.G., Arribas F., Lopez-Gil M., Palacios J (1996). Atrial flutter mapping and ablation. I. Studying atrial flutter mechanisms by mapping and entrainment. [Review] [39 refs]. PACE. 19:841-53.

Cosio F.G., Lopez G.M., Goicolea A., Arribas F. (1992) Electrophysiologic studies in atrial flutter. Clin Cardiol.; 61:667-73.

Coumel P (1996). Autonomic influences in atrial tachyarrhythmias. J Cardiovasc Electrophysiol. 7:999-1007.

Coumel P., Attuel P. (1974) Reciprocating tachycardia in overt and latent preexcitation: Influence of bundle branch block on the rate of the tachycardia. Eur J Cardiol.; 1:423-36.

Coumel P., Cabrol C., Fabiato A., Gourgon R., Slama R. (1967) Tachycardie permanent part rhythme r,coprique. I. Preuves du diagnostic par stimulation auriculaire et ventriculaire. Arc Mal Coeur Vaiss.; 60:1830-64.

Coumel P., Leclerq J.P., Slama R. (1985) Repetitive monomorphic idiopathic ventricular tachycardia. In: Cardiac Electrophysiology and Arrhythmias, Zipes D.P., Jalife J., eds. Orlando, FL: Grune and Stratton, pp. 455-66.

Cox J.L. (1993) Evolving applications of the maze procedure for atrial fibrillation. Ann Thorac Surg.; 55:578-80.

Cox J.L., Ad N., Palazzo T., et al. (2000) Current status of the Maze procedure for the treatment of atrial fibrillation. Seminars in Thoracic & Cardiovascular Surgery.; 12:15-9.

Critelli G., Gallagher J.J., Monda V., Coltorti F., Scherillo M., Rossi L. (1984) Anatomic and electrophysiologic substrate of the permanent form of junctional reciprocating tachycardia. JACC.; 4:610-.

Danse P.W., Garratt C.J., Mast F., Allessie M.A (2000). Preferential depression of conduction around a pivot point in rabbit ventricular myocardium by potassium and flecainide. J Cardiovas Electrophys. 11:262-73.

D'Avila A., Nellens P., Andries E., Brugada P. (1994) Catheter ablation of ventricular tachycardia occurring late after myocardial infarction: a point-of-view. [Review]. Pace - Pacing & Clinical Electrophysiology.; 17:532-41.

De Mello W.C (1996). Renin-angiotensin system and cell communication in the failing heart. Hypertension. 199 27:1172-7.

De Mello W.C., Altieri P.I (1992). The role of the renin-angiotensin system in the control of cell communication in heart: Effects of angiotensin II and enalapril. J Cardiovasc Pharmacol. 20:643-51.

De Mello W.C., Jan Danser A.H (2000). Angiotensin II and the Heart: On the intracrine renin-angiotensin system. Hypertension. 35:1183-8.

De Mello.(1977) Passive electrical properties of the atrio-ventricular node. Pfluegers Arch .371:135-9.

DeFelice L.J., Challice C.E. (1969) Anatomical and ultrastructural study of the electrophysiological atrioventricular node of the rabbit. Circ Res.; 24:457-74.

Delecretaz E., Stevenson W.G., Ellison K.E., et al. (2000) Mapping and radiofrequency catheter ablation of the three types of sustained monomorphic ventricular tachycardias in nonischemic heart disease. J Cardiovas Electrophys.; 11:11-7.

Delgado C., Steinhaus B., Delmar M., Chialvo D.R., Jalife J (1990). Directional differences in excitability and margin of safety for propagation in sheep ventricular epicardial muscle. Circ Res. 67:97-110.

Delmar M., Michaels D.C., Johnson T., Jalife J (1997). Effects of Increasing Intercellular Resistance on Transverse and Longitudinal Propagation in Sheep Epicardial Muscle. Circ Res. 60:780-5.

Denes P., Wu D., Amat-y-Leon F., Dhingra R., Wyndham C.R., Rosen K.M. (1977) The determinants of atrioventricular nodal re-entrance with premature atrial stimulation in patients with dual A-V nodal pathways. Circ. 56:253-9.

Denes P., Wu D., Dhringra R.D., Chuquimia R., Rosen K.M. (1973) Demonstration of dual A-V nodal pathways in patients with paroxysmal supraventricular tachycardia. Circ. 48:549.

Denton T.A., Diamond G.A., Helfant R.H., Khan S., Karagueuzian H (1990): Fascinating rhythm. A primer on chaos theory and its application to cardiology. Am Heart J. 120:1419-40.

Dillon S.M., Allessie M.A., Ursell P.C., Wit A.L. (1988) Influences of anisotropic tissue structure on reentrant circuits in the epicardial border zone of subacute canine infarcts. Circ Res.; 63:182-206.

DiMarco J.P., Lerman B.B., Kron I.L., Sellers T.D. (1985) Sustained ventricular tachyarrhythmias within 2 months of acute myocardial infarction: results of medical and surgical therapy in patients resuscitated from the initial episode. JACC.; 6:759-68.

Disertori M., Inama G., Vergara G., Guarniero M., Del Favero A., Furlanello F (1983). Evidence of a reentry circuit in the common type of atrial flutter in man. Circulation. 67:434-40.

Dominguez G., Fozzard H.A (1970). Influence of extracellular K+ concentration on cable properties and excitability of sheep cardiac Purkinje fibers. Circ Res. 26:565-74.

Draper M.H., Mya-Tu M (1959). A comparison of the conduction velocity in cardiac tissues of various mammals. Quar J Exp Physiol. 44:91-109.

Eloff BC, Lerner DL, Yamada KA, Schuessler RB, Saffitz JE, Rosenbaum DS. (2001) High resolution optical mapping reveals conduction slowing in connexin43 deficient mice. Cardiovascular Res. ;51:681-690.

El-Sherif N., Smith R.A., Evans K. (1981) Canine ventricular arrhythmias in the late myocardial infarction period. 8. Epicardial mapping of reentrant circuits. Circ Res.; 49:255-65.

Elvan A., Huang X.D., Pressler M.I., Zipes D.P (1997). Radiofrequency catheter ablation of the atria eliminates pacing-induced sustained atrial fibrillation and reduces connexin43 in dogs. Circulation. 96:1675-85.

Engelmann T.W (1875). Uber die Leitung der Erregung im Herzmuskel. Pflugers Arch. 11:465-80.

Engelmann T.W (1877). Vergleichende Untersuchungen zur Lehre von der Muskel- und Nervenelectricitat. Pfluegers Arch Physiol. 15:116-48.

Evans G.T., Scheinman M.M., Zipes D.P. (1986) The percutaneous cardiac mapping and ablation registry: summary of results. Pace - Pacing & Clinical Electrophysiology.; 9:923-6.

Falk R.H(2001). Atrial fibrillation. N Engl J Med. 344:1067-78.

Fananapazir L., Tracy C.M., Leon M.B., Winkler J.B., Cannon R.O. 3d., Bonow R.O., Maron B.J., Epstein S.E. (1989) Electrophysiologic abnormalities in patients with hyperrophic cardiomyopathy. A consecutive analysis in 155 patients. Circulation. 80:1259-68.

Fareh S., Benardeau A., Thibault B., Nattel S (1999). The T-type Ca(2+) channel blocker mibefradil prevents the development of a substrate for atrial fibrillation by tachycardia-induced atrial remodeling in dogs. Circ. 100:2191-7.

Fareh S., Benardeau A., Thibault B., Nattel S (2001). Differentiall efficacy of L-and T-type calcium channel blockers in preventing tachycardia-induced atrial remodeling in dogs. Cardiovasc Res. 49:762-70.

Feld G., Fleck R.P., Chen P.S., Boyce K., Bahnson T., Stein J.B., Calisi C.M., Ibarra M. (1992) Radiofrequency catheter ablation for the treatment of human type I atrial flutter. Identification of a critical zone in the reentrant circuit by endocardial mapping techniques. Circ.; 86:1233-40.

Feng J., Yue L., Wang Z., Nattel S (1998). Ionic mechanisms of regional action potential heterogeneity in the canine right atrium. Circ Res. 83:541-51.

Ferguson T.B. Jr., Cox J.L. (1995) Surgery for atrial fibrillation. In: Cardiac Electrophysiology: From Cell to Bedside, (ed 2nd) Zipes D.P., Jalife J., eds. Philadelphia: W.B. Saunders Company, , p. 1567.

Fischer B., Haissaguerre M., Garrigues S., Poquet F., Gencel L., Clementy J., Marcus F.I (1995). Radiofrequency catheter ablation of common atrial flutter in 80 patients. JACC.; 25:1365-72.

Fisher J.D. (2001) Bundle branch reentry tachycardia: Why is the HV interval often longer than in sinus rhythm? The critical role of anisotropic conduction. J Intervent Cardiac Electrophys.; 5:173-6.

Fisher J.D., Cohen H.L., Mehra R., Altschuler H., Excher D.J., Furman S. (1977) Cardiac pacing and pacemakers. II. Serial electrophysiologic testing for control of recurrent tachyarrhythmias. Am Heart J.; 93:658-68.

Fitzgerald D.M., Friday K.J., Wah J.A., Lazzara R., Jackman W.M. (1988) Electrogram patterns predicting successful catheter ablation of ventricular tachycardia. Circ. 77:806-14.

Fozzard H.A., Schoenberg M (1972). Strength-duration curves in cardiac Purkinje fibres: Effects of liminal length and charge distribution. J Physiol (Lond). 226:593-618.

Frustaci A., Chimenti C., Bellocci F., Morgante E., Russo M.A., Maseri A (1997). Histological substracte of atrial biopsies in patients with lone atrial fibrillation. Circ. 96:1180-4.

Fujimura O., Klein G.J., Yee R., Sharma A.D.(1990) Mode of onset of atrial fibrillation in the Wolff-Parkinson-White syndrome: how important is the accessory pathway? JACC.; 15:1082-6.

Gallagher J.J., Sealy W.C. (1978) The permanent form of junctional reciprocating tachycardia: Further elucidation of the underlying mechanism. Eur J Cardiol.; 8:413-30.

Gallagher J.J., Sealy W.C., Kasell J., Wallace A.G. (1984) Multiple accessory pathways in patients with the pre-excitation syndrome. Circ. 54:571-91.

Garan H., Ruskin J.N. (1988) Reproducible termination of ventricular tachycardia by a single extrastimulus within the reentry circuit during the ventricular effective refractory period. Am Heart J.; 116:546-50.

Gardner P.I., Ursell P.C., Fenoglio J.J. Jr., Wit A.L (1985). Electrophysiologic and anatomic basis for fractionated electrograms recorded from healed myocardial infarcts. Circulation. 72:596-611.

Gepstein L., Evans S.J. Electroanatomical mapping of the heart: Basic concepts and implications for the treatment of cardiac arrhythmias. PACE. 198; 21::1268-78.

Gibbons R.J., Alpert J.S., Antman E.M., et al. ACC/AHA/ESC Guidelines for the Managment of Patients with Atrial Fibrillation. Circulation. (In Press).

Gillette P.C., Garson A. Jr., Cooley D.A., McNamara D.G. (1982) Prolonged and decremental antegrade conduction properties in right anterior accessory connections: Wide QRS antidromic tachycardia of left bundle branch block pattern without Wolff-Parkinson-White configuration in sinus rhythm. Am Heart J. 103:66-74.

Ginsburg K., Arnsdorf M.F. (1995 Cardiac excitability, gap junctions, cable properties and impulse propagation. In: Physiology and Pathophysiology of the Heart, (ed 3rd) Sperelakis N., ed. Boston: M. Nijhoff,), pp. 153-99.

Goldberger A.L., Rigney D.R. (1991) Nonlinear Dynamics at the Bedside. In: Theory of Heart: Biomechanics, Biophysics, and Nonlinear Dynamics of Cardiac Function, Glass L., Hunter P., McCulloch A., eds. New York: Springer, pp. 584-605.

Goldstein S.S., Rall W (1974). Changes in action potential shape and velocity for changing core conductor geometry. Biophys J. 14:731-57.

Gonska B.D., Cao K., Schaumann A., Dorszewski A., von zur Muhlen F., Kreuzer H. (1994) Catheter ablation of ventricular tachycardia in 136 patients with coronary artery disease: results and long-term follow-up. JACC.; 24:1506-14.

Gonska B.D., Cao K., Schaumann A., Dorszewski A., von zur Muhlen F., Kreuzer H. (1994) Management of patients after catheter ablation of ventricular tachycardia. [Review]. Pace - Pacing & Clinical Electrophysiology.; 17:542-9.

Gourdie R.G., Green C.R., Severs N.J (1991). Gap junction distribution in adult mammalian myocardium revealed by an anti-peptide antibody and laser scanning confocal microscopy. J Cell Sci. 99:41-55.

Gourdie R.G., Green C.R., Severs N.J., Thompson R.P (1992). Immunolabeling patterns of gap junction connexins in the developing and mature rat heart. Anat Embryol (Berlin). 185:363-78.

Gray R.A., Pertsov A.M., Jalife J (1996). Incomplete reentry and epicardial breakthrough patterns during atrial fibrillation in the sheep heart. Circ. 94:2649-61.

Grogin H.R., Lee R.J., Kwasman M., Epstein L.M., Schamp D.J., Lesh M.D., Scheinman M.M. (1994) Radiofrequency catheter ablation of atriofascicular and nodoventricular Mahaim tracts [see comments]. Circ. 90:272-81.

Guevara M.R., Glass L., Shrier A (1981). Phase locking, period-doubling bifurcations, and irregular dynamics in periodically stimulated cardiac cells. Science. 214:1350-3.

Guiraudon C.M., Ernst N.M., Yee R., Lein G.J (1992). The pathology of drug resistant lone atrial fibrillation in eleven surgically treated patients. In: Atrial Fibrillation: A Treatable Disease, Kingma J.H., Hernel N.M., Lie K.I., eds. Kluwer Academic Publishers: Dordrecht, pp. 41-57.

Gupta K.B., Ratcliffe M.B., Fallert M.A., Edmunds L.H. Jr., Bogen D.K (1994). Changes in passivemechanical stiffness of myocardial tissue with aneurysm formation. Circulation. 89:2315-26.

Gussak I.B., Antzelevitch C., Hammill S.C., eds. Cardiac Repolarizatoin: Bridging Basic and Clinical Sciences, (ed 1st). Totowa,NJ: Humana Press, In Press.

Gutstein DE, Morley GE, Tamaddon H, Vaidya D, Schneider MD, Chen J, Chien KR, Stuhmann H, Fishmann GI. (2001) Conduction slowing and sudden arrhythmic death in mice with cardiac - restricted inactivation of connexin43. Circ Res ;16:333-339.

Hagendorff A., Schumacher B., Kirchhof S., et al (1999). Conduction disturbances and increased atrial vulnerability in connexin40-deficient mice analylzed by transesophageal stimulation. Circ. 99:1508-15.

Haissaguerre M., Jais P., Shah D.C., et al (1998). Spontaneous initiation of atrial fibrillation by ectopic beats originating tin the pulmonary veins. N Engl J Med. 339:659-66.

Heidenheim M (1901). Uber die Structur des menschlichen Herzmuskels. Anat Anz. 20:3-79.

Henthorn R.W., Okumura K., Olshansky B., Plumb V.J., Hess P.G., Waldo A.L (1988). A fourth criteria for transient entrainment: The electrogram equivalent of progressive fusion. Circulation. 77:1003-12.

Hiramatsu Y., Buchanan J.W., Knisley S.B., Gettes L.S (1988). Rate-dependent effects of hypoxia on internal longitudinal resistance in guinea pig papillary muscles. Circ Res. 63:923-9.

Ho S.Y., Kilpatrick L., Kanai T., Germroth P.G., Thompson R.P., Anderson R.H. (1995) The architecture of the atrioventricular conduction axis in dog compared to man: its significance to ablation of the atrioventricular nodal approaches. J Cardiovas Electrophys.; 6:26-39.

Hodgkin A.L., Rushton W.A.H (1946). The electrical constants of a crustacean nerve fibre. Proc Roy Soc B. 133:444-79.

Hoyt R.H., Cohen M.L., Saffitz J.E (1989). Distribution and three-dimensional structure of intercellular junctions in canine myocardium. Circ Res. 64:563-74.

Huang D.T., Monahan K.M., Zimetbaum P., Papageorgiou P., Epstein L.M., Josephson M.E. (1998) Hybride pharmacologic and ablative therapy: A novel and effective approach for the management of atrial fibrillation. J Cardiovasc Electrophysiol.; 9:462-9.

Huang S.K., Messer J.V., Denes P. (1983) Significance of ventricular tachycardia in idiopathic dilated cardiomyopathy. Observations in 35 patients. Am J Cardiol; 51:507-12.

Inoue H., Matsuo H., Takayanagi K., Murao S(1981). Clinical and experimental studies of the effects of atrial extrastimulation and rapid pacing on the atrial flutter cycle. Evidence of macro-reentry with an excitable gap. Am J Cardiol. 48:623-31.

Jackman W.M., Nakagawa H., Heidbuchel H., Beckman K., McClelland J., Lazzara R (1995). Three forms of atrioventricular nodal (junctional) reentrant tachycardia: Differential diagnosis, electrophysiological characteristics and implications for anatomy of the reentrant circuit. In: Cardiac Electrophysiology: From Cell to Bedside, (ed Second) Zipes D.P., Jalife J., eds. Philadelphia: W. B. Saunders Company, pp. 620-37.

Jahangir A., Munger T.M., Packer D.L., Crijns H.J.G.M(2001). Atrial fibrillation. In: Cardiac Arrhythmia: Mechanisms, Diagnosis and Management, (ed 2nd) Podrid P.J., Kowey P.R., eds. Philadelphia: Lippincott, Williams & Wilkins, pp. 457-500.

Jais P., Haissaguerre M., Shah D.C., et al (1997). A focal source of atrial fibrillation treated by discrete radiofrequency ablation. Circ.. 95:572-6.

Jalife J (1984). Mutual entrainment and electrical coupling as mechanisms for synchronous firing of rabbit sino-atrial pacemaker cells. J Physiol (London). 221-243:1984.

Jalife J., Michaels D.C (1985). Phase dependent interactions of cardiac pacemakers as machanisms of control and sychronization in the heart. In: Cardiac Electrophysiology and Arrhythmias, Zipes D.P., Jalife J., eds. Orlando, FL: Grune and Stratton, pp. 109-19.

Jalife J., Moe G. K (1979). A biologic model of parasystole. Am J Cardiol. 43:761-72.

Jalife J., Slenter V.A.J., Salata J.J., Michaels D.C (1983). Dynamic vagal control of pacemaker activity in the mammalian sinoatrial node. Circ Res. 52:642-56.

James T.N. (1961) Morphology of the human atrioventricular node with remarks pertinent to its electrophysiology. Am Heart J.; 62:756.

Janse M.J., van Capelle F.J.L., Freud G.E., Durrer D. (1971) Crcus movement within the AV node as a basis for supraventricular as shown by microelectrode recording in the isolated rabbit heart. Circ Res.; 28:403-14.

Jazayeri M.R., Deshpande S., Dhala A., Blanck Z., Sra J., Akhtar M (1994). Transcatheter mapping and radiofrequency ablation of cardiac arrhythmias. [Review]. Current Problems in Cardiology. 19:287-395.

Jongsma H.J., Wilders R., van Ginneken A.C.G., Rook M.B (1991). Modulatory effect of the transcellular electrical field on gap junction conductance. In: Biophysics of Gap Junction Channels, Peracchia C., ed. Boca Raton: CRC Press, pp. 163-72.

Josephson M. E., Horowitz L. N., Farshidi A., Kastor J. A. (1978) Recurrent sustained ventricular tachycardia. 1. Mechanisms. Circulation.; 57:431-40.

Josephson M.E. Clinical Cardiac Electrophysiology: Techniques and Interpretations, (ed 2nd). Philadelphia: Lea & Febiger, 1993.

Josephson M.E., Waxman H.L., Cain M.E., Gardner M.J., Buxton A.E. (1982) Ventricular activation during ventricular endocardial pacing. II: role of pace-mapping to localize origin of ventricular tachycardia. Am J Cardiol.; 50:11-20.

Kalman J.M., Lee R.J., Fisher W.G., Chin M.C., Ursell P., Stillson C.A., Lesh M.D., Scheinman M.M. (1995) Radiofrequency catheter modification of sinus pacemaker function guided by intracardiac echocardiography. Circ. 92:3070-81.

Kalman J.M., Olgin J.E., Karch M.R., Lesh M.D(1996). Regional entrainment of atrial fibrillation in man. J Cardiovas Electrophys. 7:867-76.

Kalman J.M., Olgin J.E., Saxin L.A., Lee R.J., Scheinman M.M., Lesh M.D(1997). Electrocardiographic and electrophysiologic characterization of atypical atrial flutter in man: Use of activation and entrainment mapping and implications for catheter ablation. J Cardiovas Electrophys. 8:121-44.

Kalman J.M., Olgin J.E., Saxon L.A., Fisher W.G., Lee R.J., Lesh M.D(1996). Activation and entrainment mapping defines the tricuspid annulus as the anterior barrier in typical atrial flutter [see comments]. Circ. 94:398-406.

Kaprielian R.R., Gunning M., Dupont E., et al (1998). Downregulation of immunodetectable connexin43 and decreased gap junction size in the pathogenesis of chronic hibernation in the human left ventricle. Circulation. 97:651-60.

Kawamura K., James T.N.(1971) Comparative ultrastructure of cellular junctions in working myocardium and the conduction system under normal and pathologic conditions. J Mol Cell Cardiol.; 3:31-60.

Keener J.P., Panfilov A.V (1995). Three-dimensional propagation in the heart: The effects of geometry and fiber orientation on propagation in myocardium. In: Cardiac Electrophysiology: From Cell to Bedside, (ed Second) Zipes D.P., Jalife J., eds. Philadelphia: W. B. Saunders Company, pp. 335-47.

Kim Y.H., O'Nunain S., Ruskin J.N., Garan H. (1993) Nonpharmacologic therapies in patients with ventricular tachyarrhythmias. Catheter ablation and ventricular tachycardia surgery. [Review]. Cardiology Clinics.; 11:85-96.

Kinoshita O., Fontaine G., Rosas F., Elias J., Iwa T., Tonet J., Lascault G., (1995) Frank R. Time- and frequency-domain analyses of the signal-averaged ECG in patients with arrhythmogenic right ventricular dysplasia. Circ.; 91:715-21.

Kirkorian G., Moncada E., Chevalier P., Canu G., Claudel J.P., Bellon C., Lyon L., Touboul P. (1994) Radiofrequency ablation of atrial flutter. Efficacy of an anatomically guided approach. Circ.; 90:2804-14.

Kleber A.G., Fleischhauer J., Cascio W.E (1995). Ischemia-induced propagation failure in the heart. In: Cardiac Electrophysiology: From Cell to Bedside, (ed Second) Zipes D.P., Jalife J., eds. Philadelphia: W. B. Saunders Company, pp. 174-81.

Kleber A.G., Janse M.J (1990). Impulse Propagation in Myocardial Ischemia. In: Cardiac Electrophysiology: From Cell to Bedside, (ed 1st) Zipes D.P., Jalife J., eds. Philadelphia: W. B. Saunders, pp. 156-61.

Klein G.J., Guiraudon G., Guiraudon C., Yee R. (1994) The nodoventricular Mahaim pathway: an endangered concept? [editorial; comment]. [Review]. Circ. 90:636-8.

Klein G.J., Guiraudon G.M., Kerr C.R., Sharma A.D., Yee R., Szabo T., Wah J.A. (1988) "Nodoventricular" accessory pathway: evidence for a distinct accessory atrioventricular pathway with atrioventricular node-like properties. JACC. 11:1035-40.

Klein G.J., Guiraudon G.M., Sharma A.D., Milstein S(1986). Demonstration of macroreentry and feasibility of operative therapy in the common type of atrial flutter. Am J Cardiol. 57:587-91.

Klein L.S., Miles W.M (1995). Ablative therapy for ventricular arrhythmias. [Review] [51 refs]. Progr Cardiovasc Dis. 37:225-42.

Klein L.S., Miles W.M., Hackett F.K., Zipes D.P. (1992) Catheter ablation of ventricular tachycardia using radiofrequency techniques in patients without structural heart disease. Herz.; 17:179-89.

Konings K.T.S., Kirchhof C.J., Smeets J.R., Wellens H.J.J., Penn O.C., Allessie M.A (1994). High-density mapping of electrically induced atrial fibrillation in humans. Circ. 89:1665-80.

Kootsey J.M (1991). Electrical Propagation in Distributed Cardiac Tissue. In: Theory of Heart: Biomechanics, Biophysics, and Nonlinear Dynamics of Cardiac Function, Glass L., Hunter P., McCulloch A., eds. New York: Springer, pp. 391-403.

Kosakai Y. (2000) Treatment of atrial fibrillation using the Maze procedure: The Japanes experience. Seminars in Thoracic & Cardiovascular Surgery.; 12:44-52.

Kottkamp H., Kindricks G., Chen X., Brunn J., Willems S., Haverkamp W., Block M., Breithardt G., Borggrefe M. (1995) Radiofrequency catheter ablation of sustained ventricular tachycardia in idiopathic dilated cardiomyopathy. Circ.; 92:1159-68.

Kovacs S.J. (1991) A Clinical Perspective on Theory of Heart. In: Theory of Heart: Biomechanics, Biophysics, and Nonlinear Dynamics of Cardiac Function, Glass L., Hunter P., McCulloch A., eds. New York: Springer, pp. 609-11.

Kowey P.R., Eisenberg R., Engel T.R.(1984) Sustained arrhythmias in hypertrophic obstructive cardiomyopathy. N Engl J Med.; 310:1566-9.

Kramer J.B., Saffitz J.E., Witkowski F.X. (1985) Intramural reentry as a mechanism of ventricular tachycardia during evolving canine myocardial infarction. Circ Res; 56:736-54.

Kuchar D.L., Ruskin J.N., Garan H. (1989) Electrocardiographic localization of the site of origin of ventricular tachycardia in patients with prior myocardial infarction. JACC.; 13:893-903.

Kuck K.H., Friday K.J., Kunze K.P. (1990) Sites of conduction block in accessory pathway conduction during the induction of orthodromic reciprocating tachycardias. Circ. 82:407-17.

Kuck K.H., Kunze K.P., Geiger M., Costard A., Schluter M. (1987) Programmed electrical stimulation in patients with hypertrophic cardiomyopathy. Zeitschrift fur Kardiologie.; 76:131-6.

Kuck K.H., Kunze K.P., Schluter M., Nienaber C.A., Costard A. (1988) Programmed electrical stimulation in hypertrophic cardiomyopathy. Results in patients with and without cardiac arrest or syncope. [Review]. Eur Heart J.; 9:177-85.

Lal R., Arnsdorf M.F (1992). Voltage-dependent gating and single channel conductance of adult mammalian atrial gap junctions. Circ Res. 71:737-43.

Landau M., Lorente P., Michaels D., Jalife J (1990). Bistabilities and annihilation phenomena in electrophysiological cardiac models. Circ Res. 66:1658-72.

Lardo A.C., McVeigh E.R., Jumrussirkul P., Berger R.D., Calkins H., Lima J., Halperin H.R. (2000) Visualization and temporal/spatial characterization of cardiac radiofrequency ablation lesions using magnetic resonance imaging. Circ.; 102:698-705.

Lawrie G.M., Pacifico A. (1995) Surgery for ventricular tachycardia. In: Cardiac Electrophysiology: From Cell to Bedside, (ed 2nd) Zipes D.P., Jalife J., eds. Philadelphia: W. B. Saunders, , pp. 1547-52.

Lee R.J., Kalman J.M., Fitzpatrick A.P., Epstein L.M., Fisher W.G., Olgin J.E., Lesh M.D., Scheinman M.M. (1995) Radiofrequency catheter modification of the sinus node for "inappropriate" sinus tachycardia. Circ. 92:2919-28.

Leitch J.W., Klein G., Yee R., Guiraudon G. (1991) Sinus node-atrioventricular node isolation: Long term results with the "corridor" operation for atrial fibrillation. JACC.; 17:970-5.

Lerman B.B., Belardinelli L., West G.A., Berne R.M., DiMarco J.P. Adenosine-sensitive ventricular tachycardia: evidence suggesting cyclic AMP-mediated triggered activity. Circ.(1986) ; 74:270-80.

Lesh M.D., Kalman J.M., Olgin J.E(1996). New approaches to treatment of atrial flutter and tachycardia. [Review]. J Cardiovas Electrophys. 7:368-81.

Lesh M.D., Spear J.F., Moore E.N (1990). Myocardial anisotropy: Basic electrophysiology and role in cardiac arrhythmias. In: Cardiac Electrophysiology: From Cell to Bedside, Zipes D.P., Jalife J., eds. Philadelphia: W. B. Saunders Company, pp. 364-76.

Levy M.N., Martin P.J., Lano T.H., Zieske H (1969). Paradoxical effect of vagus nerve stimulation on heart rate in dogs. Circ Res. 25:303-14.

Lewis M.A., P Grindrod (1991): One-way blocks in cardiac tissue. A mechanism for propagation failure in Purkinje fibers. Bull Math Biol. 53:881-99.

Li D., Fareh S., Leung T.K., Nattel S (1999). Promotion of atrial fibrillation by heart failure in dogs: Atrial modeling of a different sort. Circulation. 137:494-9.

Li H.G., Klein G.J., Thakur R.K., Yee R. (1994) Radiofrequency ablation of decremental accessory pathways mimicking "nodoventricular" conduction. Am J Cardiol.; 74:829-33.

Lindemans F.W., Denier Van der Gon J.J (1978). Current thresholds and liminal size in excitation of heart muscle. Cardiovasc Res. 12:477-85.

Lloyd E.A., Zipes D.P., Heger J.J., Prystowsky E.N. (1982) Sustained ventricular tachycardia due to bundle branch reentry. Am Heart J.; 104:1095-7.

Lorente P., Davidenko J (1990). Hysteresis phenomena in excitable cardiac tissues. Ann NY Acad Sci. 591:109-27.

Lown B., Ganong S.A., Levine S.A.(1952) The syndrome of short P-R interval, normal QRS complex and paroxysmal rapid heart action. Circ. 5:693.

Luke R.A., Safitz J.E (1991). Remodeling of Ventricular Conduction Pathways in Healed Canine Infarct Border Zones. J Clin Invest. 87:1594-602.

Marino T.A. (1979) The atrioventricular node and bundle in the ferret heart: A light and quantitative electron microscopic study. Am J Anat.; 154:365-92.

Maron B.J., Bonow R.O., Cannon R.O., Leon M.B., Epstein S.E. (1987) Hypertrophic cardiomyopathy: Interrelations of clinical manifestations, pathophysiology and therapy (Part 1). N Engl J Med.; 316:780-9.

Maron B.J., Bonow R.O., Cannon R.O., Leon M.B., Epstein S.E. (1987) Hypertrophic cardiomyopathy: Interrelations of clinical manifestations, pathophysiology and therapy (Part 2). N Engl J Med.; 316:844-52.

Maurer P., Weingart R (1987). Cell pairs isolated from adult guinea pig. effects of [Ca++]i on nexal membrane resistance. Pflugers Arch. 409:394-402.

McCarthy P.M., Gillinov A.M., Castle L., Chung M., Cosgrove D. III. (2000) The Cox-Maze procedure: The Cleveland Clinic experience. Seminars in Thoracic & Cardiovascular Surgery.; 12:25-9.

McClelland J.H., Wang X., Beckman K.J., Hazlitt H.A., Prior M.I., Nakagawa H., Lazzara R., Jackman W.M. (1994)Radiofrequency catheter ablation of right atriofascicular (Mahaim) accessory pathways guided by accessory pathway activation potentials. Circ.; 89:2655-66.

McGuire M.A., Bourke J.P., Robotin M.C., Johnson D.C., Meldrum-Hanna W., Nunn G.R., Uther J.B., Ross D.L (1993). High resolution mapping of Koch's triangle using sixty electrodes in humans with atrioventricular junctional (AV nodal) reentrant tachycardia. Circ. 88:2315-28.

McGuire M.A., Janse M.J., Ross D.L (1993). "AV nodal" reentry: Part II: AV nodal, AV junctional, or atrionodal reentry? J Cardiovas Electrophys. 4:573-86.

McKenna W.J., Franklin R.C., Nihoyannopoulos P., Robinson K.C., Deanfield J.E. (1988) Arrhythmia and prognosis in infants, children and adolescents with hypertrophic cardiomyopathy. JACC. 11:147-53.

Meinertz T., Hofmann T., Kasper W., Treese N., Bechtold H., Stienen U., Pop T., Leitner E.R., Andresen D., Meyer J. (1984) Significance of ventricular arrhythmias in idiopathic dilated cardiomyopathy. Am J Cardiol.; 53:902-7.

Mendez C., Moe G.K.(1966) Some characteristics of transmembrane potentials of AV nodal cells during propagation of premature beats. Circ Res.; 19:993-1010.

Mendez C., Mueller W.J., Urquiaga X (1970). Propagation of impulses across the Purkinje fiber-muscle junctions in the dog heart. Circulation. 26:135-50.

Michaels D.C., Matyas E.P., Jalife J (1984). A mathematical model of the vagal control of sinoatrial pacemaker activity. Circ Res. 55:89-101.

Michaels D.C., Matyas E.P.al, Jalife J (1989). Experimental and mathematical observations on pacemaker interactions as a mechanisms of synchronization in the sinoatrial node. In: Cardiac Electrophysiology: From Cell to Bedside, Zipes D.P., Jalife J., eds. Philadelphia: W.B. Saunders Co., pp. 182-214.

Michaels D.C., Slenter V.A., Salata J.J., Jalife J (1983). A model of dynamic vagus-sinoatrial node interactions. Am J Physiol. 245:H1043-1053.

Mobley B.A., Page E (1972). The surface area of sheep cardiac Purkinje fibers. J Physiol. 220:547-63.

Moe G.K (1962). On the multiple wavelet hypothesis of atrial fibrillation. Arch Int Pharmacodyn Ther. 140:183-8.

Moe G.K., Abildskov J.A (1959). Atrial fibrillation as a self sustaining arrhythmia independent of cocal discharge. Am Heart J. 58:59-70.

Moe G.K., Preston J.B., Burlington H.J(1956). Physiologic evidence for a dual A-V transmission system. Circ Res. 4:357-75.

Mont L., Sexas T., Brugada P., Simonis F., Kriek E., Smeets J.L., Wellens H.J. (1992) The electrocardiographic, clinical and electrophysiologic spectrium of idiopathic monomorphic ventricular tachycardia. Am Heart J.; 124:746-53.

Morady F., Frank R., Kou W.H., Tonet J.L., Nelson S.D., Kounde S., De Buitleir M., Fontaine G.(1988)Identification and catheter ablation of a zone of slow conduction in the reentrant circuit of ventricular tachycardia in humans. JACC.; 11:775-82.

Morady F., Scheinman M.M., Kou W.H., Griffin J.C., Dick M. 2d., Herre J., Kadish A.H., Langberg J (1989). Long-term results of catheter ablation of a posteroseptal accessory atrioventricular connection in 48 patients. Circ. 79:1160-70.

Nakagawa H., Beckman K.J., McClelland J.H., Wang X., Arruda M., Santoro I., Hazlitt H.A., Abdalla I., Singh A., Gossinger H., et al. (1993) Radiofrequency catheter ablation of idiopathic left ventricular tachycardia guided by a Purkinje potential. Circ.; 88:2607-17.

Nakagawa H., Lazzara R., Khastgir T., Beckman K.J., McClelland J.H., Imai S., Pitha J.V., Becker A.E., Arruda M., Gonzalez M.D., Widman L.E., Rome M., Neuhauser J., Wang X., Calame J.D., Goudeau M.D., Jackman W.M (1996). Role of the tricuspid annulus and the eustachian valve/ridge on atrial flutter. Relevance to catheter ablation of the septal isthmus and a new technique for rapid identification of ablation success [see comments]. Circ. 94:407-24.

Nath S., Mounsey J.P., Haines D.E., DiMarco J.P. (1995) Predictors of acute and long-term success after radiofrequency catheter ablation of type 1 atrial flutter. Am J Cardiol.; 76:604-6.

Nattel S., Li D(2000). Ionic remodeling in the heart: Pathophysiological significance and new therapeutic opportunities for atrial fibrillation. Circ Res. 87:440-7.

Nattel S., Li D., Yue L (2000). Basic mechanisms of atrial fibrillation - Very new insights into very old ideas. Annual Review of Physiology. 62:51-77.

Neus H., Schlepper M., Thormann J. (1975) Analysis of re-entry mechanisms in three patients with concealed Wolff-Parkinson-White syndrome. Circ. 51:75-81.

Okumura K., Henthorn R.W., Epstein A.E., Plumb J.V., Waldo A.L. (1986) "Incessant" atrioventricular (AV) reciprocating tachycardia utilizing left lateral AV bypass pathway with a long retrograde conduction time. PACE.; 9:332-42.

Okumura K., Matsuyama K., Miyagi H., Tsuchiya T., Yasue H. (1988) Entrainment of idiopathic ventricular tachycardia of left ventricular origin with evidence for reentry with an area of slow conduction and effect of verapamil. Am J Cardiol.; 62:727-32.

Okumura K., Olshansky B., Henthorn R.W., Epstein A.E., Plumb V.J., Waldo A.L (1987). Demonstration of the presence of slow conduction during sustained ventricular tachycardia in man: Use of transient entrainment of the tachycardia. Circ. 75:369-78.

Olgin J.E., Kalman J.M., Fitzpatrick A.P., Lesh M.D(1995). Role of right atrial endocardial structures as barriers to conduction during human type I atrial flutter. Activation and entrainment mapping guided by intracardiac echocardiography. Circ. 92:1839-48.

Olshansky B., Okumura K., Hess P.G., Waldo A.L. (1990) Demonstration of an area of slow conduction in human atrial flutter. JACC.; 16:1639-48.

Parkinson J., Papp C. (1942) Repetitive paroxysmal tachycardia. Br Heart J.; 10:241-62.

Peters N.S., Coromilas J., Severs N.J., Wit A.L (1997). Disturbed connexin43 gap junction distribution correlates with the locations of reentrant circuits in the epicardial border zone of healing canine infarcts that cause ventricular tachycardia. Circulation. 95:988-96.

Peters N.S., Green C.R., Poole-Wilson P.A., Severs N.J (1993). Reduced content of connexin43 gap junctions in ventricular myocardium from hypertrophied and ischemic human hearts. Circulation. 88:864-75.

Peters N.S., Wit A.L (1998). Myocardial architecture and ventricular arrhythmogenesis. Circulation. 97:1746-54.

Polontchouk L., Haefliger J.A., Ebelt B., Schaefer T., Stuhlmann D., Mehlhorn U., Kuhn-Regnier F., De Vivie E.R., Dhein S (2001). Effects of chronic atrial fibrillation on gap junction distribution in human and rat atria. JACC. 38:883-91.

Poty H., Saoudi N., Abdel Aziz A., Nair M., Letac B. (1995) Radiofrequency catheter ablation of type 1 atrial flutter. Prediction of late success by electrophysiological criteria. Circ.; 92:1389-92.

Poty H., Saoudi N., Haissaguerre M., Daou A., Clementy J., Letac B (1996). Radiofrequency catheter ablation of atrial tachycardias. Am Heart J. 131:481-9.

Pressler M.L (1984). Cable analysis in quiescent and active sheep Purkinje fibres. J Physiol (Lond). 352:739-57.

Pressler M.L., Munster P.N., Huang X (1995). Gap junction distribution in the heart: Functional Relevance. In: Cardiac Electrophysiology: From Cell to Bedside, (ed Second) Zipes D.P., Jalife J., eds. Philadelphia: W. B. Saunders Company, pp. 144-81.

Pritchett E.L.C., Gallagher J.J., Sealy W.C., Anderson R., Campbell R.W., Seller T.D. Jr., Wallace A.G. (1978) Supraventricular tachycardia dependent upon accessory pathways in the absence of ventricular preexcitation. Am J Med.; 64:214-20.

Pritchett E.L.C., Prystowsky E.N., Benditt D.G., Gallagher. (1980) "Dual atrioventricular nodal pathways" in patients with Wolff-Parkinson-White syndrome. Br Heart J.; 43:7-13.

Prystowsky E.N., Klein G.J. Cardiac Arrhythmias: An Integrated Approach for the Clinician, . New York: McGraw-Hill,Inc, 1994.

Ritchie A.H., Kerr C.R., Qi A., Yeung-Lai-Wah J.A. (1989) Nonsustained ventricular tachycardia arising from the right ventricular outflow tract. Am J Cardiol.; 63:594-8.

Roark S.F., McCarthy E.A., Lee K.L., Pritchett E.L. (1901) Observations on the occurrence of atrial fibrillation in paroxysmal supraventricular tachycardia. American Journal of Cardiology 1986 Mar.; 57:571-5.

Robert E., Aya A.G., De la Coussaye J.E., Peray P., Juan J.M., Brugada J., Davy J.M., Eledjam J.J. (1999) Dispersion-based reentry: Mechanism of initiation of ventricular tachycardia in isolated rabbit hearts. Am J Physiol. 276:H413-423.

Rodriguez L.M., Smeets J.L., Timmermans C., Wellens H.J. (1997) Predictors for successful ablation of right- and left-sided idopathic ventricular tachycardia. Am J Cardiol.; 79:309-14.

Rothman S.A., Hsia H.H., Cossu S.F., et al. (1997) Radiofrequency catheter ablation of postinfarction ventricular tachycardia: Long-term success and the significance of inducible nonclinical arrhythmias. Circ. 96:3499-508.

Roy D., Waxman H.L., Boxton A.E., Josephson M.E. (1983) Horizontal and longitudinal dissociation of the A-V node during atrial tachycardia. PACE.; 6:569-76.

Saffitz J.E., Laing J.G., Yamada K.A (2000). Connexin expression and turnover: Implications for cardiac excitability. Circ Res. 86:723-8.

Saffitz JE, Kanter HL, Green KG, Tolley TK, Beyer EC. (1994)Tissue-specific determinants of anisotropic conduction velocity in canine atrial and ventricular myocardium. Circ Res ;74:1065-70.

Sandoval N., Velasco V.M., Orjuela H., Caicedo V., Santos H., Rosas F., Carrea J.R., Melgarejo I., Morillo C.A. (1996) Concomitant mitral valve or atrial septal defect surgery and the modified Cox-maze procedure. Am J Cardiol.; 77:591-6.

Sasyniuk B., Mendez C (1971). A mechanism for reentry in canine venricular tissue. Circ Res. 28:3-15.

Schaff H.V., Dearani J.A., Daley R.C., Orszulak T.A., Danielson G.K. Cox-(2000) Maze procedure for atrial fibrillation: Myo Clinic experience. Seminars in Thoracic & Cardiovascular Surgery.; 12:30-7.

Scheinman M.M., Basu D., Hollenberg M. (1974) Electrophysiologic studies in patients with persistent atrial tachycardia. Circ. 50:266-73.

Schmitt C., Miller J.M., Josephson M.E (1998). Atrioventricular nodal supraventricular tachycardia with 2:1 block above the the bundle of His. PACE. 11:1018-23.

Schoenberg M., Dominguez G., Fozzard H.A (1975). Effect of diameter on membrane capacity and conductance of sheep cardiac Purkinje fibers. J Gen Physiol. 65:441-58.

Sepulveda N.G., Walker C.F., Heath R.G (1983). Finite element analysis of current pathways with implanted electrodes. J Biomed Eng. 5:41-8.

Severs N.J (1994). Pathophysiology of gap junctions in heart disease. J Cardiovas Electrophys. 5:462-75.

Shakespeare C.F., Keeling P.J., Slade A.K., McKenna W.J. (1992) Arrhythmia and hypertrophic cardiomyopathy. Archives des Maladies du Coeur et des Vaisseaux.; 85 Spec No 4:31-6.

Sharma A.D., Klein G.J., Guiraudon G.M., Milstein S. (1985) Atrial fibrillation in patients with Wolff-Parkinson-White syndrome: incidence after surgical ablation of the accessory pathway. Circ. 72:161-9.

Sie H.T., Beukema W.P., Misier A.R., Elvan A., Ennema J.J., Haalebos M.M., Wellens H.J.(2001) Radiofrequency modified maze in patients with atrial fibrillation undergoing concomitant cardiac surgery. J Thorac Cardiovasc Surg.; 122:212-5.

Simonson E (1961). Differentiation Between Normal and Abnormal in Electrocardiography, . St. Louis: C.V. Mosby.

Sjostrand F.S., Andersson E (1954). Electron microscopy of the intercalated discs of cardiac muscle tissue. Experientia. 10:369-72.

Smith J.H., Green C.R., Peters N.S., Rothery S., Severs N.J (1991). Altered patterns of gap junction distribution in ischemic heart disease. Am J Pathol. 139:801-21.

Smith J.M., Cohen R.J (1984). Simple finite-element model accounts for wide range of cardiac dysrhythmias. Proc Natl Acad Sci USA. 81:233-7.

Smith W.M., Broughton A., Reiter M.J., Benson D.W. Jr., Grant A.O., Gallagher J.J. (1983) Bystander accessory pathway during AV node reentrant tachycardia. PACE.; 6:537-47.

Sommer J.R., Johnson E.A (1979). Ultrastructure of cardiac muscle. In: The Handbook of Physiology, I: The Cardiovascular System., Berne R.M., ed. Baltimore: The American Physiological Society, Williams and Wilkins, pp. 113-86.

Sommer J.R., Scherer B (1985). The geometry of intercellular communication in cardiac muscle with emphasis on cell and bundle appositions. Am J Physiol. 17:H792-803.

Spach M.S (1995). Microscopic basis of anisotropic propagation in the heart: The nature of current flow at a cellular level. In: Cardiac Electrophysiology: From Cell to Bedside, (ed Second) Zipes D.P., Jalife J., eds. Philadelphia: W. B. Saunders Company, pp. 204-15.

Spach M.S (1991). Anisotropic Structural Complexities in the Genesis of Reentrant Arrhythmias (Editorial Comment). Circulation. 84:1447-50.

Spach M.S., Boineau J.P (1997). Microfibrosis produces electrical load variations due to loss of side-to-side cell connections: A major mechanism of structural heart disease arrhythmias. PACE. 20:397-413.

Spach M.S., Dolber P.C (1990). Discontinuous anisotropic propagation. In: Cardiac Electrophysiology: A Textbook, Rosen M., Janse M.J., Wit A.L., eds. Mt Kisco: Futura Publishing Company, pp. 517-34.

Spach M.S., Dolber P.C., Heidlage J.F (1988). Influence of the passive anisotropic properties on directional differences in propagation following modification of the sodium conductance in human atrial muscle. A model of reentry based on anisotropic discontinuous propagation. Circ Res. 62:811-32.

Spach M.S., Dolber P.C., Heidlage J.F (1990). Properties of Discontinuous Anisotropic Propagation at a Microscopic Level. Ann NY Acad Sci. 591:62-74.

Spach M.S., Dolber PC (1986): Relating extracellular potentials. Evidence for electrical uncoupling of side-to-side fiber connections with increasing age. Circ Res. 58:356-71.

Spach M.S., Heidlage J.F (1995). The stochastic nature of cardiac propagation at a microscopic level: Electrical description of myocardial architecture and its application to conduction. Circ Res. 76:366-80.

Spach M.S., Heidlage J.F., Dolber P.C., Barr R.C (2000). Electrophysiologic effects of remodeling cardiac gap junctions and cell size: Experimental and model studies of normal cardiac growth. Circ Res. 86:302-11.

Spach M.S., Kootsey J.M., Sloan J.D (1982). Active modulation of electrical coupling between cardiac cells of the dog. A mechanism for transient and steady state variations in conduction velocity. Circ Res. 51:347-62.

Spach M.S., Miller W.T., Dolber P.C., Kootsey J.M., Sommer J.R., Mosher C.E. Jr (1982). The functional role of structural complexities in the propagation of depolarization in the atrium of the dog. Cardiac conduction disturbances due to discontinuities of effective axial resistivity. Circ Res. 50:175-91.

Spach M.S., Miller W.T., Geselowitz D.B., Barr R.C., Kootsey J.M., Johnson E.A (1981). The discontinuous nature of propagation in normal canine cardiac muscle. Evidence for recurrent discontinuities of intracellular resistance that affect membrane currents. Circ Res. 48:39-54.

Spirito P., Chiarella F., Carratino L., Berisso M.Z., Bellotti P., Vecchio C. (1989) Clinical course and prognosis of hypertrophic cardiomyopathy in an outpatient population. N Engl J Med.; 320:749-55.

Spooner P.M., Joyner R.W., Jalife J., eds (1997). Discontinuous conduction in the Heart, . Armonk, NYH: Future Publishing Company, Inc.

Steinberg J.S., Prasher S., Zelenkofske S., Ehlert F.A. (1995) Radiofrequency catheter ablation of atrial flutter: procedural success and long-term outcome. Am Heart J.; 130:85-92.

Stevenson W.G (1995). Catheter mapping of ventricular tachycardia. In: Cardiac Electrophysiology: From Cell to Bedside, (ed 2nd) Zipes D.P., Jalife J., eds. Philadelphia: W. B. Saunders Company, pp. 1093-112.

Stevenson W.G., Delacretaz E. (2000) Radiofrequency catheter ablation of ventricular tachycardia. Heart.; 84:553-9.

Stevenson W.G., Friedman P.L., Kocovic D., et al. (1998 Radiofrequency catheter ablation of ventricular tachycardia after myocardial infarction. Circ. 98:308-14.

Stevenson W.G., Khan H., Sager P., Saxon L.A., Middlekauff H.R., Natterson P.D., Wiener I. (1993) Identification of reentry circuit sites during catheter mapping and radiofrequency ablation of ventricular tachycardia. Circ. 88:1647-70.

Stevenson W.G., Sager P.T., Friedman P.L (1995). Entrainment techniques for mapping atrial and ventricular tachycardias. [Review]. J Cardiovas Electrophys. 6:201-16.

Stevenson W.G., Sager P.T., Natterson P.D., Saxon L.A., MiddlekauffH.R., Wiener I.
    (1995) Relation of pace mapping QRS configuration and conduction delay to
    ventricular tachycardia reentry circuits in human infarct scars. JACC.; 26:481-
    8.
Strickberger S.A., Man K.C., Daoud E.G., et al. A prospectives evaluation of catheter
    ablation of ventricular tachycardia as adjuvant therapy in patients with
    coronary artery disease and an imploantable cardioverter-defibrillator. Circ.
    1997; 96:1525-31.
Sung R.J. (1983) Incessant supraventricular tachycardia. PACE; 6:1306-26.
Sung R.J., Castellanos A., Mallon S.M., Bloom M.G., Gelband H., Myerburg R.J.
    (1977) Mechanisms of spontaneous alternation between reciprocating
    tachycardia and atrial flutter-fibrillation in the Wolff-Parkinson-White
    syndrome. Circ. Sep; 56:409-16.
Tai C.T., Chen S.A., Tzeng J.W., Kuo B.I., Ding Y.A., Chang M.S., Shuy L.Y (2001).
    Prolonged fractionation of paced right atrial electrograms in patients with
    atrial flutter and fibrillation. JACC. 37:1651-7.
Tchou P., Jazayeri M., Denker S., Dongas J., Caceres J., Akhtar M. (1988)
    Transcatheter electrical ablation of right bundle branch. A method of treating
    macroreentrant ventricular tachycardia attributed to bundle branch reentry.
    Circ.; 78:246-57.
Touboul P., Saoudi N., Atallah G., Kirkorian G. (1989) Electrophysiologic basis of
    catheter ablation in atrial flutter. Am J Cardiol.; 64:79J-85J.
Ursell P.C., Gardner P.I., Albala A., Fenoglio J.J. Jr., Wit A.L (1985). Structural and
    electrophysiological changes in the epicardial border zone of canine
    myocardial infarcts during infarct healing. Circ Res. 56:436-51.
Ursell P.C., Gardner P.I., Albala A., Fenoglio J.J.J., Wit A.L. (1985) Structural and
    electrophysiological changes in the epicardial border zone of canine
    myocardial infarcts during infarct healing. Circ Res.; 56:436-51.
Valderrabano M., Lee M.-H., Ohara T., Lai A.C., Fishbein M.C., Lin S.-F.,
    Karagueuzia H.S., Chen P.-S. (2001) Dynamics of intramural and transmural
    reentry during ventricular fibrillation in isolated swin ventricles. Circ Res.
    88:839-48.
Van der Velden H.M., Ausma J., Rook M.B., et al (2000). Gap junctional remodeling
    in relation to stablization of atrial fibrillation in the goat. Cardiovasc Res.
    46:476-86.
Van der Velden H.M., Van Kempen M.J., Wijffels M.C., et al (1998). Altered pattern
    of connexin40 distribution in persistent atrial fibrillation in the goat. J
    Cardiovasc Electrophysiol. 46:476-86.
van Hemel N.M., Defauw J.J., Kingma J.H., Jaarsma W., Vermeulen F.E., de Bakker
    J.M., Guiraudon G.M. (1994) Long-term results of the corridor operation for
    atrial fibrillation [see comments]. Brit Heart J.; 71:170-6.

Van Wagoner D.R., Nerbonne J.M (2001). Molecular mechanisms of atrial
    fibrillation. In: Heart Physiology and Pathophysiology, (ed 4th) Sperelakis N.,
    Kurachi Y., Terzic A., Cohen M.V., eds. New York: Academic Press, pp.
    1107-24.

Varnava AM, Elliott PM, Baboonian C, Davison F, Davies MJ, McKenna WJ.
    (2001) Hypertrophic cardiomyopathy; histopathological features of sudden
    death in cardiac troponin T disease. Circulation ;104:1380-1384.

Veenstra R.D (1991). Physiological modulation of cardiac gap junction channels. J
    Cardiovasc Electrophysiol. 2:168-89.

Veenstra R.D., Joyner R.W., Rawling D.A (1984). Purkinje and ventricular activation
    sequences of canine papillary muscle. Circ Res. 54:500-15.

Verheule S., van Batenburg C.A., Coenjaerts F.E., et al (1999). Cardiac conduction
    abnormalities in mice lacking the gap junction protein connexin40. J
    Cardiovas Electrophys. 10:1380-9.

Waki K., Saito T., Becker A.E(2000). Right atrial fluter isthmus revisited: normal
    anatomy favors nonuniform anisotropic conduction. J Cardiovas Electrophys.
    11:90-4.

Waldo A.L (1995). Atrial flutter: Mechanisms, clinical feature and management. In:
    Cardiac Electrophysiology: From Cell to Bedside, (ed 2nd) Zipes D.P., Jalife
    J., eds. Philadelp;hia: W. B. Saunders Company, pp. 666-81.

Waldo A.L. (2000) Treatment of atrial flutter. Heart.; 84:227-32.

Waldo A.L., Maclean W.A.H., Karp R.B., Kochoukos N.T., James T (1977).
    Entrainment and interruption of atrial flutter with pacing; Studies in man
    following open heart surgery. Circ. 56:737-45.

Wang J., Liue L., Feng J., Nattel S (1996). Regional and functional factors
    determining induction and maintenance of atrial fibrillation in dogs. Am J
    Physiol. 271:H148-58.

Ward D.E., Bennett D.H., Camm J. (1984) Mechanisms of junctional tachycardia
    showing ventricular pre-excitation. Br Heart J.; 52:369-76.

Ward D.E., Camm A.J. (1982) Ventriculo-atrial conduction over accessory pathways
    exhibiting decremental properties. Eur Heart J.; 3:267-75.

Ward D.E., Nathan A.W., Camm A.J. (1984) Fascicular tachycardia sensitive to
    calcium antagonists. Eur Heart J.; 5:896-905.

Wathen M., Natale A., Wolfe K., Yee R., Klein G. (1993) Initiation of atrial
    fibrillation in the Wolff-Parkinson-White syndrome: the importance of the
    accessory pathway. Am Heart J.; 125:753-9.

Watson R.M., Josephson M.E(1980). Atrial flutter. I. Electrophysiologic substrates
    and modes of initiation and termination. Am J Cardiol. 45:732-41.

Weh S.-J., Yamamoto T., Lin F.-C., Wu D (1990). Atrioventricular block in the
    atypical form of junctional reciprocating tachycardia: Evidence supporting the
    atrioventricular node as the site of reentry. JACC. 15:385-92.

Weingart R., Maurer P (1988). Action potential transfer in cell pairs isolated from adult rat and guinea pig ventricles. Circ Res. 63:72-80.

Weingart R., Rudisli A., Maurer P (1990). Cell to cell communication. In: Cardiac Electrophysiology: From Cell to Bedside, (ed 1st) Zipes D.P., Jalife J., eds. Philadelphia: W. B. Saunders, pp. 122-7.

Wellens H.J. (1994) Atrial fibrillation--the last big hurdle in treating supraventricular tachycardia [editorial; comment]. N Engl J Med.; 331:944-5.

Wellens H.J., Duren D.R., Lie K.I. (1976) Observations on mechanisms of ventricular tachycardia in man. Circ.; 54:237-44.

Wellens H.J.J. (1971) The preexcitation syndrome. In: Electrical Stimulation of the Heart, Wellens H.J.J., ed. Baltimore, MD: University Park Press, pp. 97-109.

Wellens H.J.J., Durrer D. (1973) Combined conduction distrubances in two AV pathways in patients with Wolff-Parkinson-White syndrome. Eur J Cardiol.; 1:23-8.

Wen M.S., Yeh S.J., Wang C.C., Lin F.C., Chen I.C., Wu D. (1994) Radiofrequency ablation therapy in idiopathic left ventricular tachycardia with no obvious structural heart disease. Circ.; 89:1690-6.

Wijffels M.C., Kirchhoff C.J., Dorland R., Allessie M.A (1995). Atrial fibrillation begets atrial fibrillation: A study in awake chronically instrumented goats. Circ. 92:1954-68.

Wikswo J.P (1995). Tissue anisotropy, the cardiac biodomain, and the virtual cathode effect. In: Cardiac Electrophysiology: From Cell to Bedside, (ed Second) Zipes D.P., Jalife J., eds. Philadelphia: W. B. Saunders Company, pp. 348-62.

Wilber D.J., Baerman J., Olshansky B., Kall J., Kopp D. (1993) Adenosine sensitive ventricular tachycardia: Clinical characteristics and response to catheter ablation. Circ.; 87:126-34.

Wilensky R.L., Yudelman P., Cohen A.I., Fletcher R.D., Atkinson J., Virmani R., Roberts W.C. (1988) Serial electrocardiographic changes in idiopathic dilated cardiomyopathy confirmed at necropsy. Am J Cardiol.; 62:276-83.

Winfree A.T (1980). The Geometry of Biological Time, . New York: Springer-Verlag

Wit A.L., Dillon S.M., Coromilas J (1995). Anisotropic reentry as a cause of ventricular tachycarrhythmias. In: Cardiac Electrophysiology: From Cell to Bedside, (ed Second) Zipes D.P., Jalife J., eds. Philadelphia: W. B. Saunders Company, pp. 511-26.

Wit A.L., Rosen M.R (1989). Cellular electrophysiological mechanisms of cardiac arrhythmias. In: Comprehensive Electrocardiology:Theory and Practice in Health and Disease, (vol 2) MacFarlane P.W., Veitch T.D., Lawrie, eds. New York: Pergamon Press, pp. 801-41.

Wolk R., Cobbe S.M., Hicks M.N., Kane K.A (1999). Functional, structural and dynamic basis of electrical heterogeneity in healthy and diseased cardiac muscle: Implications for arrhythmogenesis and anti-arrhythmic drug therapy. Pharmacology & Therapeutics. 84:207-31.

Wood M.A., Brown-Mahoney C., Kay G.N., Ellenbogen K.A. (2000) Clinical outcomes after ablation and pacing therapy for atrial fibrillation: A meta-analysis. Circ.; 101:1138-44.

Wu E.B., Chia H.M., Gill J.S. (. 2000) Reversible cardiomyopathy after radiofrequency ablation of lateral free wall pathway-mediated incessant supraventricular tachycardia. PACE; 23:1308-10.

Yee R., Guiraudon G.M., Gardner M.J., Gulamhusein S.S., Klein G.J (1984). Refractory paroxysmal sinus tachycardia: Management by subtotal right atrial exclusion. JACC. 3:400-4.

Zipes D.P., Foster P.R., Troup P.J., Pederson D.H. (1979) Atrial induction of ventricular tachycardia: Reentry versus triggered activity. Am J Cardiol.; 44:1-8.

Index